The Complete B
of Chinese Health
and Healing

D0383941

Books by Daniel Reid

The Complete Book of Chinese Health and Healing: Guarding the Three Treasures

The Complete Guide to Chi-Gung: Harnessing the Power of the Universe

The Essence of Chi-Gung: A Handbook of Basic Forms for Daily Practice

A Handbook of Chinese Healing Herbs

Harnessing the Power of the Universe: A Complete Guide to the Principles and Practice of Chi-Gung

The Shambhala Guide to Traditional Chinese Medicine

The
COMPLETE BOOK
of
CHINESE HEALTH
and
HEALING

Guarding the Three Treasures

DANIEL REID

Illustrated by
Dexter Chou and Jony Huang

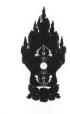

SHAMBHALA
Boston
1995

This book is not intended to replace the services of a licensed health care provider in the diagnosis or treatment of illness or disease. Any application of the material set forth in the following pages is at the reader's discretion and sole responsibility.

Shambhala Publications, Inc.
Horticultural Hall
300 Massachusetts Avenue
Boston, Massachusetts 02115
www.shambhala.com

© 1994 by Daniel Reid
All rights reserved. No part of this book may be
reproduced in any form or by any means, electronic or
mechanical, including photocopying, recording, or by any
information storage and retrieval system, without
permission in writing from the publisher.

22   21   20   19   18   17   16   15   14

Printed in the United States of America
⊗ This edition is printed on acid-free paper that meets the
American National Standards Institute Z39.48 Standard.
♻ This book is printed on 30% postconsumer recycled paper.
For more information please visit www.shambhala.com.
Distributed in the United States by Penguin Random House LLC
and in Canada by Random House of Canada Ltd

Library of Congress catalogues the hardcover edition of this work as follows:

Reid, Daniel P., 1948—
The complete book of Chinese health and healing/Daniel Reid;
illustrations by Dexter Chou and Jony Huang.—1st ed.
p.   cm.
Includes index.
ISBN 978-0-87773-929-6 (hardcover)
ISBN 978-1-57062-071-3 (pbk.)
1. Medicine, Chinese.   I. Title.
R601.R34   1994   93-26702
615.5′3′0951—dc20   CIP

for
Chou Tung

Contents

Preface

This is the second book I've written on traditional Taoist systems for cultivating health, vitality, and spiritual awareness. Although both books discuss all three facets of the 'Three Treasures' of human life—essence, energy and spirit—*The Tao of Health, Sex, and Longevity* (hereafter referred to as *The Tao of HS&L*) deals mainly with the physical and biochemical factors of essence, while *The Complete Book of Chinese Health and Healing* focuses more on the dynamic and functional manifestations of energy. In order to avoid redundancy, information and ideas discussed in detail in *The Tao of HS&L* are only briefly mentioned in this book. Therefore, readers who wish to study and practise the whole system should read both books, though not necessarily in the order they were written. Together the two books cover the essence and the energy of the matter, which constitute the basic pillars of practice. I hope the proficiency of my own practice will progress sufficiently to produce eventually a third volume that uncovers the spirit of Taoist metaphysical science, or 'alchemy'. That spirit sprouts from the seed of your own original inspiration to cultivate the Tao, is nourished by the essence and energy of your basic practices, and finally blossoms up to 'heaven' from its roots in 'earth', like a lotus blooming towards the sky from its roots in muddy waters.

Western science and philosophy adopt a dualistic view of such apparent contradictions as body and mind, heaven and earth, sacred and profane, scientific and spiritual, magic and mundane, and thus divide them into mutually exclusive realms. Taoists view and deal with opposite forces and phenomena as complementary aspects of the same basic polarity that runs throughout the entire manifest universe and is known as the 'Great Principle of Yin and Yang'. That's why there's no fixed boundary between science and philosophy, physical and spiritual, yin and yang in Taoist tradition. In addition to viewing opposite forms and forces in terms

of complementary polarity rather than antagonistic duality, Taoists also regard polar opposites as being mutually transmutable
and actively interdependent. The dynamic balance, functional
harmony, and cyclic transformations among these basic forms and
forces are what make the world go round. They're also the basis of
the 'internal alchemy' which lies at the heart of *chee-gung*, meditation, herbal medicine, sexual yoga, and other traditional Taoist
practices.

As modern transportation and communication breach the borders of time and space which once divided the human species
into isolated enclaves, the cultural and philosophical boundaries
separating East from West are also being slowly but surely erased,
despite the stubborn opposition of die-hard traditionalists in both
camps. Nowhere are the walls falling faster than in the field of
human health, for it is becoming abundantly obvious that the
traditional healing arts of the East and modern medical technology
of the West are complementary branches of the same tree, and that
together they provide a far more complete picture of human health
and offer far more effective therapies for human disease than either
one can possibly do alone.

Disease and degeneration recognize no boundaries, and neither
should the therapies used to treat them. What counts in medicine is
its utility in practice, not its theoretical agreement with culturally
conditioned concepts. In the light of the health crisis spreading
throughout the world today, physicians as well as patients can use
all the help they can get, regardless of whether it comes from
science or philosophy, ancient or modern times, China or America.

This book presents the traditional Taoist approach to human
health in terms of its own classical philosophy as well as the latest
findings of modern Western medical science. As in *The Tao of HS&L*,
all research was done from primary Chinese and Western sources,
and all programmes and practices recommended herein are based
as much on my own personal experience as on scholarly research.
Except where otherwise indicated, translations are based on my
own interpretations of the original Chinese materials.

The Complete Book of Chinese Health and Healing was inspired by
the enthusiastic response to its forerunner, and written with the
hope that it steers readers onto the 'Great Highway' of health,
longevity, and spiritual discovery.

Here's to your health!

Daniel P. Reid

Ping River, Chiang Mai, Thailand
November 1992

Acknowledgments

Thanks to the illustrators, Dexter Chou and Jony Huang; Ma Jun, for the cover illustration, Mr Chou Yun-yu, who did the Chinese calligraphy; Master Luo Teh-hsiou, for his inspiring discourses on the Tao; and Ingrid von Essen, for her fine copy-editing.

The Three Treasures

The body is the temple of life. Energy is the force of life. Spirit is the governor of life. If one of them goes off balance, all three are damaged. When the spirit takes command, the body naturally follows it, and this arrangement benefits all Three Treasures. When the body leads the way, the spirit goes along, and this harms all Three Treasures.

Wen-tzu Classic (first century BC)

All humans are born into this world endowed with the three precious treasures of life, by virtue of which we are able to exist, function, and think. These treasures compose our inherent natural legacy, and the degree to which we protect and preserve them determines the state of our health and the span of our lives. Those who squander and abuse the precious treasures of life suffer the poverty of chronic disease and premature death, while those who cultivate and conserve them enjoy the riches of health and longevity.

The Taoist tradition of China contains the world's longest on-going record of scientific inquiry, spanning a period of at least 5,000 years. Since ancient times, health and longevity have always ranked among the foremost fields of interest studied by Taoist adepts, who view the human organism as a microcosm of the universe, complete with its own internal 'heaven' and 'earth', its own 'climate' and 'seasons', its own cyclic transformations and natural interplay of universal energies.

In the Taoist view, the Three Treasures upon which life depends are essence (*jing*), energy (*chee*), and spirit (*shen*). Essence refers to the physical body of blood and flesh, including all its basic material constituents, particularly the essential fluids such as hormones, enzymes, and neurotransmitters. Energy is the primal life force which suffuses every cell and tissue of the living body and activates its vital functions. Spirit encompasses all aspects of the mind, both human and primordial, including awareness and cognition, thought and feeling, will and intent. Together the Three Treasures (*san bao*), also known as the Three Marvels (*san chee*), function as a single organic unit.

Each of the Three Treasures has two fundamental aspects, known in Taoist terminology as 'prenatal' (*hsien-tien*) and 'postnatal' (*hou-tien*), or primordial and temporal. The prenatal aspects are the pure qualities which precede birth and infuse the fertilized embryo at the moment of conception. The postnatal aspects are the temporal manifestations which develop after birth, beginning at the moment the umbilical cord is cut and the infant draws its first breath of air. Prenatally, the Three Treasures are a formless, indivisible unit, but after birth they separate and take on their respective temporal aspects, thereby becoming vulnerable to depletion and decay. One of the primary purposes of Taoist alchemy is to restore the prenatal unity and primordial purity of essence, energy, and spirit in order to prevent disease and degeneration of the postnatal human organism, retard the aging process, and prolong life.

There is really no great mystery to Taoist alchemy. It is simply a matter of learning how to employ the mind to harness energy and thereby regulate essential biochemical transformations and vital organ functions in the body. Most people passively permit environmental, emotional, and physical stimuli to govern their essence and energy; Taoists actively use their minds to master their energy, and their energy to control their essence. By regaining access to the latent primal powers of our minds, we can learn how to apply 'mind over matter' in order to guard the health and longevity of our bodies.

Taoist alchemy reverses the constant, debilitating depletion of essence, energy, and spirit caused by ordinary life in the material world and transforms it into a process of accretion that preserves the Three Treasures and prolongs life. This is a process which anyone can learn and practise, but it requires a basic familiarity with the universal principles that govern human life and its natural environment. The only qualifications required to become a Taoist adept are the will and the discipline to take full command of your own energy, full control of your own body, and full responsibility for your own life. The rest is simply a matter of method.

Essence

Essence refers to the most highly refined substances which constitute the human body, the basic stuff of corporeal life. Also translated as 'vitality', essence is a form of potential energy, like battery fluid, from which the body draws energy as required. In prenatal aspect, essence is the primal creative force of the cosmos, the universal urge to procreate and perpetuate. Each individual receives a fixed measure of this prenatal essence from the fusion of sperm and ovum provided by father and mother. After birth, as the body develops, this primal essence is stored in what the Chinese call the 'kidney glands' (adrenal cortex) as well as in male and female sexual secretions and reproductive organs. It is passed on to the next generation through sexual reproduction and is therefore regarded as immortal and self-perpetuating.

Postnatal essence is refined and synthesized from nutrients extracted from food and water and is stored primarily in the liver, blood, and marrow. It takes form as very pure and potent fluids such as hormones, enzymes, neurotransmitters, cerebrospinal fluid, lymphatic fluid, blood plasma, and other biochemical essences. It manifests itself as gender and sexuality, provides strength, vitality, and immunity, and is most easily depleted in men through excessive loss of semen, in women through menstruation, and in both genders through chronic stress, malnutrition, and illness. Postnatal essence resides in the sacrum and is closely associated with sexual and digestive functions.

Energy

Energy is the vital force that activates every function and drives every process in the human body, voluntary as well as involuntary. It is like the electric current running through a computer: without it none of the functions works. In prenatal aspect, energy is the primal power that pervades the entire universe, where it manifests itself as heat, light, motion, and other universal energies. Postnatal energy manifests itself in humans as the various energies associated with the major organ systems, and as body heat, breath, pulse, and other forms of bioenergetics. Postnatal energy is polar and electromagnetic and is characterized by constant activity and transformation.

Humans derive primal prenatal energy from two sources. One is from the transformation of the prenatal essence stored in the adrenal cortex and sexual glands. This is called *yuan-chee* ('primordial energy'), and every individual is born with a limited supply of it. Converting prenatal glandular essence into primal energy requires an advanced form of Taoist alchemy known as *nei-gung* ('internal work'). The other source of prenatal energy is called *tien* ('heaven'), which refers to the sky and the cosmos beyond. Cosmic energies from the sky enter the body through the top of the head, while light is assimilated through the skin and eyes.

The source of postnatal energy is called *dee* ('earth'), which refers to food, water, herbs, and other material supplements, as well as air. Dietary elements are digested to extract vital nutrients, which the body then transforms into energy. Energy from the air is absorbed through the lungs and may be cultivated with a simple form of Taoist breathing exercise called *chee-gung* ('energy work'). When air energy from the lungs blends in the blood with earth energy from the digestive system, it forms what is known as 'True Human Energy', the fundamental force of temporal human life.

Human energy resides in the chest and is closely associated with breathing and blood circulation, heart and lungs. Taoist medical texts state that 'energy leads blood', which means that blood flows wherever energy goes and that blood circulation may therefore be controlled by regulating breath. This is a fundamental principle of *chee-gung* practice.

Spirit

Spirit refers to the mind and all its various facets and functions. Prenatal spirit is the primordial 'mind of Tao', the immortal soul, the original light of consciousness. It is the eternal spark of awareness which 'is not born and does not die'. It is immaterial, luminous, and resides in the heart.

Postnatal spirit manifests itself as thought and sensory awareness, psyche and personality, ego and the notion of self. Although the original mind of Tao is open, undifferentiated, non-dualistic, and perfectly still, its temporal manifestation in the human mind is closed, discriminating, dualistic, and ever agitated. The postnatal human mind resides in the head and expresses itself through the cerebral functions of the brain.

Every human being possesses the primordial mind of Tao within his or her heart, but very few are aware of it. Because of the self-deluding obscurations the human mind creates from sensory perceptions and conflicting emotional reactions, most people remain blind to the light of their own primordial spirit until the moment of death, when everyone gets a sudden glimpse of it. The higher stages of esoteric Taoist alchemy and meditation teach us how to control our senses, calm our emotions, and balance our energies, so that we may look tranquilly inwards beyond the human mind in order to restore awareness of the primordial mind of Tao. This awareness enhances life and also prepares us for death. Since primordial spirit is the only aspect of mind that 'is not born and does not die', those who know it do not fear death, and this knowledge gives them perfect freedom and equanimity in life.

The Taoist sage Lu Tung-ping, who lived during the Tang dynasty (AD 618 – 905) and is still revered as one of the great progenitors of Taoist philosophy, described the Three Treasures as follows, translated here by Thomas Cleary:

> *Vitality*: In heaven, vitality is the Milky Way, it is the light of the sun, moon, and stars, it is rain and dew, sleet and hail, snow and frost. On earth it is water, streams, rivers, oceans, springs, wells, ponds, and marshes. In people it is vitality, the root of essence and life, the body of blood and flesh.

> *Energy*: In heaven, energy is substance and form, yin and yang, the movement of the sun, moon, and stars, the processes of waxing and waning; it is clouds, mist, fog, and moisture; it is the heart of living beings, evolution and development. On earth, it is power, fuel, the pith of myriad beings, the source of mountain streams; it is life-giving and killing, activating and storing; it is the passage of time, flourishing and decline, rising and falling, sprouts and sprout sheaths. In humans it is energy, phys-ical movement, activity, speech, and perception; it is use of the body, the gateway of death and life.

> *Spirit*: In heaven, spirit is the pivot, the true director, the silent mover; it is the essence of the sun, moon, and stars; it is the wind blowing, thunder pealing; it is compassion and dignity; it is the force of creation, the basis of the origin of beings. On earth, it is ability, communion, open-ing; it is the shapes of myriad species, mountains and waters; it is peace and quietude, the source of stability; it is calm, warmth, and kindness. In humans, it is the spirit, the light in the eyes, thought in the mind; it is wisdom and intelligence, innate knowledge and capacity; it is the

government of vitality and energy, awareness and understanding; it is the basis of the physical shell, the foundation of the life span.

Trinity

The Three Treasures are one aspect of the fundamental trinity which runs throughout Taoist philosophy and esoteric practices. Anatomically, the Three Treasures of essence, energy, and spirit 'reside' in the sacrum, thorax, and brain, where they manifest respectively as fluids, breath, and thought. Energetically, the Three Treasures are associated with three power points known as 'elixir fields' (dan-tien), which are the focal points of esoteric Taoist alchemy. Essence pools in the Lower Elixir Field, located behind and a bit below the navel, and its alchemical name is 'water'. Energy collects in the Middle Elixir Field in the chest and is associated with breath, pulse, and speech. Its alchemical identity is 'fire'. Postnatal spirit is housed in the Upper Elixir Field, located behind the point between the eyebrows, and is associated with the pituitary and pineal glands and the hypothalamus. In Taoist alchemy it is known as the 'embryo'.

Metaphysically, the Three Treasures originate in the 'Three Powers' of heaven, earth, and humans. Heaven is the source of spirit, and earth is the source of the essential elements which constitute the human body. Humans, who stands between heaven and earth, are the source of the unique force known as True Human Energy, which fuses the spirit of heaven with the essence of earth to form the human body and manifest the human mind.

Alchemy

All humans are born replete with the full potential of their innate primordial powers. During the ordinary course of life on earth, the demands and distractions of the temporal postnatal world gradually deplete essence, dissipate energy, and exhaust spirit, undermining health and hastening death. Most people are constantly distracted by the demands of the body and its insatiable appetites for food, sex, and entertainment. Rather than treasuring their bodies as 'temples of the spirit', they abuse them to satisfy their animal appetites. Indeed, most people these days take better care of their cars than they do of their bodies, spend money more carefully than they spend energy, and devote more time and attention to television than to their own minds. They pollute their essential bodily fluids with denatured foods and toxic drugs, deplete their energy with chronic stress and emotional turmoil, and exhaust their spirits with the myriad distractions and desires of worldly life. Even those who profess interest in spiritual life often fail to make significant progress simply because they neglect to take the first crucial step of cleaning up their acts on the levels of essence and energy. When essence is polluted and energy unbalanced, spirit grows dim and weak.

Taoist alchemy reverses this process of depletion first by purifying and preserving essence, then by balancing and conserving energy, and finally by cultivating and concentrating spirit. Through an esoteric alchemical process known as 'Triplex Unity', purified essence is converted into energy, which is then raised and refined through the higher energy centres until it reaches the brain, where it is again transformed to nurture spirit. *The Classification of Therapies*, a Taoist medical text written 2,000 years ago, states: 'Spirit is sustained by energy, and energy is obtained from the transformation of essence. Essence transforms into energy, and energy transforms into spirit.' When sufficiently clarified, energized, and rejuvenated, the human mind is able to restore its long-lost connection with its own primordial powers, thereby recharging the postnatal aspects of the Three Treasures with their prenatal antecedents. This is called 'returning to the source'. Through careful control and patient cultivation of the temporal aspects of essence, energy, and spirit manifested in human life, the adept of Taoist alchemy restores a direct link with the infinite primordial power of the universal mind of Tao.

Balance and harmony

Balance and harmony are pivotal points in the Taoist way of life. Health and longevity depend entirely upon the maintenance of optimum balance and harmony among the Three Treasures, among the energies of the vital organs, and between the human body and its natural environment.

According to the Taoist view, disease and degeneration are caused not so much by external invasion as by 'letting down one's guard'. Germs, toxins, and 'evil energies' are ever present in our environment, but they can only gain entry and cause damage to a body whose immunity and resistance are impaired by negligence and improper lifestyle. Health and longevity are sustained not by doctors and drugs but by carefully guarding the Three Treasures of life, and the onset of any disease is a clear indication of one's own failure to maintain a strong defence system.

The way to balance and harmony is to live in accord rather than in conflict with nature. The universal principles of the primordial Tao manifest themselves on earth in the form of Mother Nature, who flawlessly follows and clearly reflects the Tao's cyclic patterns. Therefore, Taoists learn the Way by observing and emulating nature. Those who conform to nature and learn how to harness its powers flourish and live long. Those who defy nature and try to pervert its powers for profit and pleasure degenerate and die early.

The primary principle of nature is constant change and ceaseless flux. These changes and fluctuations are neither arbitrary nor chaotic. They are cyclic and follow predictable patterns. The universal principles of yin and yang, the Three Treasures, the Five Energies, and other cyclic patterns manifest themselves clearly throughout nature, and by studying them the adept learns how to adapt himself or herself to the world and thrive through thick and thin. Rigid attachment to habitual behaviour, material objects, and fixed ideas runs contrary to the Tao and blocks one's capacity to adapt to an ever-changing world. Flexibility, spontaneity, and complete freedom of thought and action are the only ways to respond successfully to the constant flux of nature and thus live in accord with the Tao.

The modern world operates under the foolish misconception that science and technology can 'conquer nature', thereby permitting human beings to indulge their every whim and fancy. We cut down forests and plunder the seas, pollute the air we breathe and poison the water we drink, contaminate our bodies with artificial foods and synthetic drugs, and stunt our minds with trivial distractions and unnatural notions. The net result of this battle between nature and humans is a hostile environment that subverts rather than supports human life, and the ultimate losers are humans. The human body is a highly evolved product of nature, so it is obvious that if we destroy our natural habitat we also destroy ourselves, and no degree of science or technology can save us from such self-destruction. Our only hope is to call a truce and restore our long-disrupted harmony with nature, and this is how the ancient Tao can best serve the modern world. The Tao provides us with all we need to know to live in accord with nature, to benefit from the trinity of heaven, earth, and humans, and to protect the precious treasures of essence, energy, and spirit upon which our lives depend.

Unfortunately, most people spend their entire lives travelling the path of dissipation, without ever realizing that it is the quickest short-cut to the grave. As the sage Lu Tung-pin put it:

> The human body is composed entirely of essence, energy, and spirit. If you do not cherish your essence and dissipate it recklessly, it is like pouring water into a cracked cup. Instead of filling the cup, it will leak away until it is depleted to the last drop. If you do not cherish your energy and dissipate it carelessly, it is like putting incense on hot coals and continuously adding fuel to the fire until the incense has burned to ashes. If you do not cherish your spirit and dissipate it indiscriminately, it is like setting a lamp out in the wind unprotected and letting the wind blow on the flame until it is extinguished.

The Tao offers a viable alternative to the self-destructive behaviour of 'life in the fast lane', an alternative path that leads to health and longevity, prevents disease and degeneration, cultivates wisdom, and protects the Three Treasures. The Taoist way of life need not be boring or ascetic; in fact, Taoists usually get a lot more out of life than ordinary people, including the pleasures of food and sex, precisely because they understand both the limitations and the full possibilities of nature. Yet few people follow this path, not because it is hidden or obscure, but because it is a path that must be travelled slowly, step by step, entirely under one's own power, driven only by virtue of one's own discipline and determination. It is a path of total freedom and independence, but few people are willing to exercise the sort of self-restraint and self-reliance which such freedom demands. As Hu Szu-hui, physician to the emperor of China, wrote in his medical manual in 1330:

> Men of high antiquity knew the Tao and patterned their lives on the harmony of yin and yang, living in complete accordance with the rhythms of nature. They observed moderation in food and drink, regularity in their daily lives, and they did not recklessly overstrain themselves. Consequently they lived long lives. But people today are different. Their daily lives are irregular, they eat and drink indiscriminately without knowing what to avoid, and they do not observe moderation. They give themselves over to dissipation, indulge freely in richly flavoured foods, ignore the Golden Mean, and are

perpetually dissatisfied with what they have. Consequently most people today are ruined before the age of fifty.

The Taoist tree of health

The Taoist tradition of China contains the world's most complete and effective system of preventive health care, based on thousands of years of empirical observation and scientific experimentation. This ancient system of health and longevity is like a grand old tree rooted deeply in the fertile soil of traditional Taoist philosophy. Regardless which branch of the tree you cultivate, they all sprout from the same roots, and each branch bears fruit that contains the seed of the entire tree.

The roots of this venerable tree are the fundamental philosophical principles of the primordial Tao and its earthly manifestations. These theoretical roots include the Great Principle of Yin and Yang, the Three Treasures of life, the Four Foundations of health, the Five Energies, and so forth, and they are elucidated in this book in Part I: The Roots.

From these roots the tree branches upwards to form the three great limbs of the Taoist trinity: the Three Treasures of essence, energy, and spirit. Each of these limbs branches further into the various stems of practice, such as diet and nutrition, herbs and acupuncture, breathing and exercise, dual and solo sexual yoga, meditation and internal alchemy. These are discussed in detail in Part II: The Branches.

From the branches and stems of the tree grow the healthy fruits of practice, the beneficial results obtained by cultivating the Taoist way of life. This rich harvest includes health and vitality, physical longevity and spiritual immortality, mental clarity and emotional equanimity. They are covered in Part III: The Fruits.

In addition, there are chapters on modern hybrids of the ancient tree, such as the 'New Medicine' and 'New Alchemy', and a section on 'Precious Prescriptions', including formulas for Chinese herbal tonics to enhance essence and elevate energy, therapeutic foods for health and longevity, and a selected list of Chinese patent medicines that provide safe and effective relief for common ailments.

In Chinese tradition, health is a branch of philosophy rooted in the same universal principles that govern cosmology and chemistry, agriculture and astronomy, physics and pharmacology, and all other natural sciences. The human body is viewed as a self-contained microcosm of the universe, and various parts and appendages are treated more in terms of their functional relationships than their anatomical forms. In the Taoist system of thought, insights into such fundamental natural phenomena as solar and lunar cycles and seasonal changes also provide parallel insight into the workings of the human body. The common denominator which links all natural phenomena and balances all equations is energy, the dynamic power of the universe. Energy is the force which gives form its function, the link between mind and matter, the medium through which humans interact with the invisible powers of heaven and their visible manifestations on earth. It is the pervasive force and transformational power of energy that binds all objects and activities in nature into one organic system of form and function. That universal system is simply called the 'Way', or 'Tao', and human life flourishes or declines to the extent that it stays on or strays from the Way.

PART I

The Roots:
Theoretical Foundations

CHAPTER 1

The One Source

The Tao gave birth to the one source,
The one gave birth to two things,
Then to three things,
Then to ten thousand . . .

Tao Teh Ching (third century BC)

The Chinese word 'Tao' (pronounced 'dao', as in Dow Jones) is cropping up with growing frequency throughout the Western world. There are books on the 'Tao of Physics' and the 'Tao of Art', the 'Tao of Health' and the 'Tao of Sex', the 'Tao of Wall Street' and the 'Tao of Politics', even the 'Tao of Winnie-the-Pooh'. Yet few Western readers actually know what Tao means or understand why it applies to so many different topics.

The Chinese ideogram for 'Tao' means 'path' or 'way' and consists of two symbols: 'walk' and 'head' (Fig. 1). In other words, the Tao is a path one walks by following one's head rather than feet, a way of life guided by mind rather than body. '*Tao*' is also a verb which means 'to say' or 'to guide', implying that unless you've found the one and only 'Way', you're misguided and don't have much to say.

Fig. 1 **Chinese ideogram for 'Tao', combining symbols for 'head' (right) and 'walk' (left and bottom).**

The Chinese word for 'to know' is a combination of two ideograms: 'know' and 'Tao'. This implies that the only true knowledge is knowledge of the Tao, and that the Tao is the only source of true knowledge. When you say 'I know' in Chinese, what you're literally saying is 'I know the Way'.

The Tao then is the original source of all knowledge, the grand highway from which all byways branch, the fountainhead from which all streams spring, the root from which all branches grow. The Tao is the singular source of ultimate as well as relative reality, of the primordial as well as the temporal aspects of the universe, of nirvana (enlightened awareness) as well as samsara (cyclic existence). Formless, without sound or substance, the Tao is nevertheless omniscient, omnipotent, and omnipresent throughout the universe. 'Tao never does,' states the *Tao Teh Ching*, 'but through it all things are done.' Though it cannot be named of described in words, it can be known intuitively by contemplating its myriad manifestations, and it can be experienced in life by practising its principles. The terse verse of the 5,000-word *Tao Teh Ching* ('The Way and its Power'), of which more than a hundred different translations have been published, states: 'The name which can be named is not the real Name.' It also says:

> There was something formless yet complete
> That existed before heaven and earth . . .
> One may think of it as the mother
> Of all things under heaven.
> Its true name I do not know;
> 'Tao' is the nickname I give it.

'Returning to the source'

Other nicknames for the Tao are *Tai-Chi* ('Supreme Ultimate'), *Tai-Hsu* ('Supreme Void'), and *Tai-Yi* ('Supreme Mover'). As the supreme and ultimate source of all substance, energy, and awareness, the Tao itself is an undifferentiated continuum without boundaries in time and space, as infinite, formless, and luminous as awareness itself. However, in order to manifest its power in form and function, the primordial Tao must polarize its energy into 'two things', yin and yang, which in turn give birth to 'three things, then to ten thousand'. Since all the myriad manifestations of the Tao spring from the same singular source, 'the One', life flourishes to the extent that it accords with the natural universal principles of the

Tao and declines the further we stray from the Way. Owing to the elegance and literary sophistication of the classical Chinese language, the terms and metaphors in which the ancient masters couched their teachings are consistently allegorical and symbolic, but the principles and practices to which they allude are as natural as eating and breathing, as perennial as sun and moon, and as fundamental as fire and water.

Studying and practising the Tao is not an esoteric hobby or strange occult pastime, but rather a very practical and effective way to promote health, maintain sanity, and prolong life on earth, while at the same time paving the way to the ultimate goal of spiritual enlightenment, of 'returning to the source'. Like following a winding stream uphill into the mountains in order to discover its source, or watering the roots of a tree in order to insure a bountiful harvest of fruit from its branches, practising the Tao is an effort which rewards the adept with the sweet fruits of health and longevity, while also providing the deeper long-term satisfaction of spiritual discovery.

The Taoist way of life permits us to work with what we have on earth here and now – body, breath, and mind – in order to recover our original treasures of primordial essence, energy, and spirit. It teaches us how to use the temporary assets of temporal life to restore the eternal treasure of primordial awareness, how to reach for the infinite by extending the finite, how to refine the purity of heaven from the pollution of earth, how to live simply in a complex world, and how to achieve mental calm and clarity amid the confusion of corporeal life. Followed to the ultimate goal of enlightenment, the Tao endows us with the spiritual insights required to transcend death and escape the endless cycle of rebirth which marks corporeal existence, qualifying us instead for entry into the simple, pure, crystal-clear realms reserved for the spiritually enlightened. That, however, is a lofty goal which only a few deeply disciplined, highly talented adepts reach, and then only after long lifetimes of diligent practice and unwavering intent. For most of us, the Tao points out a simple, pure, and clear way of life here on earth, allowing us to enjoy fully the carnal birthrights of our corporeal existence, while simultaneously freeing us of our animal fear of death and preparing us for a shot at the ultimate goal of enlightenment in a future lifetime.

Whether you aim high or low, roam far abroad or stay close to home, aspire to the ultimate heavenly goal of spiritual enlightenment, or the more modest earthly goals of health and longevity, the Tao will guide you to your destined goal as directly and unerringly as an express train delivers passengers to their various destinations along its route. All you have to do is select your own itinerary, then climb on board and stay on track. It's as simple as that.

As the master Chang Po-tuan said a thousand years ago: 'The words are simple, and the way is easy. It's like finding the source by following the stream'. Whether you follow the stream all the way back to its ultimate source in this life or the next, in one lifetime or a hundred, doesn't really matter. As long as you stay on course and don't get sidetracked en route, you will get there sooner or later. Meanwhile, the journey itself is half the fun, and the Tao teaches us how to enjoy the trip without exhausting all our resources and forfeiting our chance of one day 'going all the Way' back to the sole source of creation, returning fully conscious back to where we once belonged.

The Tao of Complete Reality

Many branches, including aberrant deviations, sprouted from the root source of the Tao in early Chinese history, giving rise to feuding sects and conflicting doctrines. Wizards and alchemists, martial artists and medical therapists, ascetic hermits and religious leaders all claimed to carry the torch of the true Tao. By the fifth century AD, when Taoism was already at least 3,000 years old in China, it had become a colourful collage of bizarre characters and outlandish ideas that in many cases had drifted off the Great Highway of the Tao. 'Great highways are safe and easy,' states the *Tao Teh Ching*, 'but men love byways.'

Then along came Bodhidharma (Ta Mo), a scowling monk cowled in rags who walked from his native India all the way to China, arriving there at the height of Taoist sectarianism (Fig. 2). Bodhidharma was an adept of the 'crazy wisdom' Tantric school of Buddhism that was sweeping across India at the time, and he was a character so eccentric that even the weirdest wizards of aberrant Taoism stood up and took note of his uninvited presence. It is said, for example, that in order to prevent himself from dozing off during the marathon meditations he practised, he sliced-off his own eyelids, and that before consenting to teach the Chinese anything, he first insisted on practising nine years of solitary meditation facing a stone wall in a monastery, 'listening to the ants scream'. Among the many lessons which Bodhidharma subsequently taught the Chinese was *pranayama*, the science of breathing practised by Indian yogis. This he blended with indigenous forms of Chinese

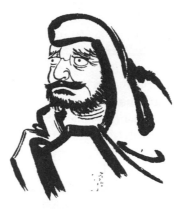

Fig. 2 **Ta Mo (Bodhidharma), the monk from India who became first patriarch of Chan (Zen) Buddism in China and progenitor of *chee-gung* and martial arts.**

calisthenics, thereby giving birth to *chee-gung* exercise and Chinese martial arts as we know them today. The two classic texts that form the basis for almost all Chinese health and longevity exercises are attributed to him and will be discussed later in the chapter on 'Energy'.

Bodhidharma was also the founder and first patriarch of Chan, a Chinese style of Buddhism heavily influenced by Taoist thought, which became Zen in Japan. Bodhidharma thus began the long syncretic process of reweaving the tangled threads of Taoism together with strong strands of Buddhist thought, including karma and reincarnation, to form a sturdy tapestry whose patterns truly reflected 'everything under heaven', or 'complete reality'.

This melding process continued during the Tang dynasty (AD 618–905), the great Golden Age of Chinese civilization, when the adept Lu Tung-pin appeared on the scene and engendered a school of thought which became known as the Tao of 'Complete Reality' (*chuan-jen*). Complete Reality Taoism transcended sectarian divisions and dispensed with doctrinaire debates, not only among Taoists but also between Taoists and followers of other mystical traditions such as Buddhism. Instead, it focused attention directly on rigorous spiritual practice and the spontaneous experience of intuitive insight. Known to later generations of followers as 'Ancestor Lu' for his pivotal role as progenitor of the Complete Reality school, Lu Tung-pin was later elevated to divine status as one of the legendary 'Eight Immortals' (*ba-hsien*) of Taoism.

During the following Sung dynasty (960–1279), the torch of Complete Reality Taoism was taken up again by two of the greatest Tao masters in Chinese history: Chang Po-tuan and Wang Che. In the introduction to his famous treatise on Taoist alchemy, called *Understanding Reality*, Chang Po-tuan had this to say about the futility of sectarian debate, translated here by Thomas Cleary:

> Is it not a fact that the doctrines [of Taoism, Buddhism, and Confucianism] may be three, but the Way is ulti-mately one? But that hasn't stopped the priesthoods of later generations from sole devotion to their own sects and repudiation of others, causing the basic essentials of all three philosophies to be lost in false distinctions, so that they cannot be unified and end up at the same goal.

Taoism, Buddhism, and Confucianism were the three prevailing -isms' of thought in ancient China, and Chang Po-tuan refined the essence of each in order to reveal their common source of truth. 'Both Lao-tzu [legendary author of the *Tao Teh Ching*] and Buddha elucidated effective techniques for applying the sciences of nature and destiny in order to teach people how to cultivate the embryonic seed by which to escape the cycles of birth and death,' he wrote in his introduction to *Understanding Reality*. By extending Chang's view to the entire world today, one might just as easily follow other streams of thought, such as Christianity, Hinduism, or Zoroastrianism, back to the original source of all creation, 'the mother of all things under heaven', for the true Tao has no borders and is not conditioned by cultural biases.

Chang Po-tuan spent his entire life seeking the one source of 'complete reality', and when he was already in his early eighties, he finally met a fully realized 'True Human', who kindly transmitted to him the 'precious oral secret' that filled in all the gaps in his practice, resolved all his doubts, and completely illuminated his mind. 'Having finally encountered the true explanation,' he wrote, 'how could I dare to conceal it from others?' So, before he 'ascended to heaven in broad daylight' to join the ranks of the immortals at the age of a hundred, he wrote several out-standing alchemical texts that are still regarded as indispensable reading by all serious adepts of Complete Reality. These works include *The Secret of Opening the Passes*, *The Four-Hundred-Character Treatise on the Golden Elixir*, and his greatest work of all, *Understanding Reality*, a condensed version of which has been trans-lated into English by Thomas Cleary under the title *The Inner Teachings of Taoism*. In his introduction to *Understanding Reality*, Chang wrote: 'My purpose in writing this is so that when people who share similar aspirations read it, they will understand the roots by observing the branches and abandon their illusions in order to pursue reality.'

Wang Che was a warrior as well as an erudite scholar from northern China who gave up his ranks and honours at the age of forty-seven in order to become a Taoist adept. He later became master to seven disciples who vigorously spread the influence of the Complete Reality school far and wide throughout China, erasing the 'false distinctions' of sectarian debate and rejuvenating the original Taoist premise that 'the Way is ultimately one'. One of the most brilliant of his seven disciples was Sun Pu-er, the 'Immortal Sister' who became the most famous female adept of the Tao in Chinese history. The story of their apprenticeship to Wang Che and the remarkable accomplishments of their practices was recorded in the novel *Seven Taoist Masters*. Its authorship is unknown but it has been translated into English by Eva Wong.

During the Mongol Yuan dynasty (1260–1368) which followed the collapse of the Sung empire, Complete Reality Taoism received another big boost with the advent of Chang San-feng, who further erased arbitrary doctrinaire distinctions among the great schools of thought in China and stressed instead the overriding importance of personal practice and spontaneous insight. Master of meditation, medicine, and martial arts, Chang San-feng was the quintessential 'True Human' or 'Man of Tao', an adept whose mastery of the One Way gave him the key to accomplishment in all ways. He wrote extensively on many subjects and is said to be the original founder of the *tai-chi-chuan* system of exercise and martial arts. Here are a few words of wisdom on spiritual practice attributed to his brush, translated by Thomas Cleary:

> The mind is like an eye – if even a tiny hair gets in an eye, the eye is uncomfortable. Similarly, if even a small matter concerns the mind, the mind will be disturbed. Once afflicted by disturbance, it is hard to concentrate.

> Just as an enormous tree grows from a tiny sprout, the stabilization of the spirit and attainment of enlightenment comes about through accumulated practice.

> Luxurious food and clothing, social distinction, and material riches are all extraneous likes of psychological desire, not good medicines that enhance life. When people pursue them, they bring about their own destruction. What could be more confused?

Nonetheless, the body that practices the Way must be sustained by food and clothing. There are some matters that cannot be neglected, some things that cannot be abandoned . . . Social relations and the necessities of life are a boat for us – if we want to cross the sea, we need the aid of a boat.

Every meal, every nap, is a potential source of gain or loss; every act, every word, can be a basis of calamity or fortune.

One's deeds are done by oneself, but destiny is bestowed by heaven. The relation of deeds to destiny is like shadows and echoes following form and sound.

If you want to practice the way to attain reality, first get rid of warped behavior.

There are people who are serene and free, following natural reality, whom others consider lazy, but I consider at peace.

There are people who conduct themselves simply and have very stable personalities, whom others consider uncultured, but I consider unspoiled.

To those who want to know the way to deal with the world, I suggest, Love People.

During the Manchu Ching dynasty (1644–1911), China's last imperial reign, there appeared yet another great master of Complete Reality Taoism – the adept and writer Liu I-ming, who wrote several important commentaries on the works of Chang Po-tuan, *The Book of Change (I-Ching)*, and other essential Taoist classics. Born in an age of decadence and decline in China, Liu left home in search of the Tao at the age of eighteen, and by the time of his death around the age of ninety he is said to have attained the 'spiritual immortality' of full enlightenment. Liu I-ming was a superb writer whose works remain among the clearest, most lucid explanations of the Tao on record. A collection of his best writing on the Tao, composed when he was nearly eighty years old, has been translated into equally lucid English by Thomas Cleary under the title *Awakening to the Tao*, a must on the reading list of every Western Taoist. Here are a few excerpts from *Awakening to the Tao* which clearly reflect the blend of Taoist and Buddhist thought that characterizes the Complete Reality school:

There is no deception in the Tao – even a little bit of false-hood already set you far astray. It is essential to detach from the energies of wine, physical beauty, and material goods. Aggression, greed, and stupidity should all be eliminated.

The Tao is in the body. Within the body is hidden another person, who always accompanies you, whatever you do. Awake or asleep, it is always there; looking, listening, talking, walking, it is very very close. This is not the awareness of conditioned knowledge, it is the original sane energy, vitality, and spirit. If you seek this in terms of form or shape, you are mistaking the servant for the master.

The Tao is unique, without duality – why do deluded people divide it into high and low? The great ultimate is originally a name for complete awareness, ultimate sincerity is itself the form of the gold pill. When you recognize that the principles of the sages are the same, you will realize that Taoism and Buddhism are alike. If you do not understand this and seek elsewhere, you will get involved in sidetracks, wasting your life in vain imagining.

The Complete Reality school of Taoism continues to flourish without fanfare in our own age, thanks to the ongoing tradition of personal transmission handed down through the ages from accomplished masters to trusted disciples, and it is this stream of Taoist thought that concerns us here, for not only does it point directly to the One Source of all truth and reflect clearly the primordial Way of all ways, it also suits the increasingly syncretic world we live in. Nonsectarian, non-nationalistic, and non-ethnocentric, Complete Reality Taoism transcends the petty squabbles of warring states and feuding factions and encompasses one and all along with 'everything under heaven' within its vast embrace. In today's world, Complete Reality Taoism could become a powerful force for international peace, harmony, and understanding, as well as the swift path for inner development that it has always formed for individual seekers fortunate enough to discover it in time to put it into practice.

CHAPTER 2

The Two Poles

The yang transforms and the yin conserves. The yang and the yin manifest as movement and rest: yang moves to its utmost, then rests; yin rests to its utmost, then moves. Therefore, yin rests within yang, and yang moves within yin; the two are inseparably interwoven. It is thus as a single unit that they are one with the Tao.

Chu Hsi (eleventh century AD)

Polarity is the most pervasive principle of the manifest material universe, providing the boundless dynamic force which makes the world go round. Although indivisible unity is the ultimate law of the primordial Tao at its highest spiritual levels, polarity is the means by which the primal power of the universal Tao expresses itself in the temporal world of essence and energy. Without polarity material worlds and physical bodies could not exist, and without polar fields energy could not function, essence could not take form, and the rhythmic cycles of nature could not transpire.

In Taoist parlance, polarity is known as the Great Principle of Yin and Yang. This is not an occult concept or esoteric mystery but rather a highly scientific paradigm which applies to every process and phenomenon in the universe, from the macrocosmic to the microscopic. It explains the mystery of transformation and demonstrates that all change in the universe is cyclical rather than linear and therefore predictable. Cyclic change is the salient principle in the 3,000-year-old Chinese manual of divination called *The Book of Change (I-Ching)*, which shows how to predict change according to the cyclic interplay of yin and yang.

The principle of polarity applies equally to human energy and electric energy, the circulation of blood in veins and the flow of water in rivers, the rotation of planets around the sun and of electrons around the nucleus of an atom. It is a law with no loopholes, a rule without exceptions, and therefore those who understand and apply it in their lives enjoy the distinct advantage of being on 'the right side of the law', living in harmony with the entire universe, and acting in accord rather than in conflict with nature's cyclic patterns.

Throughout the ages, Taoist sages have left us prolific written records elucidating the Great Principle of Yin and Yang, and these books remain of timeless utility. The classic book of strategy called *The Art of War*, for example, written 2,000 years ago by the Taoist philosopher Sun-tzu, was used by Mao Tse-tung in his long campaign to unify China, and it is still studied today to obvious advantage by Japanese corporate executives as a basis for their global economic strategies. The medical treatise called *The Yellow Emperor's Classic of Internal Medicine*, written at least 2,000 years ago, is also based on the principle of yin and yang, and to this day it remains an indispensable text in the study and practice of Chinese medicine. The Tao never goes out of date.

The Great Principle of Yin and Yang was formulated in prehistoric China as a way of explaining natural phenomena which had formerly been attributed to the caprice of spirits and demons. It is the earliest instance in human history of rational scientific principle replacing blind superstitious belief. Observing that all phenomena in nature occur in opposite pairs, the ancient Chinese deduced the natural law of complementary polarity and applied it to 'everything under heaven'. By contemplating the movements of planets and stars, the rhythmic cycles of seasons and weather, the sexual behaviour of animals and humans, and the parallel patterns of day and night, life and death, growth and decay, they realized that polarity creates the dynamic field in which energy moves and change transpires.

The terms 'yin' and 'yang' first appeared in *The Book of Change* around 1250 BC. The ideogram for 'yin' means 'the shady side of a hill' while 'yang' means 'the sunny side of a hill'. Not only do these contrasting images denote polarity, they also indicate the cyclic transformations of one into the other, for as the earth rotates from sunrise to sunset, the shady side of a hill becomes the sunny side and the sunny side falls into shadow. *The Book of Change* states:

> The ceaseless interplay of heaven and earth gives form to all things. The sexual union of male and female gives life to all things. This interaction of yin and yang is called the Way [Tao], and the resulting creative process is called change.

Today, the Chinese still apply the principle of yin and yang to their daily lives, in geomancy (*feng shui*) and astrology, medicine and cooking, arts and crafts, and other traditions. Yin and yang polarity is also the underlying principle in the binary system used in computer technology, in the flux of quantum physics, in aero-dynamics and the thrust of rockets, and in other modern sciences.

The nature of yin and yang

Contrary to common misconceptions, yin and yang are not two different types of energy, but rather two complementary poles of the same basic energy, like the positive and negative poles of an electric current or a magnetic field. Yin and yang are reciprocal states of cyclic change, polar phases in the rhythmic transfor-mations of energy. Depending on the phenomenon involved, the interplay of yin and yang shows in various ways: active and passive, overt and covert, expansive and contractive, radiant and concentrated, ascending and descending. These are phases of activity, not static entities. The concepts commonly used to repre-sent yin and yang – such as male and female, hot and cold, night and day – are oversimplifications and can be misleading because they imply static states rather than dynamic processes.

Man and woman, for example, each contain aspects of both yin and yang. Women are said to be yin on the outside (soft, yielding) but yang on the inside (firm, resilient), while men are yang on the outside but yin on the inside. These two aspects shift and interact until they strike a relative balance that is most suitable for each individual. In fact, some women are more assertive and yang than men, and this type of woman tends to gravitate towards a man who is more yielding and yin than others. Similarly, extremely macho men tend to prefer more docile, yielding women.

Nothing is absolutely yin or yang, and everything tends to seek a complementary opposite that strikes the most stable balance relative to itself. Take for example water, which is often invoked as a symbol of yin but which also has its own yang phases. When the sun (yang) heats water (yin) to a sufficient degree, it transforms into vapour (yang) and rises upwards (a yang direction). High in the sky, vapour cools and condenses to form clouds, and when this yin process of condensation reaches its utmost stage, yang vapour transforms into yin water and falls down (a yin direction) as rain. Stars are formed when the yin process of coalescence acts upon yang gases until they become yin matter, after which they begin the yang process of radiating yang heat and yang light outwards until they burn out and the process starts over again.

In breathing, inhalation is the yin phase, accumulating and concentrating air inwards while exhalation is the yang phase, releasing and expanding air outwards. In the nervous system, the sympathetic circuit is the active yang phase, preparing the body for action and putting all yin functions on hold. The parasympathetic circuit, in which energy is conserved and the body is calmed, is triggered by stillness and rest and forms the yin phase of the nervous system.

Yin and yang are therefore measures of relative polarity and degrees of activity, not fixed qualities. When it is said that energy is either too yin or too yang, it means that the energy is too strong or too weak, too hot or too cold, too light or too dark, with respect to a particular condition or reference point. In human health, that point of reference is the particular individual and his or her own optimum point of balance. The heat of midsummer in the tropics, for example, may be far too yang for a person born and raised in Scandinavia, but just right for a native of India or Africa. A Thai or Tahitian, however, might find even the mildest autumn weather in Canada to be much too yin, while a Canadian would feel perfectly comfortable.

Contrary to superficial appearances, the polarity of yin and yang is always complementary, not conflicting. Yin and yang are opposite slopes of the same hill, two sides of the same coin, and neither one could exist without the presence of the other, for there are no one-sided coins in nature. Furthermore, when you flip a coin, either side can turn up, indicating the mutual interchangeability of both sides. Yin and yang are therefore two complementary aspects of the same energy, and they both come from the same source. As Lao-tzu wrote in the *Tao Teh Ching*; 'The One [Source] gave birth to two things [yin and yang].'

Mutual transmutation is a fundamental aspect of the law of yin and yang. Each carries within itself the seed of the other, as indicated in the classical Chinese Symbol (Fig. 3). Whenever either yin or yang reaches its most extreme phase, it spontaneously transmutes itself to the other pole, thereby re-establishing optimum balance in relation to the particular circumstances. When a fever (yang) gets too hot, the body bursts out in sweat (yin), which carries the excess heat out of the body and thereby re-establishes equilibrium. When your body gets too cold, it starts to shiver, and these involuntary muscular contractions help generate body heat to balance the cold.

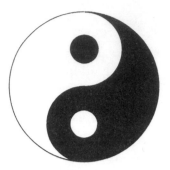

Fig. 3 **Tai-Chi (pronounced 'tai-jee'), the 'Supreme Ultimate': ancient Taoist symbol depicting the primordial unity, interdependence, and constant flux of yin and yang.**

When something obstructs the normal cyclic transformations of yin and yang and they are unable to establish and maintain relative balance, the extreme degree of one or the other causes abnormal conditions. In nature, extreme imbalances in the energies of sky and earth cause such abnormal phenomena as hurricanes, forest fires, floods, and earthquakes. In humans, energy imbalances cause fevers, indigestion, headaches, high blood pressure, constipation, and other disorders, and if such conditions are not corrected, they lead to degeneration and death.

The relative balance of yin and yang in humans is closely related to emotions, which unleash powerful energy currents that have profound physiological side effects. In English, the word 'emotion' is best understood as a contraction of the phrase 'energy in motion'. When you lose your temper, for example, you 'fume' and get 'steaming mad', an extreme yang condition. Your breath becomes short and fast, with stronger exhalations than inhalations. Since exhalation is the yang phase of breathing, your body employs it to expel the excess yang accumulated by anger, thereby rebalancing internal energy. When you're sad, you feel 'down' and 'low' (yin directions), and your energy swings towards yin, causing you to sigh, a yin breathing mode that deepens inhalation and shortens exhalation. This condition of extreme yin is thus balanced by assimilating extra energy from air, which raises the level of yang. Extreme emotions invariably upset the delicate balance of energies within the human system, and in Chinese medicine they are regarded as root causes of disease and degeneration.

Practical applications

In philosophy, the Great Principle of Yin and Yang provides the measure which determines all values and qualities. 'Hot' (yang) has no degree of heat without 'cold' (yin) to contrast it. 'Good' (yang) has no significance without the concept of 'bad' (yin) as counterpoint. 'Beauty' without 'ugliness' to compare it remains invisible. Realizing that temporal life on earth is always a matter of relative balance, Taoist philosophy always includes the other side of the story and takes no rigid stand or absolute view on any worldly issue. Every object and idea has both its front and back sides, its up and down directions, its positive and negative aspects, and as relative phases of yin and yang they have no fixed values. As Lao-tzu points out in the *Tao Teh Ching*: 'Long and short compare one another; high and low determine one another.' Unlike the dualistic philosophy of the West, which separates everything into two exclusively opposite and mutually hostile camps, such as 'good' and 'evil', 'right' and 'wrong', Taoist philosophy links all opposites as relative values according to the principle of yin and yang. In Taoist terms, 'good' and 'bad', 'right' and 'wrong' function as complementary pairs, as singular units with two interchangeable phases. Therefore, Taoists take a 'both/and' rather than an 'either/or' approach to life's dualistic decisions.

Taoists also stress the importance of flexibility in thought and behaviour. Rigid patterns of thought and inflexible attachment to habitual modes of behaviour run counter to the law of yin and yang, creating conflict among humans and disharmony between humans and their natural habitats. Only flexibility in thought and behaviour permits spontaneous adaptation to the constant cyclical change of nature and life. This spontaneous adaptability is the true meaning of Darwin's term 'survival of the fittest'. The 'fittest' are not necessarily the strongest, but rather those who 'fit' most successfully into their environments. In fact, the strongest are often the first to perish because of their stubborn insistence on asserting themselves over their environment rather than conforming to it: 'The bigger they come, the harder they fall.' Similarly, the tree with the hardest wood is the first to be felled by the woodcutter's axe and the first to crack in hurricane winds, and the hardest stone is slowly but surely ground to sand by soft, yielding, ever adaptable water.

Bamboo has always been a Taoist symbol of longevity because it bends in the strongest winds without breaking and therefore survives, while rigid plants break and die. The Taoist way of life combines external flexibility (yin) with internal firmness (yang). Remaining firm in their inner goals, Taoists take a very flexible approach to the methods they employ in achieving those goals. They regard goals as eternal ideals engendered by spirit and drawn from 'heaven', which is yang, and view methods as practical techniques dependent upon the changing conditions and natural limitations of life on earth, which is yin. It is therefore appropriate to hold firmly to one's goals while remaining flexible in one's methods. What works well for one person does not necessarily work well for another: 'different strokes for different folks'. Stubborn insistence on always doing things the same way, regardless of changing external conditions, causes conflict between humans and nature. Similarly, spiritual vacillation and ambivalent goals lead nowhere. One reason Taoists have such deep respect for the female yin principle is that it is like water, adapting itself flexibly to all conditions without losing its own essential nature. Women adapt more successfully to the world and live longer than men because, while remaining internally firm and resilient, they adapt readily to external changes.

In human health and medical science, yin and yang have abundant practical applications, based on the principle 'like macrocosm, like microcosm'. In Chinese, this concept is expressed with the phrases: 'Heaven and humans mutually reflect each other.' Every human being has his or her own 'microcosmic' electromagnetic energy field, with the positive pole in the head and the negative pole in the sacrum, and this field interacts with the earth's own electromagnetic field. Celestial energy from the sky enters the human energy system through the head, while earth energy enters through the 'yin confluence' (hui yin) point in the perineum. These energies circulate within the human system through an energy circuit called the Microcosmic Orbit (Fig. 4).

It is through the parallel convergence of the electromagnetic fields of the earth and humans that elemental environmental energies such as weather, the cyclic changes of seasons, solar and lunar phases, and other external energies have direct impacts on human energy. Western medical science is just beginning to recognize these natural rhythmic shifts in human energy as 'biorhythms', but Taoist science has known about it for thousands of years. Each day, for example, is divided into its own yang phase (midnight till noon) and yin phase (noon till midnight), and human energy shifts accordingly. Thus early morning (yang) has always been associated with high energy, and midafternoon (yin) siesta time. Each month also has its yin and yang phases, with yin rising

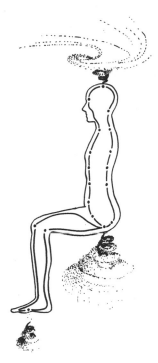

Fig. 4 **The Microcosmic Orbit: cosmic energies of heaven and earth enter into orbit within the human system via energy channels and power points.**

from the full moon till the new moon, and yang rising from the new moon till the full moon. Women's menstrual cycles are the most obvious human reflection of the earth's lunar cycles, but men as well as women are influenced by the moon's cycles in more subtle ways, such as moods, emotions, and general vitality. The year shifts rhythmically between yin and yang in terms of seasons, with new yang arising in spring and reaching full yang maturity in summer and new yin developing in autumn and maturing in the full yin of winter. Taoists always adjust their diets, sexual activity, and other habits to fit appropriately with these shifting seasonal energies. Although the Western medical establishment has been very reluctant to accept the results of recent scientific research on human energy and biorhythms, some Western scientists are nevertheless forging full steam ahead in this field, as evidenced by the following passage written in 1971 by Dr Bertram S. Brown of the US National Institute of Mental Health:

> From the moment of conception until death, rhythm is as much a part of our structure as our bones and flesh. Most of us are dimly aware that we fluctuate in energy, mood,

well-being, and performance each day, and that there are longer, more subtle behavioral alterations each week, each month, season, and year.

Through studies of biological rhythms, many aspects of human variability – in symptoms of illness, in response to medical treatment, in learning, and job performance – are being illuminated. Already, some of our changes of moods and vulnerabilities to stress and illness, our peaks of strength and productivity, can be anticipated . . . Timing promises to become an important factor in preventive health programs and medicine . . .

When we're healthy and environmental conditions are normal, our bodies adjust automatically to the cyclic changes of seasons, days, months, and weather. However, when human vitality is weak from energy stagnation or illness, or when environmental changes are extreme, the human system often fails to adjust properly to fluctuation in external energies. These 'evil energies' can then invade the human energy system and upset the internal balance of yin and yang, causing all sorts of diseases and discomforts.

In human physiology, yin and yang govern the dynamics of form and function in every organ, gland, tissue, and vital fluid in the body. Yin is regarded as 'solid' and therefore governs form, while yang is 'hollow' and governs function. Yin assimilates and stores, yang transforms and transports. Thus the vital organs are all divided into matched pairs according to yin and yang: the 'solid' yin organs are the heart, liver, kidneys, lungs, and spleen; their respective yang partners are the small intestine, gall bladder, bladder, large intestine, and stomach. Blood is yin, energy is yang; the endocrine system is yin, the nervous system is yang; digestion is yin, excretion is yang; and so forth. In biochemistry, alkaline is yin and acid is yang, and their relative equilibrium is expressed in terms of pH balance.

In Chinese medicine, the diagnosis and pathology of disease is analysed first in terms of yin and yang balance. The *Internal Medicine Classic* states; 'Physicians who excel in diagnosis first check complexion and pulse, then analyse the condition in terms of yin and yang.' Just as maintenance of optimum yin-yang balance is the key to health, correct analysis of yin-yang imbalance is the first step in diagnosis of disease. Symptoms of excess yang, for example, include fever, sweating, constipation, chronic thirst, dry lips and mouth, dark urine, heavy breathing, rapid pulse, and irritability. Excess yin is reflected in such symptoms as chills, cold hands and feet, loose bowels, lack of thirst, shallow breathing, slow pulse, and lethargy. Chinese therapy focuses not on the temporary relief of these various external symptoms, as modern Western medicine does, but rather on correcting the basic internal imbalance of yin and yang which causes the external symptoms. When the root cause is corrected, all symptoms disappear naturally. This is called 'treating the root, not the symptom'.

All Chinese herbs are categorized according to the degree of therapeutic influence they have on the balance of yin and yang in the human energy system. Extremely yang herbs are labelled 'hot', moderately yang are 'warm'. Extremely yin herbs are 'cold', moderately yin are 'cool'. Herbs with equally balanced yin-yang energies are called 'neutral'. The *Internal Medicine Classic* states; 'If it is hot, cool it down; if it is cold, warm it up.' Therefore, cooling yin herbs such as rhubarb and senna are prescribed for acute constipation, which is a 'hot' yang condition. Warming yang herbs such as cayenne and ginger are given for such 'cold' yin conditions as colds, flu, poor circulation, and indigestion. 'Cool' coriander soothes the excess yang responsible for urinary tract discomfort, such as cystitis and the heartburn of hyperacidity, while 'warm' ginseng balances the excess yin that causes fatigue and anaemia. Some yang herbs cause internal energy to ascend, thereby counter-acting yin conditions of descending energy such as diarrhoea. Certain yin herbs induce internal energy to descend, thereby balancing yang symptoms of 'rebellious ascending energy' such as headaches and irritability. The permutations and combinations are endless, and it requires many years of clinical experience to learn how to juggle all the relevant internal and external factors in the great balancing act of yin and yang.

Yin and yang provide Taoists with a convenient and accurate measure with which to calibrate and adjust their daily habits in order to guard the Three Treasures of life. During the cold yin conditions of winter, Taoists adjust their diets to include more warming yang foods, and males sharply reduce their frequency of ejaculation in order to preserve the precious warming yang essence of semen. If a Taoist feels hot and feverish (yang), he will consume plenty of fruits and fluids (yin) to cool down his excess body heat. Today, hypertension is a very common condition of yang excess caused by chronic stress. An easy and effective antidote that requires neither drugs nor doctors is simply to practise a few minutes of deep abdominal breathing and sit in stillness and silence for a while. This automatically switches the nervous system over from the active yang phase of the sympathetic circuit to the calming, restorative yin phase of the parasympathetic circuit. Taking 'uppers' and 'downers' (amphetamines and barbiturates) to whip up or bludgeon down the nervous system provides only temporary symptomatic relief for nervous disorders without correcting the root causes. The toxic side effects of such drugs further impair the body's capacity to restore balance between the sympathetic yang and parasympathetic yin circuits, thereby causing a vicious cycle of drug dependency. This sort of therapy, which prevails in Western allopathic medicine, causes more problems than it cures and runs contrary to the fundamental principles of human health.

By taking appropriate measures to maintain optimum balance of yin and yang both internally and externally, you can prevent the extreme conditions of energy imbalance which cause disease and accelerate the degenerative aging process. You don't need to be a doctor to practise such basic preventive health care, and if you practise it diligently, you won't need doctors. All you need to do is familiarize yourself with the universal principles of polarity, trinity, and other fundamental forces that make heat rise and rain fall, winds blow and rivers flow, then apply those principles creatively to the microcosmic universe within yourself.

CHAPTER 3

The Three Powers

Heaven is clear and calm; earth is stable and tranquil.
Humans who reject these virtues perish, while those who
adopt them thrive.

Huai-nan-tzu (first century AD)

Heaven (*tien*), earth (*dee*), and humans (*ren*) are known in Taoist
alchemy as the 'Three Powers'. These three powers intersect and
interact, weaving the mental and material threads of life into the
warp and woof of the human body and mind. Humans thrive to
the extent that they conform to the forces which mould and
nurture them. From heaven they receive the treasure of spirit and
the awareness it confers, and from earth they obtain the essential
elements that constitute their bodies. The fusion of spirit and
essence generates the energy with which humans conduct their
lives. When human energy remains in harmony with the primal
forces of heaven and earth, it flourishes and protects the health of
the body. When human energy runs counter to the laws of heaven
and earth, it soon exhausts itself, and the body degenerates and
perishes. The laws of heaven are sometimes referred to as 'destiny',
while the laws of earth are called 'nature'. The harmony of destiny
and nature is the Tao, the Great Way, and manifests its highest form
in humans. Consequently, humans who follow the Tao fulfil their
spiritual destiny while also enjoying the fruits of their earthly
nature.

The Taoist way of life taps the energies of heaven and earth and
blends them harmoniously with human energy in order to cultivate
and conserve the Three Treasures. The enhanced power derived by
the practice of Taoist alchemy is called *Tao teh*, 'the virtue of Tao',
because it springs from prenatal sources of postnatal essence,
energy, and spirit. In other words, to obtain the health-giving, life-
prolonging 'virtue of Tao', one must balance the eternal ways of

heaven with the temporal nature of earth and harmonize them with human life.

'Heaven' refers to the sky and stars, to the sun, moon, and planets, and to all the cosmic energies which rain down on earth from these celestial sources. It also refers to the 'Source' – the infinite, ineffable, invisible, indivisible fount of primordial spirit and mental awareness. Externally, heaven's most obvious manifestation is weather, which in Chinese is called 'celestial energy' (*tien chee*). Heaven manifests its power in human life not only in thought and consciousness, but also in the mysterious force of fate and destiny (*ming*). It is therefore associated with the Taoist sciences of astrology and divination.

'Earth' refers to the planet we inhabit, the material world of continents and oceans, mountains and rivers, forests and plains. It is the source of the essential elements of which our physical bodies are composed and the wellspring of the postnatal energy we extract from food, water, and air. Earth manifests its power in the forces of nature (*hsing*), a term which in Chinese is synonymous with 'sex'. In human as well as other forms of life, nature expresses itself primarily in the fundamental appetites for food and sex, the two basic drives which sustain and propagate all species. The earthly aspect of human existence is neatly summarized in the old Taoist equation: food + sex = nature. Earth is thus associated with the sciences of nutrition and medicine, physical exercise and sexual yoga, geomancy and geophysics.

Macrocosmically, the term 'humanity' includes the entire human condition in all its various physical and spiritual manifestations, 'covered by heaven above and supported by earth below'. The human realm is the source of our human heritage and of the specific genetic attributes which distinguish us among the many species with whom we share the earth. Humanity is the mould that forms the expression of our energy and the way it interacts with the energies of heaven and earth.

Human energy is engendered at the moment of conception and sustained postnatally by blending the energy derived from food with the energy extracted from air to form the True Human Energy of life. Humans exist between heaven and earth and must therefore harness and harmonize the powers of heaven and earth to survive and propagate the species. Heaven is the source of spirit and generates the human mind; earth is the source of essence and generates the human body. These two powers flow together in humanity and are regulated by human energy.

Long ago, Taoist sages noticed a fundamental difference in the energy coming down from the sky and the energy radiating up from the ground. They labelled these contrasting yet complementary forces as 'yang' and 'yin' and named their sources as 'heaven' and 'earth'. They discovered that heaven and earth project their forces into the human realm as formless but highly functional emanations of pure energy and that the yang of heaven and the yin of earth create the dynamic polar field in which human energy functions. The *Internal Medicine Classic* states: 'The principle of yin and yang is the foundation of the entire universe and the basis of all creation. Heaven was created by the accumulation of yang. Earth was formed by the accumulation of yin. Yin and yang are the primal sources of all power and the wellsprings of all creation.'

Thus the yang forces of heaven and the yin forces of earth meet and mix in humans as well as in all other forms of life on earth. Yin and yang are kept in balance by human energy, which also harmonizes the Five Elemental Energies of nature. The lower species of animals adapt to nature by natural instinct and apply their energy entirely to physiological survival and propagation of their species. Owing to the superior awareness bestowed by heaven, humans are endowed not only with earthly instinct but also with spiritual insight, and therefore humans are the only species on earth with conscious access to the transcendental powers of heaven. This pivotal position between heaven and earth, spirit and flesh, allows humans the privilege of free will. For humans, the conduct of life on earth is a matter of choice, ranging from the base animal instincts and sensual gratifications of the hedonist to the higher spiritual aspirations and ascetic disciplines of the sage and yogi.

Heaven and earth, spiritual and sensual, will and instinct – these compose the fundamental dichotomy of corporeal human life and define the human condition. It is the task of each individual to balance these polar forces as he or she forges a path through life. In Taoist terminology, the earthly physical pole of human life is called 'nature' (*hsing*) and the heavenly spiritual pole is called 'destiny' (*ming*). The manner in which an individual juggles these forces determines the direction and focus of his or her life and forms another fundamental Taoist equation: Nature + destiny = human life. The Taoist way of life is neatly summarized in the ancient Chinese phrase '*hsing ming shuang hsiou*', which means 'to cultivate nature and destiny together'.

Most of the world's religious and mystical traditions separate heaven and earth into two irreconcilable realms, thereby forcing humans to choose one and forfeit the other. The hedonist who cleaves to the sensory gratifications of earth is condemned as a sinner and denied a berth in heaven, while the ascetic who aspires to heaven is revered as a saint but deprived of the sensual pleasures on earth. This dualistic division of body and mind cuts against the grain of human nature and denies humans the opportunity to develop and express their full potential. Splitting humanity into the hostile camps of saints and sinners, believers and infidels, the elect and the losers, has been responsible for much of the pride and prejudice, spiritual anxiety and physical frustration, persecution and warfare that have marked human history. Only the Tao combines heaven and earth on a single path that integrates destiny with nature and taps the powers of both for the physical as well as spiritual fulfilment of human life.

The Three Powers have macrocosmic as well as microcosmic aspects, external as well as internal manifestations, and Taoist alchemy applies the principles of the former towards the cultivation and conservation of the latter. On the internal micro-cosmic level, the forces of heaven, earth, and humanity express themselves within the body and mind of every individual human being, and it is these forces that are manipulated in the esoteric Taoist alchemy called *nei-gung* ('internal work'). The head is associated with the spiritual qualities and cosmic forces emanating from heaven, the sacrum houses vital essence and draws upon the energies of earth, and the chest expresses True Human Energy through breath, speech, and emotions. The human body has its own internal 'weather' and 'seasons', its 'winds' and 'waves', 'rivers' and 'mountains', and the vital organs are governed by the Five Elemental Energies of Fire, Water, Wood, Metal, and Earth. The body has its yang pole above and its yin pole below, its own geography and cosmology, flora and fauna, heaven and earth, forming a complete world unto itself (Fig. 5).

By studying the cyclic patterns of earth and invoking the spiritual guidance of heaven, the Taoist adept forges a syncretic path which balances the powers of heaven and earth and harmonizes them with human life. On this path, the finite limitations of temporal life on earth become vehicles for the expression of the infinite spiritual awareness of heaven, and human life conforms harmoniously with nature as well as destiny.

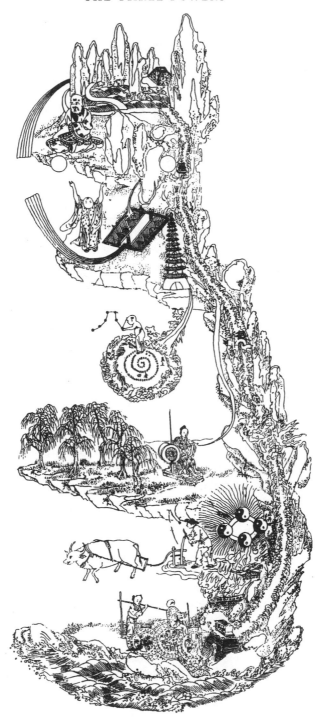

Fig. 5 **Classical Taoist illustration of universal forces at work within the human system, harmonized and transformed by the internal alchemy of meditation.**

CHAPTER 4

The Four Foundations

Blood and nourishment are yin and circulate internally;
they are protected by yang. Energy and resistance are
yang and emanate externally; they are nourished by yin.
The Yellow Emperor's Classic of Internal Medicine
(second century BC)

The Four Foundations of health are blood (*hsueh*), energy (*chee*),
nourishment (*ying*), and resistance (*wei*). Physiologically functional
manifestations of yin and yang, they are interactive and mutually
dependent, and their condition and relative balance determine the
state of one's health and the strength of one's resistance to disease
and degeneration. Among the Four Foundations, the continuous
and unimpeded circulation of blood and energy forms the basis
and the vehicle for the nourishment and resistance of the entire
organism. As the *Internal Medicine Classic* states: 'Blood and energy
flow constantly as water in a stream, revolve continuously as the
sun and moon, turn endlessly as a circle.'

Blood is the circulatory vehicle for nourishment. Both belong
to yin and are forms of essence. The fluid biochemical forms of
nourishment circulate within the blood vessels, while the pure
bioenergetic potency derived from nourishment, which is called
'nourishing energy' (*ying chee*), flows within the energy meridians.

Similarly, energy is the circulatory vehicle for resistance.
Both belong to yang and are functional manifestations of
energy. The type of energy which generates resistance is
called 'protective energy' (*wei chee*) and circulates through
the subcutaneous tissues around the surface of the body.
Protective energy and the resistance it provides circulate
outside the blood vessels and energy meridians. The interrelationships among the Four Foundations are summarized in the
following chart:

vehicle	function	pole	treasure	location	path	role
blood	nourishment	yin	essence	internal	within vessels	internal nourishment
energy	resistance	yang	energy	external	outside vessels	external protection

The functions of the Four Foundations

Blood

The term 'blood' includes all the essential elements of which blood is composed and for which blood serves as a circulatory vehicle, including red and white blood cells, T- and B-lymphocytes and scavenger cells, enzymes and hormones, glucose and nutrients. It also refers to the overall condition of the bloodstream – its degree of purity or toxicity, acid or alkaline pH balance, its capacity to carry oxygen and nutrients, and its circulatory efficiency. Blood depends on the heart for circulation, on the liver for filtering out toxins and replenishing nutrients, and on the marrow for fresh supplies of red and white blood cells. Among the Four Foundations, blood is the factor most directly responsible for the nourishment and overall welfare of the physical body, and its condition influences the other three foundations through the complementary interplay of yin and yang. For example, since blood (yin) nourishes energy (yang) and carries nourishment (yin), weak or toxic blood cannot sustain high energy and cannot circulate sufficient nourishment to meet the body's needs. In turn, insufficient nourishment (yin) cannot nurture high resistance (yang), and low energy provides a poor vehicle for resistance. In the alchemy of the Four Foundations, blood is the primary ingredient and regulator of health.

Energy

'Energy' refers to all the various types of bioenergy associated with human health and vitality, including the elemental energies of the vital organs, the nourishing energy which circulates in the meridians, the protective energy which suffuses the surface of the body, and the neuro-active energy of the nervous system. Energy is associated with the lungs through breathing, which extracts external energy from air and blends it in the bloodstream with the internal energy extracted by digestion from food and water. The resulting blend is the basis for human energy and metabolism. Energy also refers to the relative balance and condition of the body's collective energies, as measured on four polar scales: yin and yang; cold and hot; deficient and excessive; internal and external. Since 'energy commands blood' and also generates resistance, deficient or stagnant energy impedes circulation of blood, depriving the entire body of adequate nourishment, and lowers resistance.

Nourishment

'Nourishment' is a functional extension of blood, upon whose unimpeded circulation it depends for delivery. It obtains vital nutrients from the stomach and associated digestive organs and vital fluids from the glands. The nourishing elements circulated in the blood include such basic nutrients as vitamins, minerals, amino acids, and glucose (blood sugar), as well as essential secretions such as hormones and enzymes. 'Nourishment' refers primarily to the vital biodynamic functions of blood, rather than to nutrients and other forms of essence themselves. In addition to circulating internally as biochemicals within the blood vessels, a more pure and potent form of nourishment extracted from essential substances and called 'essential energy' (*jing chee*) or 'vitality' circulates internally within the twelve major meridians associated with the vital organs. The essential elements of nourishment depend upon adequate diet and nutrition, efficient digestion and assimilation of nutrients, and sufficient secretions of essential hormones and enzymes.

Resistance

Resistance is a functional manifestation of the protective energy which flows along the surface of the body, outside the energy meridians. It depends on the kidneys and adrenal glands as a primary source of energy and is related to sexual vitality and sexual hormones. Resistance radiates outwards from the surface of the body and beyond, forming a protective shield which guards the body from invasion by the 'Six Evils' of excessive environmental energies – wind, cold, dampness, and so forth. It manifests itself as vitality and is reflected in the condition of skin, pores, and hair. Its primary indicator in Chinese diagnosis is called *chee-seh* (literally 'energy colour'), a term which refers to an individual's vitality as reflected in the tone and colour of his or her facial complexion, ears, eyes, and tongue. A bright, rosy complexion, clear eyes, pink tongue, and well-flushed ears indicate flourishing vitality and strong resistance, while a pallid complexion, dull eyes, dark tongue, and pale ears reflect low vitality and weak resistance. Resistance is therefore a sort of radiant energy which suffuses and surrounds the entire surface of the body, protecting it from negative external energies. Since 'blood follows where energy leads', strong protective energy draws blood to the surface, especially in the face, where its sufficiency or deficiency is reflected in the 'energy colour' of complexion.

Immunity

Collectively, the Four Foundations of health constitute the complex defence mechanisms of the human immune system. In Western medicine, immunity is attributed solely to the presence of certain forms of 'vital essence' in the bloodstream, such as T-cells from the thymus gland, white blood cells from the marrow, scavenger cells such as leukocytes, and a variety of enzymes. In Chinese medicine, the immunological role of these essential secretions is also fully recognized, but they are regarded as basic components in a larger defence system, not as the body's sole immunity factors. A highly toxic or acidified bloodstream, for example, is a poor conductor for immune factors such as T-cells, and if energy is deficient, circulation will be insufficient to distribute those factors uniformly throughout the body. In the Taoist system of health, energy is even more important to immunity than essence, especially the radiant energy of protective *wei chee* which envelops the surface of the body. Unfortunately, even though the existence of human energy has been conclusively established by modern technology, conventional Western medicine still does not recognize its immunological role in human health and therefore does not know how to manipulate it as a tool in curative and preventive health care. Because of the rapidly spreading phenomenon of acquired immune deficiency syndrome (AIDS) throughout the world, the pathology of human immune deficiency is of paramount importance these days, and energy medicine could play a key role in the cure and prevention of this acquired condition.

Immune deficiency

In traditional Chinese medicine, there are four fundamental forms of immune deficiency, each associated with one of the Four Foundations of health, as follows:

Blood deficiency

The primary symptom of blood deficiency is anaemia, or 'weak blood'. It can be caused by blood toxicity, hyperacidity of the bloodstream, insufficient haemoglobin, and poor circulation. It is also associated with low red and white blood-cell count, deficiency of certain protective antioxidant enzymes such as superoxide dismutase (SOD), and malnutrition. It impairs the blood's 'house-cleaning' functions as well as its nourishing distribution of nutrients, oxygen, enzymes, and other essential elements.

Energy deficiency

Primary symptoms of energy deficiency include chronic fatigue, physical lassitude, mental lethargy, low libido, and 'low spirits'. It can be caused by a variety of conditions, including obstructions in the energy meridians, inefficient digestion and poor assimilation of nutrients, cellular metabolic disorders, shallow or erratic breathing patterns, emotional excess, and dysfunction of the adrenal glands due to chronic stress. Energy deficiency impairs immunity by depressing blood circulation, impeding vital functions such as digestion, metabolism, and excretion, and weakening the radiant shield of protective energy which guards against harmful external energies.

Yin deficiency

Associated with nourishment and vital fluids, yin deficiency results in insufficient secretions of essential hormones and enzymes, deficient digestion, and impairment in the protective cleansing functions of the lymphatic system and mucous membranes. Common symptoms of yin deficiency include dry skin, chronic thirst, and aversion to heat.

Yang deficiency

Yang deficiency is directly related to resistance and results in a weakening of the body's protective shield of radiant energy. It is often caused by deficiency in the kidneys, especially the adrenal glands, which in Chinese medicine are regarded as the 'Root of Life' because they store the body's precious supplies of primordial energy. In middle-aged men, this condition, which is called *shen-kui* ('deficient kidneys'), is often caused by excessive loss of semen due to frequent ejaculation, which puts a tremendous strain on the adrenals. Chronic stress and emotional strain, which also distress the adrenals, are causes of yang deficiency in both men and women. Aversion to cold, lack of thirst, cold hands and feet, and chronic fatigue are common symptoms of yang deficiency.

As mentioned above, blood is the cornerstone of the Four Foundations, and its condition determines the degree of one's resistance to negative external energies as well as immunity to disease. Cancer, for example, is regarded as a 'blood disease' in traditional Chinese medicine, because weak, toxic, or otherwise impaired blood is unable to perform its vital functions of nourishing and cleansing bodily tissues. Deficient blood permits cellular wastes and pollutants to accumulate in tissues, until they become so toxic that they fester and ferment like rotting flesh, forming malignant tumours which spread to other tissues. Conventional Western therapy treats cancer with surgery, radiation, and toxic chemicals, attacking the symptomatic tumours but doing nothing whatsoever to correct the extreme toxicity of blood and imbalance of energy which causes the problem in the first place. Indeed, such radical therapy further weakens blood and depletes energy, so that even if a temporary remission is achieved by removing or destroying a few tumours, the cancer usually recurs in even more virulent form.

The proper preventive as well as curative therapy for cancer is first to detoxify and purify the blood, then rebuild it with proper nutrition and appropriate supplements and circulate it with deep breathing and rhythmic exercise. Scavenger cells, enzymes, and other immune factors carried by healthy blood will then attack the cancerous tissues, digest and dissolve the tumours, and dispose of the debris through the excretory organs. There are many documented examples of people who have conquered cancer naturally by rebuilding the Four Foundations, and countless cases of those who died prematurely by permitting doctors to cut, burn, or poison their tumorous tissues; yet natural cancer therapies remain illegal in the United States and many other industrialized countries, despite the failure of conventional Western medicine to deal successfully with this fatal condition, which continues to spread.

The acute immune deficiency associated with AIDS is another example of what happens when modern lifestyles erode the Four Foundations of health. Immune deficiency is not simply caused by a virus but by environmental factors. If HIV were the sole cause of

AIDS, it would stand to scientific reason that everyone with symptoms of full-blown AIDS would be infected with HIV, but that is not the case. And so far, fewer than 5 per cent of those who carry HIV have developed any AIDS-related symptoms.

Meanwhile, *all* the following conditions are known to produce symptoms of immune deficiency identical to those officially attributed to AIDS and HIV: acute pesticide poisoning; chronic long-term use of antibiotics; syphilis, which is making a big comeback in the USA and Africa; exposure to nuclear waste and radiation; chronic malnutrition. Like cancer, immune deficiency can be acquired by internal and external toxicity, by pollution of the environment, by junk food and chemical drugs, by heavy metals in tap water and steroids in beef, and other public policies which promote economic growth at the direct expense of human health.

Building the Four Foundations

The key to health and longevity is to guard the Three Treasures of life, and the best way to do that is to build the Four Foundations. In this age of pernicious pollution, denatured junk-food diets, toxic chemicals, and misguided medical care, taking the initiative to guard your own health is more important than ever.

On the physical level of essence, one of the most effective ways of building blood, boosting vitality, and raising resistance is to use tonic Chinese herbal formulas regularly. There are four basic types of tonic formula, one for each of the Four Foundations.

Blood tonics
These yin potions build up the liver and heart, which are the organs primarily responsible for filtering, nourishing, and circulating blood. These formulas also enrichen blood plasma, cleanse the bloodstream, and strengthen the blood vessels.

Energy tonics
Energy tonics are yang formulas and stimulate the circulation of vital energy throughout the body's network of energy meridians, thereby enhancing both physical and mental vitality. They also improve the functions of the lungs and pancreas, the organs responsible for extracting postnatal energy from air through breathing and from food through the secretion of digestive enzymes.

Yin tonics

These formulas enhance nourishment by stimulating secretions of vital essence, including hormones and enzymes, and by improving digestion and assimilation of nutrients. They also stimulate production of spinal fluids, semen, blood, mucus, lymph, and other vital bodily fluids.

Yang tonics

Yang tonics warm up the kidneys, which store primordial essence and energy. When the kidneys are thus stimulated, they radiate protective energy to the surface of the body, where it fortifies the guardian shield of resistance and enhances the body's capacity to adapt itself quickly to environmental energy cycles. Yang tonics also boost sexual vitality and enhance potency.

Tonic herbs should be used only when your health and vitality are flourishing, never during periods of illness or debility. Further details and specific formulas are provided in Part V.

The Four Foundations may also be strengthened by marshalling energy through the daily practice of *chee-gung*. This is perhaps the most potent and effective system of preventive health care in the world. Applying the principle that 'blood follows where energy leads', *chee-gung* brings the breathing process under voluntary control in order to harness and circulate energy, which simultaneously stimulates the circulation of blood to all tissues. *Chee-gung* regulates the heart and pulse, oxygenates the bloodstream, and detoxifies blood and tissues by facilitating rapid excretion of metabolic wastes as well as toxic pollutants absorbed from the environment. It enhances energy by improving respiratory efficiency and stimulates the metabolic conversion of essence to energy. *Chee-gung* builds the foundation of nourishment by stimulating secretions of hormones from glands, increasing secretions of digestive enzymes in the pancreas and stomach, and improving metabolism. It also gives a direct boost to resistance by driving and distributing energy outwards to the surface, thereby enhancing guardian energy. This last effect is reflected in the visible improvement of *chee-seh* in the facial complexion of anyone who practises *chee-gung* for a while.

Spiritual practices such as meditation also help fortify the Four Foundations and should always be included in any well-balanced programme of preventive health care. Chronic stress severely strains the adrenals and nerves, and meditation is a quick and effective way to switch the autonomous nervous system from the stressful sympathetic circuit over to the restful, restorative parasympathetic circuit. Meditation permits the entire body to relax and the energy channels to open up, so that energy as well as blood may circulate freely throughout the system, invigorating organs, stimulating glands, and tonifying other vital tissues. It is no accident that in Eastern as well as Western traditions, paintings of monks, spiritual masters, holy men, and yogis always depict a halo around the head. That's the aura of energy which meditation generates, the pure glow of 'radiant health'. Meditation also cultivates the emotional equanimity and positive outlook which are so essential to maintaining health and promoting longevity.

Like yin and yang and the Three Treasures, the Four Foundations are mutually dependent and indivisibly complementary factors of human life. By understanding their dynamic functions and inter-actions and cultivating each in its own way, you can maintain the natural balance and harmony your body, energy, and mind require in order to survive and thrive in an increasingly hostile environment.

CHAPTER 5

The Five Energies

The Five Elemental Energies of Wood, Fire, Earth, Metal,
and Water encompass all the myriad phenomena of
nature. It is a paradigm that applies equally to humans.
The Yellow Emperor's Classic of Internal Medicine
(second century BC)

The Five Elemental Energies (*wu hsing*) represent the tangible
activities of yin and yang as manifested in the cyclic changes of
nature which regulate life on earth. Also known as the Five
Movements (*wu yun*), they define the various stages of transformation in the recurring natural cycles of seasonal change, growth
and decay, shifting climatic conditions, sounds, flavours, emotions,
and human physiology. Each energy is associated with the natural
element which most closely resembles its function and character,
and from these elements they take their names. Unlike the Western
and other systems of five elements, the Chinese system focuses on
energy and its transformations, not on form and substance. The
elements thus symbolize the *activities* of the energies with which
they are associated.

As manifestations of yin and yang on earth, the Five Elemental
Energies represent various degrees of 'fullness' and 'emptiness' in
the relative balance of yin and yang within any particular energy
system. An ancient Chinese text explains this principle as follows:

By the transformation of yang and its union with yin, the
Five Elemental Energies of Wood, Fire, Earth, Metal, and
Water arise, each with its specific nature according to its
share of yin and yang. These Five Elemental Energies
constantly change their sphere of activity, nurturing and
counteracting one another so that there is a constancy in
the transformation from emptiness to abundance and

abundance to emptiness, like a ring without beginning or end. The interaction of these primordial forces brings harmonious change and the cycles of nature run their course . . . The Five Elemental Energies combine and recombine in innumerable ways to produce manifest existence. All things contain all Five Elemental Energies in various proportions.

Let's take a look at this idea in terms of the basic seasonal cycles of nature, which influence every living thing on earth. Water is the elemental energy associated with winter, when a state of extreme yin prevails. Winter is the season of stillness and rest, during which energy is condensed, conserved, and stored. Water is a highly concentrated element containing great potential power awaiting release. In the human body, Water is associated with essential fluids such as hormones, lymph, marrow, and enzymes, all of which contain great potential energy. Its colour is black, the colour which contains all other colours in concentrated form. In nature, Water is dissipated by excess heat; in humans, Water energy is depleted by the 'heat' of stress and excess emotions. The way to conserve the potential energy of Water is to stay still and 'be cool'.

The next phase of the seasonal cycle is spring, during which the Wood element arises from the potential energy of Water, just as plants sprout from the ground in spring rains. This is the 'new yang' stage of the cycle. Wood energy is expansive, exhilarant, explosive. It is the creative energy of 'spring fever', awakening the procreative drive of sexuality. It is associated with vigour and youth, growth and development. In the human body, Wood energy is associated with the movement of muscles and the activity of tissues. Its colour is green, the vibrant colour of spring growth. Wood energy demands free expression and space for open expansion. Blocking it gives rise to feelings of frustration, anger, jealousy, and stagnation.

Just as spring develops naturally into summer, so the aggressive creative energy of Wood matures into the flourishing 'full yang' energy of Fire. This is the most overtly energetic phase of the cycle, during which the 'heat' of full yang energy is sustained. All life forms flourish in summer owing to the warm, stable glow of Fire energy. Fire is related to the heart, which is the seat of human emotions and the organ whose constant warmth and pulse keeps blood and energy moving. Its colour is red, the warm colour of fire and blood. It is associated with love and compassion, generosity and joy, openness and abundance. If blocked, it results in hypertension and hysteria, heart problems and nervous disorders.

Towards the end of summer comes an interlude of perfect balance during which Fire burns down and energy mellows, transforming itself into the elemental energy of Earth. Neither yin nor yang predominates during this period; instead they are in a state of optimum balance. This is the pivot of the cycle, the fulcrum between the yang energies of spring and summer and the yin energies of autumn and winter. The Five Elemental Energies hum in harmony at this time, providing a sense of ease, wellbeing, and completeness. The Earth energy of late summer is the phase and the feeling celebrated in the song 'Summertime, and the living is easy . . .' Its colour is yellow, the colour of sun and earth, and in human anatomy it is associated with the stomach, spleen, and pancreas, which lie at the centre of the body and nourish the entire system. If Earth energy is deficient, digestion is impaired and the entire organism is thrown off balance owing to insufficient nourishment and vitality.

As summer passes into autumn, the energy of Earth transforms into Metal. During the Metal phase, energy once again begins to condense, contract, and draw inward for accumulation and storage, just as the crops of summer are harvested and stored in autumn for use in winter. Wastes are eliminated, like winnowing chaff from wheat, and only the essence is kept in preparation for the nonproductive Water phase of winter. If the harvest fails or falls short, there may not be sufficient energy stored during Water/ winter to generate a strong and healthy new cycle in the following Wood/spring. Metal energy controls the lungs, which extract and store essential energy from air and expel wastes from the blood, and the large intestine, which eliminates solid wastes while retaining and recycling water. Its colour is white, the colour of purity and essence. Autumn is the season of retrospection and meditative insight, for shedding old skin and dumping the excess baggage of external attachments and emotions accumulated in summer, just as trees shed their leaves and bees drive drones from the hive at this time of year. Resisting this energy by clinging sentimentally to past attachments can cause feelings of melancholy, grief, and anxiety, which manifest themselves physiologically in breathing difficulties, chest pain, skin problems, and low resistance. Flus, colds, and other respiratory ailments are common indicators of blocked Metal energy, which is associated with the lungs. Just as Metal is a refined extract of Earth forged by Fire, so autumn is the season for extracting and refining essential lessons from the activities and experiences of summer, transforming them into the quiet wisdom of winter.

And so the great wheel of nature turns in a continuous cycle of elementary energies, drawing all living things in its wake and proceeding in an orderly and rhythmic sequence:

Wood >	Fire >	Earth >	Metal >	Water
new yang	full yang	balanced yin & yang	new yin	full yin
spring	summer	late summer	autumn	winter
		{pivot}		

Like yin and yang, the Five Elemental Energies maintain their internal harmony through a system of mutual checks and balances known as 'creative' and 'control' cycles. Both these cycles, which counteract and balance one another, are in constant operation, maintaining the dynamic fields of polar forces required to move and transform energies. The creative cycle is one of generation, like the relationship between mother and child. Water generates Wood by nourishing its growth; Wood generates Fire by providing its fuel; Fire generates Earth by fertilizing it with ashes; Earth yields Metal by extraction and refinement; Metal becomes liquid like Water when it is melted.

The opposite force is the control cycle, a relationship of subjugation similar to that between the victor and the vanquished in battle. The *Internal Medicine Classic* describes the control cycle as follows:

> Wood brought into contact with Metal is felled;
> Fire brought into contact with Water is extinguished;
> Earth brought into contact with Wood is penetrated;
> Metal brought into contact with Fire is dissolved;
> Water brought into contact with Earth is halted.

Whenever a particular elemental energy grows too strong, it tends to exert an excessively stimulating influence over the following element in the creative cycle, like a domineering mother over a child, and at this point the element which controls the excessive energy kicks in to subjugate it and restore harmony. For example, if Wood flourishes to excess, providing so much fuel that Fire burns out of control, Metal steps in to cut down the supply of Wood and thereby re-establish normal balance. The creative and control cycles maintain constant harmony and balance among the Five Elemental Energies, as depicted in the diagram in Fig. 6.

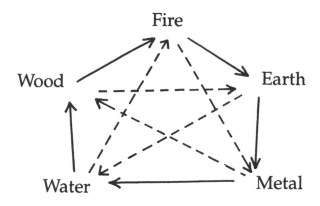

Fig. 6 **The creative (solid lines) and control (dotted lines) cycles of the Five Elemental Energies.**

Physiological applications

An ancient Chinese adage says: 'A tree grows from the roots.' Yin and yang and the Five Elemental Energies form the main roots in the Taoist tree of health, and the entire edifice of traditional Chinese medicine and physiology is based upon the foundation of these energy principles.

The Five Elemental Energies and their cycles provide a practical working model through which the interrelationships between the human body and the natural environment may be understood and controlled. They also illuminate the internal functional relationships between the body's various vital organs and explain how external elements such as foods and medicinal herbs influence the organs and their functions. All aspects of human health, including physiology and pathology, diagnosis and therapy, are rooted in this remarkably reliable system of polar forces and cyclic energy transformations.

The traditional Chinese view of human physiology differs significantly from the Western view in that the Chinese have always focused attention on the function rather than the form of the vital organs. The Western medical practice of studying human physiology based upon the anatomical locations of various organs as revealed in dissected cadavers makes no sense to Chinese physicians, because cadavers have no living energy and their organs are not functional. How can a dead body reveal anything significant about the dynamics of living energy? Furthermore, in addition to their biological functions and anatomical locations, the

Chinese concept of 'organs' also includes the specific type of energy that infuses each organ, as well as the energy meridians that channel organ energies to and from other parts of the body.

Over the ages, Chinese physicians discovered two fundamental principles which govern the vital organs and regulate their functional relationships. The first principle is that all the major organs are functionally paired according to yin and yang. The yin organs are called *dzang* or 'solid' organs and are involved primarily in functions of 'collecting and storing'. The matching yang organs are called *fu* or 'hollow' organs and deal mainly with functions of 'movement and transformation'. There are six *dzang* and six *fu*, matched in six yin/yang pairs, and each one is regulated by one of the Twelve Major Meridians.

The second principle is that each of the six pairs of organs is governed by one of the Five Elemental Energies, with Fire controlling two pairs. The creative and control cycles of these energies orchestrate the functional relationships between the organs and determine how external environmental energies influence internal conditions. Internal conditions are in turn reflected externally by the colour, tone, and texture of 'the five apertures and five tissues', such as eyes and ears, skin and hair, which thus provide handy tools for diagnosing disease.

In the Chinese system, everything ultimately boils down to energy, a view which modern Western physics is beginning to verify. Therefore, the Chinese approach to human health and physiology accounts not only for the effects of obvious visible substances such as microbes and toxins, blood and bile, but also for the invisible and even more pervasive influences of emotions and weather, solar and lunar cycles, electromagnetic forces, and other energies that have a direct impact on the human energy system. As the energy therapist Dr John Veltheim puts it: 'Science tells us that everything is energy and that matter is nothing more than energy in a different form.' The Five Elemental Energies and their cycles provide an intelligible formula for diagnosing and correcting the energy disorders that lie at the root of most human ailments, and for taking preventive measures to avoid such disruptions before they occur.

Since the Chinese view differs so significantly from the conventional Western view of human physiology, a brief review of each of the twelve vital organ systems and their functions according to traditional Chinese medical practice is in order here, so that Western readers may gain a proper working perspective on the subject. We'll run through the organs according to the Five

Elemental Energies, first describing the associated 'solid' yin organ, then its 'hollow' yang partner.

Heart: Fire-energy yin organ

The heart is called the 'King' of the organs. The *Internal Medicine Classic* states: 'The heart commands all of the organs and viscera, houses the spirit, and controls the emotions.' In Chinese, the word for 'heart' (*hsin*) is also used to denote 'mind'. When the heart is strong and steady, it controls the emotions; when it is weak and wavering, the emotions rebel and prey upon the heart/mind, which then loses its command over the body.

Physiologically, the heart controls the circulation and distribution of blood, and therefore all the other organs depend upon it for sustenance. Thoughts and emotions influence the function of various organs via pulse and blood pressure, which are controlled by the heart, where emotions arise. Internally, the heart is functionally associated with the thymus gland, which is located in the same cavity and forms a mainstay of the immune system. Extreme emotions such as grief and anger have an immediate suppressive effect on the immune system by inhibiting thymus function, a phenomenon that has long been observed but little understood in Western medicine.

Externally, the heart is related to the tongue, to which it is connected by the heart muscle. The colour and texture of the tongue thus reflect the condition of the heart. Speech impediments such as stuttering and mutism are often caused by dysfunction or imbalance in heart energy. Facial complexion, which is a direct reflection of blood circulation, is also a major external indicator of heart function. Fire energy makes the heart the dominant organ of summer, during which season the heart must increase circulation to the surface in order to dissipate excess body heat.

Small intestine: Fire-energy yang organ

Known as the 'Minister of Reception', the small intestine receives partially digested food from the stomach and further refines it, separating 'the pure from the impure', then assimilating the purified nutrients and moving the impure wastes onwards to the large intestine for elimination. Associated with the heart by Fire energy, the small intestine controls the more basic emotions, as reflected in the Chinese term *duan chang* ('broken intestines'), which is equivalent to the English term 'broken heart'. Its energy meridian runs into the head, where it influences the function of the pituitary gland, the 'master gland' whose secretions regulate growth, metabolism, immunity, sexuality, and the entire endocrine system.

Liver: wood-energy yin organ

The liver is called the 'General' or 'Chief of Staff' and is responsible for filtering, detoxifying, nourishing, replenishing, and storing blood. The liver stores large amounts of sugar in the form of glycogen, which it releases into the blood stream as glucose whenever the body requires extra infusions of metabolic energy. The liver receives all amino acids extracted from food by the small intestine and recombines them to synthesize the various forms of protein required for growth and repair of bodily tissues.

The liver controls the peripheral nervous system, which regulates muscular activity and tension. The inability to relax is often caused by liver dysfunction or imbalance in Wood energy. Liver energy also controls ligaments and tendons, which together with muscles regulate motor activity and determine physical coordination. Liver function is reflected externally in the condition of finger- and toenails and by the eyes and vision. Blurry vision is often a result of liver malfunction rather than an eye problem, and even Western medicine recognizes the symptomatic yellow eyes of liver jaundice.

Through its association with Wood energy, the liver governs growth and development, drives and desires, ambitions and creativity. Obstruction of liver energy can cause intense feelings of frustration, rage, and anger, and these emotions in turn further disrupt liver energy and suppress liver function, in a vicious self-destructive cycle.

Gall bladder: Wood-energy yang organ

Known as the 'Honourable Minister', the gall bladder is in charge of the 'Central Clearing Department'. It secretes the pure and potent bile fluids required to digest and metabolize fats and oils, and its energy provides muscular strength and vitality. It works with the lymphatic system to clear toxic by-products of metabolism from the muscular system, thereby eliminating muscular aches and fatigue. In the Chinese system, the common tension headache is caused by obstruction in the gall-bladder meridian, which runs up over the shoulders and back of the neck to the top of the head and forehead. Hence such headaches are usually accompanied by neck and shoulder tension.

The gall bladder governs daring and decisiveness. In Chinese, the word for 'daring' is *da dan* ('big gall'). The English language also acknowledges this psychophysiological relationship with the phrase 'a lot of gall'. An old Chinese adage states: 'The gall bladder is daring, the heart is careful', which reflects the stimulating generative influence of Wood to Fire.

Spleen and pancreas: Earth-energy yin organ

In Chinese medicine, the function of the spleen organ-energy system includes the pancreas. Called the 'Minister of the Granary', the spleen and pancreas control extraction and assimilation of nutrients from food and fluids by providing the digestive enzymes and energy required by the stomach and small intestine. They regulate the quantity and quality of blood in circulation and coordinate with the kidneys to control fluid balance throughout the system. Spleen energy commands extraction of energy from food as well as the transportation of this energy from stomach to lungs, where it is blended with energy from air to form True Human Energy. The spleen directly influences and is reflected by the tone and condition of muscle tissue. Weak limbs and muscular atrophy are indications of deficient spleen energy.

Spleen and pancreas condition is reflected externally by the colour and tone of the lips: reddish moist lips indicate strong spleen function; pale dry lips are a sign of weak spleen function. The mouth is the spleen's external aperture, and temperamental moodiness is its associated emotion. The Chinese term for 'bad temper' is 'bad spleen energy', a psychophysiological association also reflected in the English term 'splenetic'.

Stomach: Earth-energy yang organ

The stomach is called the 'Minister of the Mill' and is also known as the 'Sea of Nourishment'. Because it is responsible for providing the entire system with postnatal energy from the digestion of food and fluids, it is regarded as the 'Root of Postnatal Life'. In addition to digesting bulk foods and fluids and moving them onwards to the small intestine for extraction and assimilation of nutrients, the stomach also extracts pure postnatal energy from food and fluids, and in coordination with spleen energy it transports this food energy through the meridian system to the lungs, where it combines with air energy from breathing. This is a function of the stomach not acknowledged in Western medicine, which focuses only on the biochemistry of digestion and does not recognize its bioenergetic aspect.

Governed by pivotal Earth energy, the stomach is responsible for extracting and balancing all Five Elemental Energies from foods and fluids ingested through the mouth, which it shares with the spleen as its external aperture. Any dysfunction of the stomach results in an immediate deficiency or imbalance in the nourishing energy channelled from the stomach to other organs.

Lungs: Metal-energy yin organ

Known as the 'Prime Minister', the lungs control breath and energy and assist the 'King' heart with the circulation of blood. The *Internal Medicine Classic* states: 'Energy is the commander of blood; when energy moves, blood follows. Blood is the mother of energy; where blood goes, energy follows.' This intimate relationship between breath and pulse, blood and energy, is the basis of Chinese breathing exercises.

Breathing controls cellular respiration, and shallow irregular breathing is therefore a major cause of low vitality and insufficient metabolism. The lungs also control the skin, which 'breathes' via the opening and closing of pores and is responsible for adjusting body temperature through perspiration and shivering. The skin is where the radiant energy of resistance emanates, forming the first line of defence against noxious environmental energies such as heat and cold. Flu and the common cold are caused by impairment of radiant skin energy's capacity to resist external invasion, and symptoms of these diseases usually settle in the lungs and bronchial tract. Pallid skin and poor complexion are common indications of weak lungs. The nose is the external aperture of the lungs and the gate of breath. A clogged or runny nose is another indicator of ailing lungs.

Breathing directly controls the autonomous nervous system, and this relationship is the basis for almost every system of yoga and meditation. By regulating the autonomous nervous system and governing energy and pulse, breathing forms a direct bridge between body and mind and may be utilized to keep the two in balance.

Large intestine: Metal-energy yang organ

The large intestine is called the 'Minister of Transportation'. It controls the transformation of digestive wastes from liquid to solid state and transports the solids onwards and outwards for excretion through the rectum. It plays a major role in the balance and purity of bodily fluids and assists the lungs in controlling the skin's pores and perspiration.

Coupled with the lungs by Metal energy, the large intestine depends on the lungs for movement via the expansion and contraction of the diaphragm, which works like a pump to give impetus to peristalsis by regulating abdominal pressure. Thus sluggish bowels may be stimulated and constipation cured by deep diaphragmic breathing and by tonifying lung energy. Conversely, congested lungs and clogged bronchial passages may be cleared by purging the bowels.

Kidney: Water-energy yin organ

Known as the 'Minister of Power', the kidney is regarded as the body's most important reservoir of essential energy. The original prenatal energy (*yuan chee*) which forms the basis of life is stored in the kidney organ-energy system, which is why the kidneys are also known as the 'Root of Life'. In the Chinese view, the kidney organ system also includes the adrenal glands, which consist of the adrenal medulla and the adrenal cortex. These glands sit like hats on top of the kidneys and secrete a wide range of essential hormones that regulate metabolism, excretion, immunity, sexual potency and fertility. Destruction of the adrenal cortex is fatal. The kidney system also includes what the Chinese call the 'external kidneys': the testicles in men and the ovaries in women. Thus the kidneys control sexual and reproductive functions and provide the body's prime source of sexual vitality, which the Chinese regard as a major indicator of health and immunity.

The kidneys themselves are responsible for filtering waste metabolites from the blood and moving them onwards to the bladder for excretion in urine. Along with the large intestine, the kidneys control the balance of fluids in the body. In addition, they regulate the body's acid-alkaline balance (pH) by selectively filtering out or retaining various minerals.

The kidneys, particularly the adrenal glands, are especially vulnerable to damage from excessive stress and sexual abuse. In the Chinese view, such damage is a major cause of immune deficiency, low vitality, and sexual impotence.

The kidneys control the growth and development of bones and nourish the marrow, which is the body's source of red and white blood cells. Weak kidney energy is therefore a prime cause of anaemia and immune deficiency. The Chinese view the spinal cord and the brain as forms of marrow, and therefore poor memory, inability to think clearly, and backache are all regarded as indicators of impaired kidney function and deficient kidney energy.

Kidney vitality is reflected externally by the condition of head and body hair and is associated with the aperture of the ears. Tinnitus (ringing ears) is thus a sign of kidney dysfunction. The kidneys are the seat of courage and willpower, and therefore any impairment in kidney energy results in feelings of fear and paranoia. Intense fear can cause involuntary urination, a phenomenon also known to Western medicine.

Bladder: Water-energy yang organ

The bladder is called the 'Minister of the Reservoir' and is responsible for storing and excreting the urinary waste fluids passed down from the kidneys. As an organ the bladder has only this function, but as an energy system the bladder is intimately related to the functions and balance of the autonomous nervous system. That's because the bladder energy meridian runs along the back of the body from head to heel, with two parallel branches flowing along each side of the spinal column. These four branches of the bladder meridian exert a direct influence on the sympathetic and parasympathetic trunks of the autonomous nervous system, whose nerve fibres also run along the spine. Chronic stress, a common condition of modern life, overactivates the sympathetic system, causing tension and pain along the spine and its periphery. This tension and pain may be relieved by stimulating the flow of energy along the spinal branches of the bladder meridian. Such stimulation induces total relaxation by switching the autonomous nervous system over to the restful, restorative parasympathetic mode. Chinese massage therapy focuses primarily on these four spinal branches of the bladder meridian because of their direct influence over the autonomous nervous system, which regulates all the body's basic vital functions.

Pericardium: Fire-energy yin organ

Known as the 'King's Bodyguard', the pericardium is the heart's protective sack. Although it is not recognized as an organ in Western physiology, it is regarded in Chinese medicine as a Fire-energy organ whose special function is to protect the heart. Not only does the pericardium provide the heart with physical protection, its energy also protects the heart from damage and disruption by excessive emotional energies generated by the other organs, such as anger from the liver, fear from the kidneys, and grief from the lungs. In the Chinese system of health, extreme outbursts of the Seven Emotions are regarded as powerful disruptors of internal energy balance and major causes of disease. Without the pericardium to protect it, the heart would be subject to injury from the radical fluctuations in energy caused by every emotional up and down of the day.

The pericardium also helps regulate circulation in the major blood vessels that run in and out of the heart. Emotionally, pericardium energy is related to the loving feelings associated with sex, thereby linking the physical and emotional aspects of sexual activity. It does this by moderating the raw sexual energy of the kidneys with the all-embracing love generated by the heart.

Triple burner: Fire-energy yang organ

This organ-energy system, which is not recognized in Western physiology, is called the 'Minister of Dykes and Dredges' and is responsible for the movement and transformation of various solids and fluids throughout the system, as well as for the production and circulation of nourishing energy (*ying chee*) and protective energy (*wei chee*). It is not a single self-contained organ, but rather a functional energy system involved in regulating the activities of other organs. It is composed of three parts, known as 'burners', each associated with one of the body's three main cavities: thorax, abdomen, and pelvis. An ancient Chinese medical text states: 'The Upper Burner controls intake, the Middle Burner controls transformation, the Lower Burner controls elimination.'

The Upper Burner runs from the base of the tongue to the entrance to the stomach and controls the intake of air, food, and fluids. It harmonizes the functions of heart and lungs, governs respiration, and regulates the distribution of protective energy to the body's external surfaces.

The Middle Burner runs from the entrance to the stomach down to its exit at the pyloric valve and controls digestion by harmonizing the functions of stomach, spleen, and pancreas. It is responsible for extracting nourishing energy from food and fluids and distributing it via the meridian system to the lungs and other parts of the body.

The Lower Burner runs from the pyloric valve down to the anus and urinary tract and is responsible for separating the pure from the impure products of digestion, absorbing nutrients, and eliminating solid and liquid wastes. It harmonizes the functions of liver, kidney, bladder, and large and small intestines and also regulates sexual and reproductive functions.

Some medical researchers believe that the Triple Burner is associated with the hypothalamus, the part of the brain which regulates appetite, digestion, fluid balance, body temperature, heartbeat, blood pressure, and other basic autonomous functions.

While each organ in the body has its own unique structure, anatomical location, and biological activity, it is their functional interaction as a complete organic system that counts in the Chinese system of health care. Harmony among the Five Elemental Energies of the organs and balance between their yin and yang aspects form the foundation for health and vitality, while functional disharmony and energy imbalance are the prime causes of disease and debility. Unlike modern Western medicine, which treats diseases of individual organs based upon isolated symptomatic disorders, Chinese diagnosis and therapy are based on the functional interrelationships between all the organs as a whole system, in which diseases are often traced to root causes far removed from where the obvious symptoms appear. Focusing on function rather than form requires a thorough understanding of how the human energy system operates, and this in turn enables the physician to track down root causes of disease and effect lasting cures, rather than simply providing symptomatic relief.

Just as each season and each organ is governed by one of the Five Elemental Energies, so each medicinal herb in the Chinese pharmacopoeia is associated primarily with one of the Five Energies, and this association is indicated by the herb's dominant flavour. The energy and flavour of the herb determine its 'natural affinity' (*gui jing*) for the organ associated with the same energy, as well as its therapeutic effect on that organ, as follows:

Wood >	sour	>	astringent	>	liver – gall bladder
Fire >	bitter	>	energizing	>	heart – small intestine; pericardium – triple burner
Earth >	sweet	>	detoxifying & balancing	>	stomach – pancreas – spleen
Metal >	pungent	>	dispersing	>	lungs – large intestine
Water >	salty	>	diuretic	>	kidneys – bladder

The Five Flavours are also used in traditional Taoist 'Five Elements' cooking, which combines various foods and condiments according to the creative and control cycles of the Five Elemental Energies and their natural affinities with associated organs. Thus sour foods are prescribed for weak livers but proscribed for overactive livers, owing to their affinity for the Wood energy of the liver. Pungent Metal-energy foods stimulate the lungs and large intestine, salty Water-energy foods have a diuretic effect on the kidneys and bladder, and so forth. In this system, whole brown rice is regarded as the most perfectly balanced food, because it contains all the Five Elemental Energies in proper proportion.

Psychic aspects

In addition to their physiological functions in human health, the Five Elemental Energies also exert profound influences on the human psyche and personality, and this aspect is applied in Chinese astrology and fortune telling. While the physiological manifestations of the five energies are prenatally determined by human genetics, their psychic manifestations in human personality are developed postnatally according to time and place of birth as well as environmental and social influences. Because of the mutual interaction of body and mind through the medium of energy, psychic tendencies often have powerful effects on the internal organs and glands and therefore constitute important factors in health.

A strong Fire-type personality, for example, tends to overheat his or her organs and usually has an overactive heart. Such persons should avoid alcohol and stimulating yang foods and balance their excess Fire with cooling yin foods and calming Water-energy herbs. Metal-type persons tend to act impulsively and are often subject to respiratory ailments. They should therefore take special care of their lungs, practise daily *chee-gung* breathing exercises, and cultivate deliberation and restraint. If a person lacks sufficient Wood energy in his or her personality, he or she should take supplements to tonify the liver (Wood organ) and make a point of wearing green (Wood colour). One reason the Chinese are so fond of consulting fortune tellers is that they provide them with insights on their individual psychic tendencies, which may be effectively applied to promoting health and longevity and avoiding self-destructive behaviour. The link between personality and physiology is based on energy, which bridges the gap between body and mind, and the system by which the two interact and influence one another is the Five Elemental Energies, which also provides the means for manipulating various energies to promote health and longevity.

Lu Tung-pin, the great Taoist sage who founded the Complete Reality School, elucidated the effects of the Five Elemental Energies on human nature as follows, translated here by Thomas Cleary in his book *Vitality, Energy, Spirit:*

> The earthy nature is mostly turbid, and the turbid are mostly dull. The metallic nature is mostly decisive, and the decisive are mostly determined. The wooden nature is mostly kind, and the kind are mostly benevolent. The fiery nature is mostly adamant, and the adamant are mostly manic. The watery nature is mostly yielding, and the yielding are mostly docile.
>
> The docile tend to wander aimlessly. The manic tend to undergo extremes. The benevolent tend to harmonize warmly. The determined tend to be strong and brave. The dull tend to be closed in.
>
> The closed-in are ignorant; the strong and brave are unruly; those who wander aimlessly are shifty; those who harmonize warmly fall into traps; those who are adamant can endure extremes and are cruel.
>
> Therefore each of the five natures has a bias, so it is important to balance each with the others. By yielding one can overcome being adamant, by being adamant one can overcome yielding. Benevolence is balanced by effectiveness, effectiveness is balanced by benevolence. The ignorance of earthly dullness is to be overcome by developed understanding. If developed understanding is not dominant, one loses the function of yielding . . .
>
> In terms of social virtues, the water nature corresponds to wisdom, the fire nature corresponds to courtesy, the wood nature corresponds to benevolence, the metal nature corresponds to righteousness, and the earth nature corresponds to trustworthiness. In a balanced

personality, these five natures should be able to produce and control one another.

Wisdom should be able to produce benevolence. Benevolence should be able to produce courtesy. Courtesy should be able to produce trustworthiness. Trustworthiness should be able to produce righteousness. Righteousness should be able to produce wisdom.

Wisdom should control courtesy. Courtesy should control righteousness. Righteousness should control benevolence. Benevolence should control trustworthiness. Trustworthiness should control wisdom.

When these five natures produce and control each other thus in a continuous circle, then no element of personality dominates; they all interact, balancing each other, resulting in completeness of the five natures.

Thus the Five Elemental Energies provide an accurate working model as well as a meaningful symbolism, illuminating the inner mechanisms of many different aspects of life, based on the fundamental transformations of energy which activate all vital functions and drive all natural cycles. Fig. 7 shows the scope of natural phenomena and activities in which the Five Elemental Energies provide the operating mechanism. In nature, functional forces are always more important than static forms because the latter are always subject to change by the former. The Five Elemental Energies reflect the complementary nature of these forces and reveal their relationships to be cyclic and orderly rather than chaotic, thus permitting humans to predict and manipulate them to advantage.

Elemental Energy Quality	Wood	Fire	Earth	Metal	Water
yin organ	liver	heart	spleen/pancreas	lungs	kidneys
yang organ	gall bladder	small intestine	stomach	large intestine	bladder
direction	east	south	centre	west	north
flavour	sour	bitter	sweet	pungent	salty
vital functions	nervous system	blood, endocrine	digestion, lymph, muscles	respiration	reproductive and urinary systems
colour	green	red	yellow	white	black
season	spring	summer	late summer	autumn	winter
aperture	eyes	tongue/throat	lips/mouth	nose	ears
mental quality	emotion, sensitivity	willpower, creativity	clarity	intuition	spon-taneity
emotions neg/pos	anger/kindness	hate/joy	anxiety/empathy	grief/courage	fear/calmness
development phase	sprouting, leaves growing	blooming, fruit growing	ripening, harvest	seeds falling, withering	dormancy, storage
life cycle	infancy	youth	adulthood	old age	death
bodily fluid	tears	sweat	saliva	mucus	urine
expands into	nails	facial complexion	lips	body hair	head hair
hour	3–7 a.m.	9 a.m.–1 p.m.	1–3, 7–9 a.m. 1–3, 7–9 p.m.	3–7 p.m.	9 p.m.–1 a.m.
climate	windy	hot	damp	dry	cold
primal spirit	Green Dragon	Red Pheasant	Yellow Phoenix	White Tiger	Black Tortoise
Healing sound	*hsü*	*her*	*hoo*	*shee*	*chway*
energy quality	generative	expansive	stabilizing	contracting	conserving
planet	Jupiter	Mars	Saturn	Venus	Mercury
numbers	8, 3	2, 7	10, 5	4, 9	6, 1

Fig. 7 **The Five Elemental Energies and some of their associated qualities and relationships.**

CHAPTER 6

The Six Evils

When the six environmental energies of Wind, Cold, Heat, Dampness, Dryness, and Fire grow extreme or occur out of season, they become causes of disease and are known as the Six Evils.

Encyclopedia of Chinese Medicine (1978)

Ever since Louis Pasteur discovered the existence of bacteria, Western medicine has subscribed increasingly to the 'germ theory' of disease. According to this theory, human diseases are caused by germs, which enter the body through contaminated food, water, or air, or from physical contact with infected persons. Based upon this hypothesis, Western medicine represents the allopathic approach to treating disease. Allopathic medicine relies on powerful drugs to combat disease by killing the specific germs and reversing the superficial symptoms associated with a particular disease. If one drug does not work, another is prescribed, and this continues until the symptoms disappear or surgery is required, after which the patient is considered to be cured.

While there is no doubt that certain germs can cause specific diseases, certain conditions must prevail in order for any particular germ to invade the human system and multiply sufficiently to cause disease. Pasteur himself noted in his journals that each particular strain of bacteria he studied required a very specific and narrow range of temperature, moisture, light, pH balance, and other conditions in order to survive and multiply. If any of those conditions were altered or eliminated, the germ automatically perished. Any winemaker can tell you how carefully temperature, humidity, and other environmental energies must be controlled in order to get specific yeasts to ferment grapes into wine. This aspect of Pasteur's work has been played down by the Western medical and pharmaceutical industries in favour of the assumption that the same germ causes the same disease in all patients under all conditions. Consequently, modern Western medical practice relies entirely on powerful antibiotics, antifungals, antivirals, antihistamines, and other toxic chemicals to bludgeon various germs into submission, often without success and without the slightest regard for the damage such poisons do to the sensitive essences and energies of the human body. This 'chemical warfare' approach to the treatment of disease severely disturbs the subtle mechanisms which regulate vital functions and disrupts the delicate balance of energies upon which human health and vitality depend.

Modern Western medical practice ignores the influence of environmental energies on the human system and denies the possibility that exposure to certain extreme energy conditions can predispose the human body to invasion by external pathogens. In the heat and humidity of summer, when the body naturally forces circulation to the surface and opens the pores wide to dissipate internal heat, people work and sleep in air-conditioned rooms that mimic the conditions of winter, permitting cold and dry energy to chill their blood and enter their meridians. Then they wonder why they get 'summer colds', allergies, headaches, backaches, and other aches and ailments. When they go to the doctor, who works in an air-conditioned clinic, he gives them a drug to numb the pain or kill the suspected germ.

The artificial environmental energies that pervade our lives play havoc with the human body's natural energy currents and fields, particularly the radiant shield of protective energy emanating from the surface. Such 'energy pollution' renders the human system vulnerable to noxious external influences, creating the preconditions for all sorts of diseases and disorders that no drug can cure or prevent. You must either forgo modern lifestyles entirely and return to a primitive holistic way of life far from big cities, an option few people care to exercise; or else take preventive measures to prepare your body's defences to deal with the constant environmental assaults of life in the modern world.

The Six Evils

First, let's take a look at the Six Evils of extreme or unseasonal environmental conditions from the traditional Chinese point of view and see how such noxious energies influence the human system. Traditionally, these energies were associated with the seasons, as follows: wind/spring; heat/summer; dampness/late summer; dryness/autumn; and cold/winter. The sixth evil, called 'fire', can develop as a result of prolonged or intense exposure to any of the other five. Note that problems usually arise as a result of the body's own protective energy shield's failure to adjust defensively to exposure to any one or more of the Six Evils. Therefore, the greatest danger occurs during the change of seasons, during a sudden spell of unseasonal weather, or during exposure to artificially created environmental conditions which conflict with prevailing natural conditions.

Wind: The prevailing energy of spring

Wind is the environmental energy associated with the Wood element and the spring season, when under normal conditions it comes as a mild, pleasant breeze called 'harmonious wind'. However, Wind also occurs in all seasons, taking on and carrying the prevailing climatic conditions associated with each season. Thus in summer there is 'heat wind', in late summer 'damp wind', in winter 'cold wind', and in autumn 'dry wind'. Symptoms of 'wind injury' include hot spells, profuse sweating, chronic cough, and stuffy nose.

Since 'wind' is a carrier of all climatic conditions, it is said that 'wind carries the myriad ailments' and that 'wind is the chief of the Six Evils'. The Internal Medicine Classic states: 'Wind moves fast and is subject to frequent and rapid change.' Thus 'wind' injuries enter the human energy system rapidly, and its symptoms progress and change swiftly.

In addition, Chinese medical practice recognizes 'internal wind' associated with internal-organ energy. When excess energy accumulates within an organ, it moves suddenly to other organs in accordance with the creative and control cycles of the Five Elemental Energies. Such energy has a disruptive influence on the receiving organ, either overstimulating it or suppressing it, and manifests itself in various pathological symptoms. For example, when excess 'liver wind' rises to the heart and head, it causes dizziness, insomnia, blurry vision, and numbness in the fingers.

In the modern industrial world, Wind Evil takes on new forms that did not exist in traditional times, such as air conditioning, central heating, microwaves, and radiation. Such forms are even more damaging and disruptive to human organs and energies than ordinary environmental 'wind'.

Cold: The prevailing energy of winter

Associated with the Water element and winter season, 'cold' energy is created by low air temperature. When 'cold' invades the human system through defects in the body's shield of protective energy, or owing to sudden exposure, it causes such symptoms as chills and fever, cessation of sweat, headache, and body aches. If it settles in the gut, it causes gas, diarrhoea, and abdominal cramps.

'Internal cold' arises from deficient yang energy in the vital organs, resulting in loose bowels, coldness in the extremities, and sexual impotence.

In the modern world, Cold Evil arises externally from air conditioning and internally from ice-cold beverages and drugs which suppress metabolism and other vital functions, as well as excessive consumption of 'cold' yin foods.

Heat: The prevailing energy of summer

Summer 'heat', which is associated with 'fire' energy, is caused by excessively hot air temperatures over a prolonged period of time. Its symptoms include headaches, hot flushes, chronic thirst, profuse sweating, and irritability. Heat Evil also occurs in other seasons, taking on the prevailing energy of those seasons and thereby compounding its disruptive influence on human energy. Thus in late summer there is 'damp heat' and in autumn 'dry heat'.

Internal 'heat' due to overstimulation of the organs falls into the category of Fire Evil.

Central heating is an artificial modern source of Heat Evil and usually takes the form of 'dry heat'.

Dampness: The prevailing energy of late summer

Damp Evil occurs most frequently during late summer in humid climates and is associated with Earth energy. Humidity, summer rains, mould, morning mists, and damp ground are all sources of external Damp Evil, which easily seeps through the body's shield of protective energy, especially during sleep. Its symptoms include fatigue, sluggishness, cold sweats, rheumatism, and bloating. It combines easily with other environmental energies to produce 'cold dampness', 'wind dampness', and 'hot dampness', each of which manifests itself with compound symptoms.

'Internal dampness' is generally caused by excessive consumption of alcohol, coffee, tea, ice-cold fruit, sugary soft drinks, and sweets, all of which have deleterious suppressive effects on the internal organs and their vital functions. Refined white sugar can impede spleen and pancreas functions and distress the adrenal glands. Such products are major causes of diabetes, immune deficiency, and other degenerative conditions.

Dryness: The prevailing energy of autumn

Dry Evil is caused by insufficient moisture in the air and is particularly damaging to the lungs. It prevails in autumn and is associated with the elemental energy of Metal. When combined with 'cold', 'cold dryness' causes headache, aversion to cold, chronic dry cough, cessation of sweat, and stuffy nose. 'Hot dryness' results in symptoms of hot spells, profuse sweat, thirst, sore throat, and dry nose. Both forms of Dry Evil cause chapped lips, dry skin, hard stools, and constipation.

'Internal dryness' is due to an insufficiency in vital bodily fluids, resulting in constant thirst, dry throat and tongue, and nausea.

'Cold dryness' can be caused by air conditioning and 'hot dryness' by central heating. Smoking is a source of internal Dry Evil that is specifically damaging to the lungs and inhibits the body's protective energy shield, thereby lowering resistance.

Fire: The extreme energy of all seasons

If any one of the five seasonal energies becomes extreme over a prolonged period of time, it can transform into Fire Evil. 'Fire' is a term applied to any extremely abnormal environmental condition which causes the symptoms associated with the original energy to grow much worse and begin to 'burn out' the affected organ-energy system. Fire Evil rapidly depletes organ energies and can easily cause permanent damage to the associated organs.

Overstimulation or abuse of any of the internal organs creates 'internal fire'. For example, overindulgence in rich foods causes 'stomach fire', resulting in indigestion, gas, and ulcers. Alcoholism creates 'stomach fire' as well as liver 'fire', sexual excess causes 'kidney fire', frequent outbursts of anger result in 'liver fire', heavy smoking causes 'lung fire', and so forth. Prolonged 'internal fire' inevitably causes permanent damage to the primary organ affected, and can also cause serious damage to secondary organs associated with the primary organs by yin/yang and the Five Elemental Energies.

The Six Evils are all regarded as forms of 'evil energy' (*hsieh chee*), and the best antidote for evil energy is 'pure energy' (*jeng chee*). Pure energy is cultivated with *chee-gung* breathing exercises, acupuncture, meditation, and other traditional methods, but there are also modern methods of cultivating pure energy to combat modern sources of evil energy. Some of these are mentioned below. It ultimately comes down to the balance between evil and pure energies within the human energy system. As the *Internal Medicine Classic* states: 'Where evil energy gathers, weakness occurs. When pure energy collects internally, evil energy cannot cause damage to the organs. When pure energy flourishes, evil energy flees. When evil energy is driven out of the system, pure energy grows.'

Westerners are not accustomed to dealing with health problems in terms of energy, but in fact pure energy is always the best medicine and the most effective healing element. What counts in health care is results, and anyone who tries working with healing energy will find the proof in the practice. Energy medicine is especially useful today, when human energy systems are subject to constant distortion and distress from artificial industrial sources of aberrant energies.

Preventive measures

The Six Evils are even more pervasive and damaging to human health today than in the past, because of the many artificial sources of disruptive energies. Air conditioning and central heating subject the human body to abrupt and radical changes in temperature and humidity many times throughout the day, impairing the natural regulatory mechanisms of the body's radiant shield of protective energy. As a result, Hot and Cold Evils easily enter our energy meridians and disrupt our internal energy balance. Air pollution, fossil fuels, and damage to the earth's protective ozone shield have caused abnormal shifts in weather patterns and disrupted natural seasonal rhythms, further aggravating the balance of yin and yang and the harmony of the Five Elemental Energies in our internal organ-energy systems.

Electric transformers and power lines emanate powerful electromagnetic fields which disrupt and distort human energy fields, and broadcasting stations, microwave ovens, cellular phones, and scores of other electronic gadgets bombard our energy systems with nonstop showers of highly disruptive microwaves. Television and computer screens, fluorescent lights and video games emanate irritating artificial light rays which invade our eyes and travel along the optic nerve into the brain, where they suppress the pituitary gland and disturb cerebral functions. All these appliances, utilities, and toys are sources of powerful external energies which distort and upset human energy fields, impair vital organ functions, throw internal energies off balance, suppress immunity, and cause countless other symptoms. Like X-rays, they are invisible and silent, but excess exposure to them can kill.

'Internal dampness', 'cold', and 'fire' are also caused by modern lifestyles, particularly by the more than 6,000 chemical food additives, the toxic pesticides, and the denatured junk foods which the food industry foists upon the public. Many of these chemicals unleash a blitzkrieg of free radicals in the human system, a modern form of 'internal wind' which destroys cells, disrupts metabolism, and causes premature degeneration and aging of human tissues.

Among the worst offenders in modern diets are the scores of sugary soft drinks sold throughout the world. Cola drinks often also contain caffeine, which is addictive. 'Sugar-free' varieties are no better, for the highly processed artificial sweeteners used in them are just as dangerous as sugar, if not more so. The internal Damp Evil generated by concentrated forms of sugar is a major cause of diabetes, and habitual consumption leads to internal Fire Evil, which burns out the adrenal glands and leads to severe immune deficiency.

While the terminology used by traditional Chinese physicians to denote these damaging internal and external energy conditions may sound quaint to contemporary Western ears, the principles behind the terms are as valid today as in ancient times, and the problems to which they refer are deadly serious. In fact, the earthy terms used in traditional Chinese medicine, which are all drawn from nature, are much easier to understand than the long-winded technical jargon used in modern Western medicine, and once you become familiar with the basic principles and natural laws of the Tao, Chinese medical terminology becomes self-evident.

Detailed suggestions on how to prevent disease and degeneration caused by modern living are made in the chapters on essence and energy. Here is a brief list of measures you can take to ward off artificial sources of the Six Evils and prevent the awful toll they take on your health.

• Don't sleep in air-conditioned rooms. It may be difficult to avoid air conditioning at work and in public buildings, but you need not compound the damage. Air conditioning devoids the air of negative ions, which carry the vital atmospheric energy required to form True Human Energy. It creates Dry and Cold Evils, which damage the sinuses and lungs and enter the energy meridians during sleep. If it is hot at night, use a fan and keep the windows open.

• Install a negative-ion generator in your office, car, and home, especially if you live in a big city. Also called 'ionizers', negative-ion generators remove smoke, dust, and other pollutants from air, while at the same time infusing air-conditioned, centrally heated, and polluted air with a constant stream of billions of negative ions, which replenish and recharge the air you breathe with precisely the sort of energy your body needs. Negative-ion generators are compact, inexpensive, and consume very little electricity.

• Practice *chee-gung* breathing exercises daily. Twenty minutes of *chee-gung* re-establishes natural biorhythms, harmonizes the nervous and endocrine systems, switches the autonomous nervous system from the stressful sympathetic over to the restorative parasympathetic mode, and suffuses the entire body and all its tissues with oxygen-enriched blood and invigorating vital energy.

• Avoid exposure to sudden changes in temperature and humidity. If necessary, wear a sweater or vest in air-conditioned rooms, at least until your body has adjusted.

• Eliminate all soft drinks, sweets, and other foods made with white refined sugar, and cut down or eliminate white refined starch from your diet. Stay away from deep-fried foods, margarine, and anything else made with hydrogenated vegetable oil. As a rule, do not eat packaged or junk food, processed meat such as bacon, ham, and bologna, fast food, or any other food that is so heavily preserved and processed with artificial additives that it will not rot at room temperature. It's all poison to the human body, suppresses the immune system, and creates rampant free radicals that destroy human cells. As an added measure of protection against all forms of internal Dampness, Cold, and Fire Evils, take a daily course of vitamin, mineral, and herbal supplements (as detailed in a later chapter).

The steps suggested above, if faithfully followed, will suffice to eliminate most of the damage caused by artificial industrial sources of the Six Evils, both internal and external. Persons plagued by frequent bouts of flu and the common cold, allergic reactions, headaches, chronic fatigue, or yeast infections, will probably discover that by cleaning up and harmonizing their internal and external energy environments, they will have eliminated the very conditions that permit germs and aberrant energies to gain footholds in their systems and cause 'dis-ease'. As Hippocrates, the founder of Western medicine, wrote; 'One must know which diseases are caused by natural forces and which are caused by material elements.'

CHAPTER 7

The Seven Emotions

Anger causes energy to rise, joy causes energy to slow down, grief causes energy to dissipate, fear causes energy to descend, fright causes energy to scatter, exhaustion causes energy to wither, worry causes energy to stagnate.
The Yellow Emperor's Classic of Internal Medicine
(second century BC)

Conventional Western medical practice attributes emotional disturbances exclusively to the mind and usually refers emotionally disturbed patients to psychiatrists for treatment. The typical Freudian explanation for neuroses and emotional trauma is that they are a result of childhood fixations and unresolved psychological conflicts, and the Freudian approach to treating such problems is to lie the patient down on a couch and get to the root of the disturbance through endless hours of meandering conversation. As often as not, psychoanalysis turns out to be a colossal waste of time and money that provides no lasting relief for mental and emotional disturbances.

Emotions are triggered by sensory contact with the outside world, based upon the input of the five senses. Since humans relate to the phenomenal world and to each other through the five sensory organs, they remain in a state of constant emotional response. As the Chinese say: 'Contact with the external world generates internal emotions.' Therefore, the initial stimulant for each and every emotional response is external sensory contact, which at the primary stage is a physiological function of the nervous system, not a psychological process. In addition to the five physical senses, the Chinese and other Oriental traditions also recognize the temporal human mind as a sixth sense, and therefore fantasies, dreams, and other self-generated mental images function similarly to external images to engender emotional responses.

Psychology enters the picture briefly in the second stage of emotional response by interpreting and evaluating the sensory stimuli in terms of aversion or attraction, which determines the sort of emotion attached to the response. After that, the emotion leaves the realm of mind and enters the body's meridian system as a form of energy. Like all forms of human energy, emotions exert profound physiological effects on the internal organs, glands, and other tissues to which they travel through the energy channels. The word 'emotion' is best understood as a contraction of 'energy in motion', or 'e-motion'. In other words, the mind attaches a value to a physical or cerebral sensory stimulus, then sets a powerful current of emotional energy into motion through the body's energy channels. Once that energy is in motion, it takes on a life of its own.

Each emotion we generate triggers physiological reactions throughout the system, including secretions of various hormones, release of neurotransmitters in the brain and nervous system, changes in pulse and blood pressure, adjustments in breathing and respiration, and stimulation or suppression of digestion and peristalsis. When emotional responses are moderate and well balanced and are permitted to run their course swiftly and smoothly, they cause no serious harm and sometimes even provide positive stimulation to the body's organ-energy systems. But if a particular emotional response becomes extreme or explosive, and if it is prolonged or frequently repeated, it causes a series of severe physiological reactions which can seriously damage the associated organs and throw the entire human energy system off balance. When this happens, the body's radiant shield of protective energy is impaired, resistance and immunity are lowered, and the offending emotions become major internal causes of disease, degeneration, and debility.

In the traditional Chinese system of health care, extreme emotional responses are called the 'Seven Injurious Emotions' and are regarded as the primary internal causes of disease, just as the Six Evils of extreme environmental energies are regarded as the main external causes of disease. In Taoist alchemy, the five senses are called the 'Five Thieves' because they rob the adept's Three Treasures of essence, energy, and spirit and waste his precious time and energy on idle sensory distractions and emotional indulgences. The leader of this pack of thieves is emotion, which is called the 'Chief Hooligan'. If you think about it, this is a very accurate analogy, for sensory distractions and the emotions they provoke behave like a gang of vandals in your system, mugging your willpower to practise higher disciplines, assaulting your organs, glands, and nerves with stress, looting your stores of precious essence and energy, and intimidating your spirit.

The inseparable connection between emotional disturbances and physiological pathology has also been recognized by enlightened practitioners of Western medicine, but the medical establishment continues to resist their views. Wilhelm Reich, whose studies on human bioenergy during the 1950s provoked such controversy that they landed him in prison, stated that emotional 'fixations and conflicts cause fundamental disturbances of the bioelectric system and so get anchored somatically' and that 'it is impossible to separate the psychic from the somatic process'. Dr George Watson of the University of Southern California, who successfully treats all forms of mental illness and emotional disturbance solely by nutritional therapy, says; 'We have found functional mental illness to be a reflection of disordered metabolism, principally involving the malfunction of enzyme systems.'

In other words, emotional disturbances and metabolic disorders can form a vicious circle of self-sustaining disease. Frequent incidents of extreme anger, for example, damage the liver, according to Chinese medical views. After a while, the emotional energy released by anger disrupts and depresses liver function, one of the symptoms of which is irritability and short temper, which in turn predisposes a person to even more frequent outbursts of anger, thereby further damaging the liver and establishing an increasingly pernicious psycho-physiological cycle of disease and debility.

Another example is schizophrenia and chronic violence, an emotional disturbance which for many decades was relegated to the psychiatrist's couch, with absolutely no therapeutic success. Today, this dangerous emotional disorder has been successfully treated by administering a daily megadose of a single nutrient – niacin (vitamin B_3) – which has recorded an 80 per cent cure rate. This shows that a basic nutritional deficiency can impair brain function to the point of causing a severe imbalance in cerebral energy, provoking an extreme emotional response that distorts behaviour. No amount of psychoanalysis can ever unravel such a condition.

Perhaps the most dangerous physiological consequence caused by the Seven Emotions is the impairment of the immune system, which renders the human body vulnerable to opportunistic infections and degenerative diseases, many of them fatal. It is a well-known fact in Western medicine that a person who succumbs to prolonged grief after the death of a spouse becomes highly susceptible to cancer, heart disease, and other fatal ailments. In this age of chronic stress, excessive sensory stimulation, emotional insecurity, and constant anxiety, it seems incredible that Western medical scientists have not yet explored the possible connections between extreme emotional disturbances and AIDS. It may well be that HIV and other viruses associated with AIDS are more of a symptom than a cause of this condition, which is further aggravated by the immunosuppressive emotional distress it causes its victims.

In order to understand how emotional extremes can affect the vital organs and other functions, let's review the Seven Emotions according to traditional Chinese medical theory. Many of these psychophysiological correlations are also known to Western physicians, but they are neither properly understood nor correctly treated because modern Western medicine has not yet grasped the fundamental dynamics of human energy.

The Seven Emotions

Joy

The *Internal Medicine Classic* states: 'Excessive joy and laughter injure the heart and scatter the spirit.' When one indulges in extreme joy and laughter, it slows down and congests heart energy, causing the heart to flutter erratically. This not only damages the heart; since the heart houses the spirit, it also causes the spirit to scatter, so that it loses control over the body and its vital functions. Laughter is the sound associated with Fire energy, which governs the heart. People with weak hearts can easily die laughing, a phenomenon well known in Western medicine, and many people have dropped dead from heart attacks upon becoming overjoyed at unexpected good news.

Anger

Anger is the emotion associated with Wood energy and the liver. Extreme anger injures the liver's yin energy, which controls blood, bile, and other fluids associated with the liver. The resulting imbalance permits the liver's yang energy to flare up like a fire out of control. This rising liver yang energy ascends to the heart and head, causing headache, dizziness, blurred vision, and mental confusion. The English word 'bilious' refers to bad temper as well as liver dysfunction. Frequent outbursts of anger damage the liver, which in turn renders one prone to even more anger, thereby establishing a self-perpetuating cycle of destructive emotional energy.

Anxiety

The *Internal Medicine Classic* states: 'Anxiety blocks energy and injures the lungs. It congests the breathing apparatus and suppresses respiration.' Since the lungs govern energy through breathing, anxiety impairs energy circulation by inhibiting breath, and this in turns lowers resistance by weakening the body's shield of protective energy. The shallow breathing and shortness of breath experienced during periods of intense anxiety are common symptoms known to Western as well as Chinese physicians. Anxiety also impairs the large intestine, which is the lungs' coupled yang organ, and can therefore cause constipation and ulcerative colitis. In addition, chronic anxiety injures the functions of spleen, pancreas, and stomach, causing indigestion and depriving the entire system of nourishing energy, which further lowers resistance.

Concentration

Excessive concentration injures the spleen and pancreas as well as their coupled yang organ, the stomach. The term 'concentration' refers to obsessive mental fixation on a specific problem which constantly preoccupies the mind, including any sort of chronic worry. It impairs digestion, causes abdominal pain, and lowers resistance by depriving the body of nourishing energy. Western medicine also recognizes the connection between chronic worry and stomach disorders such as ulcers and indigestion.

Grief

Sustained periods of extreme grief injure the heart and lungs, and sometimes also damage the pericardium and its linked yang organ, the Triple Burner. It causes the body's stores of vital energy to dissipate rapidly, thereby severely impairing resistance. Grief-stricken people are well known in Western medical practice to be highly vulnerable to serious diseases, including cancer. In the Chinese system, the term 'grief' includes pessimism, which is particularly injurious to the heart. The *Internal Medicine Classic* states: 'People with weak heart energy are prone to grief and pessimism.' In other words, not only do grief and pessimism injure the heart, weak hearts render one prone to chronic grief and pessimism, which in turn further weaken the heart in a continuous psychophysiological circle.

Fear

Excess fear damages kidney energy and causes it to descend, sometimes causing loss of bladder control in the coupled yang organ. Conversely, states the *Internal Medicine Classic*, 'if kidney energy is weak, one is prone to chronic fear'. Chronic fear and paranoia can easily cause renal failure and permanent kidney damage. Children who wet their beds are often plagued by feelings of fear, and both the bed wetting and the fearful feelings are often the result of weak kidney energy. The solution therefore is to feed them foods and herbal tonics which boost the Water energy that governs the kidneys and bladder.

Fright

Fright is distinguished from fear by its sudden unexpected nature, which shocks the system, alarms the spirit, and causes energy to scatter. Since the heart houses the spirit, fright primarily injures the heart, particularly in its initial stage. If fright persists and becomes chronic fear, it moves to and injures the kidneys as well.

Generally, the heart is the organ most vulnerable to injury from emotional excess because it houses spirit and consciousness. However, all of the Seven Emotions are injurious and disrupt the energies of the vital organs via the creative and control cycles of the Five Elemental Energies and yin-yang balance. Furthermore, since the heart is 'King' of the internal organs, any impairment of heart energy also injures all the other organs by causing fluctuations in pulse, blood pressure, and circulation. Excessive emotional energies upset the delicate balance of yin and yang within the organ-energy systems and cause wild aberrations in the creative and control cycles of the Five Elemental Energies. Not only does this damage the affected organs, it also lowers resistance and thereby establishes the conditions for external invasion by the Six Evils of noxious environmental energies.

Owing to constant shifts in external stimuli, emotions rarely come singly but rather in contrasting series, like waves breaking on the beach. Known as 'conflicting emotions', these contrasting energies not only disrupt energy balance and injure the organs, they also confuse the mind, scatter the spirit, and create major obstacles to higher spiritual practices, which require emotional equanimity. Conflicting emotions cause constant energy disruptions which have deleterious effects on the body as well as the mind. Once they become entrenched in the organs, they perpetuate themselves by distorting organ energies and rising spontaneously to disturb the mind, even without the original external stimuli. That's why Taoists attach such importance to controlling the Five Thieves of the senses and their Chief Hooligan of emotion, for without emotional tranquillity it is difficult to maintain health and impossible to sustain the equanimity and stability required for meditation and other spiritual disciplines.

While Western medical practice still regards emotional problems as falling mainly into the domain of psychology and psychiatry, Chinese medicine treats them primarily as pathological phenomena with physiological causes and effects. Recent Western discoveries in the fields of nutrition and neurochemistry tend to verify the traditional Chinese view of emotions. The roles that neurotransmitters such as serotonin, acetycholine, and noradrenaline play in emotional stress and mental imbalance have become common knowledge in Western 'New Age' medicine, which treats many emotional disorders with high-dosage nutrients, especially the amino acids and synergistic vitamins and minerals with which the brain synthesizes various neurotransmitters. The simplicity and success of such nutritional therapy is a source of great consternation to the pharmaceutical industry, because nutrients cannot be patented, don't require prescriptions, and often work wonders where drugs fail.

Diseases that are caused neither externally by the Six Evils nor internally by the Seven Emotions fall into a miscellaneous category known as 'neither external nor internal'. This category includes such dietary factors as excess consumption of the wrong types of food and drink, malnutrition, and food poisoning, as well as other factors such as lack of exercise, epidemics, infectious wounds, insect and animal bites, parasites, and toxins. However, these miscellaneous causes are directly responsible for only a small minority of the chronic ailments and degenerative conditions which undermine human health and shorten human life. Most human disease and degeneration are caused by adverse external and internal energies created by noxious environmental conditions and extreme emotions, which lower resistance and impair immunity. By taking measures to counteract adverse environmental energies and control injurious emotions, and by cultivating pure energy, you can maintain a strong defence of resistance and immunity in order to prevent the Six Evils and Seven Emotions from disrupting your essence and energy and paving the way for invasion by germs, toxins, parasites, and other pathogens.

CHAPTER 8

The Eight Indicators

> It is easy to prescribe drugs but difficult to diagnose disease.
>
> ancient Chinese medical proverb

The proverb quoted above should be prominently displayed in every Western medical clinic and pharmacy in the world. Misdiagnosis is perhaps the most common and dangerous form of malpractice in Western medicine today, causing millions of people untold misery and needless medical complications.

For over 3,000 years, prevention of disease has been the guiding principle in traditional Chinese health care. The onset of disease was regarded as a failure of preventive medicine rather than a normal occurrence as it is today, and the use of medicinal drugs was always a last resort. The Three Treasures of body, energy, and spirit were cherished as precious assets of life and carefully guarded from damage. Health was considered to be an important individual responsibility, and disease was viewed as a failure in prevention by the individual as well as the family physician. In the old days, Chinese households retained a family physician whose duty it was to keep everyone in the household, including servants, healthy. For this service the physician received a monthly retainer. If anyone fell ill, it was the physician's responsibility to restore the patient to health at his own expense, and the monthly stipend was withheld until he affected a complete cure. This system served as a wonderfully effective deterrent to medical malpractice, because doctors profited only by keeping their patients healthy.

Today, Americans spend billions of dollars every year to maintain a strong national defence as a deterrent against external attack by foreign powers, but they fail entirely to apply the same principle of preventive defence to their own health. They eat, drink, and live indiscriminately and treat their bodies as engines of pleasure, without the slightest regard for the damage their habits inflict on their health. When they get sick, they run to the doctor or hospital for a quick fix and never imagine that their ailments are self-inflicted. Those ailments are then further compounded at the clinic, because more often than not they are not correctly diagnosed owing to the lack of a comprehensive and systematic view of the human body and human health. Western medical practice has become increasingly fragmented into narrow fields of speciality, and patients are referred to 'specialists' based entirely on what parts of the body exhibit their symptoms. It does not occur to Western medical specialists that symptoms may appear in parts of the body far removed from the root cause of the disease, although this remains a fundamental tenet of traditional Chinese medicine.

Although food should be our greatest source of health and vitality, modern diets, especially of the sort promoted by American fast-food corporations, have become a major cause of disease and physiological degeneration throughout the world today. Public food supplies have become virtually monopolized by agricultural and industrial cartels, which routinely denature them with pesticides, preservatives, artificial flavours, food colouring, and other unhealthy additives. Despite this, few Western physicians even bother to ask patients about their dietary habits, and even fewer understand anything about nutritional therapy as a cure and a preventive measure against disease.

Tap water is another example of a legally condoned public health hazard. As early as the Han dynasty (206 BC–AD 220) in China, the imperial government strictly enforced laws which required the public to clean their wells and water storage facilities regularly in order to maintain the purity of public drinking water. These laws also specified that pipes, vats, and basins used to transport and store drinking water must be made of clay, not metal, because the health hazards of heavy metals were well known to Chinese health authorities. Today, public water utilities poison our drinking water with chlorine, fluoride, aluminium salts, and other substances which they call 'purifiers', then run it through metal pipes which further contaminate the water with lead, iron, nickel, cadmium, and other metals that are extremely toxic to the human system. Public utilities and private corporations combine to poison the food, air, and water upon which we must all rely to stay alive. Orthodox Western medical practice compounds these public health hazards by ignoring them as causes of disease, then further aggravates the situation by prescribing toxic drugs, injections, vaccines, and radical surgery as cures for the ills they cause.

Modern fads and lifestyles, which are created and popularized by high-profit consumer industries, are as much to blame for the deterioration of public health as are negligent public policies. The *Internal Medicine Classic* contains a passage on detrimental lifestyle which precisely describes the way most people live today:

> Indulging their every whim and desire, people these days routinely eat and drink to excess and live indiscriminately without restraint or discipline. They indulge excessively in sex while intoxicated, deplete their brains with abnormal stress and strain, and live only for the moment's pleasure. This sort of lifestyle easily causes pure energy to dissipate and vitality to degenerate and leads to premature debility and death. Therefore, people these days begin to show signs of decrepitude and senility around the age of fifty.

Having briefly stated the case for assuming personal responsibility for one's own health and making prevention the primary principle in health care, let's see how traditional Chinese physicians approach the delicate and difficult art of diagnosis when prevention fails and disease gains entry into the human system.

The Four Diagnostics

The first step in the diagnosis of disease requires the physician to meet the patient in privacy and apply what the Chinese call the Four Diagnostics (*seh jen*). These four methods, which rely more on the physician's practical experience in the clinic than on medical manuals, are referred to as 'Interviewing', 'Observing', 'Listening', and 'Touching'.

First the physician interviews the patient in depth and detail, focusing on major symptoms and any factors of personal habit and lifestyle which may have contributed to the patient's current condition. Patients are asked to review their entire medical histories as well as those of their immediate families and to explain candidly how and when their ailments commenced, where the symptoms first appeared, and other relevant factors. Of particular interest to the physician are any alterations or transformations in the symptoms from their initial onset up to the time of the interview. Six main topics are emphasized in the diagnostic interview:

Chills and fever

The presence of chills and/or fever indicates whether the disease is primarily a yin or a yang condition. For example, fever without chills usually indicates an overabundance of yang energy, whereas chills without fever indicates a yang deficiency. Intermittent chills and fever indicate a more complex ailment which affects both yin and yang energies and which is moving inwards from the surface of the body to the interior.

Perspiration

Profuse or scant perspiration is an indicator of yin or yang deficiency and also a sign of whether the ailment is internal or external. Viscosity and odour of perspiration are also important factors.

Stool and urine

Constipation or diarrhoea are important symptoms in Chinese diagnosis, for they indicate 'hot' or 'cold' and 'full' or 'empty' energy conditions. Blood or mucus in stools are also vital clues. Scant, dark urine indicates a condition of excess 'hot' and 'full' energy, while profuse, clear urine is a sign of 'cold' and 'empty' conditions.

Diet

Dietary habits and any recent cravings for particular foods provide another source of insight into the cause and nature of the patient's ailment. Aversion to hot fluids and craving for cold drinks, for example, indicate a 'hot' type of disease. The dominant presence of any particular flavour in the mouth can indicate which organ is primarily affected through the flavour's association with one of the Five Elemental Energies and its related organ. A sour taste, for example, is related to the Wood energy of the liver.

Sleep

Oversleeping indicates a yang deficiency, while insomnia is a sign of poor circulation, excessive worry, or spleen deficiency. Rising unusually early in the morning indicates an overactive Fire energy in the heart, while fitful sleep and nightmares are signs of overindulgence in rich foods and drinks or emotional imbalance.

Sex

For men, the vital questions regarding sex are frequency of coitus and ejaculation, nocturnal emissions, impotence, and overall sexual drive. For women, the important sexual indicators are frequency and duration of menstrual cycles, colour and consistency of menstrual and other vaginal discharges, recent pregnancies and abortions, number of childbirths, and frequency of sexual intercourse.

'Observation' includes visual analysis of the patient's complexion, eyes, ears, tongue, hair, skin, and nails. The experienced physician can determine the state of a patient's energy and spirit by observing the way he or she walks, talks, breathes, and moves the limbs. The colour and tone of the patient's face, eyes, ears, and tongue provide direct reflections of the condition of the related internal organs. Chinese physicians carefully observe what they call *chee seh*, literally the 'colour of energy', which is reflected in facial complexion, the colour of the earlobes, and the condition of the facial apertures, signs which clearly indicate the state of the patient's vitality and resistance. Tongue diagnosis has been refined to a fine art in traditional Chinese medical practice, which distinguishes twenty-four different conditions based on the colour, tone, and texture of the tongue and tongue fur.

'Listening' includes 'smelling' in Chinese diagnosis; in fact, one of the Chinese ideograms which denote the verb 'to listen' also means 'to smell'. The physician listens carefully to the patient's breath, voice, and cough, as well as to the heartbeat and any sounds emanating from the stomach and bowels. He or she uses the nose to sniff and analyse the odours of the patient's breath and bodily secretions, which help determine the nature and location of the disease and the type of energy imbalance involved.

'Touching' means tactile examination of the patient's flesh, palpitation of the internal organs, and acupressure massage of the major energy meridians, especially along the spine, in order to determine which organs are affected by the disease. Particular vital points along the meridians, known as 'alarm points', become very tender and painful to touch when their associated organs are ailing, and nerve ganglia along the spine become tight and knotted when the organs they control are weak or dysfunctional.

The most important and difficult form of tactile examination is pulse diagnosis, an ancient technique whereby the physician places his or her fingertips along either side of the radial artery on each wrist and applies three different degrees of pressure. Under different pressures, these points reveal a total of twelve different pulses, one related to each of the twelve major organ-energy systems. An experienced physician with a sufficiently sensitive touch can use this method not only to diagnose correctly a current ailment in a particular organ, but also to trace past ailments in all the organs and determine what sort of residual damage remains, and to predict accurately the development of the current ailment and any other potential ailments that might be brewing in other organs. To those unfamiliar with this technique, its accuracy can seem uncanny. It can also be quite embarrassing, because it reveals habits and conditions which the patient may have failed to mention to the physician because of modesty.

After applying the Four Diagnostics to establish a basic understanding of the cause, nature, and location of a patient's disease, the physician next employs the Eight Indicators of symptomology to analyse the precise pathology and progressive development of the ailment and to determine the appropriate sort of therapy to apply at each stage of the healing process.

The Eight Indicators

Regardless of the cause or name attached to any particular disease, all diseases pollute the purity of the body's blood, bile, lymph, mucus, hormones, and other essences and provoke severe imbalances in human energy systems. Pollution of vital essences, impairment of vital functions, and imbalance in vital energies always manifest themselves in abnormal symptomatic reactions which skilled physicians are able to interpret correctly as a basis for treatment. In traditional Chinese medical practice, the Eight Indicators are symptomatic signposts which the physician follows on the road to curing a patient's disease. As a disease progresses under therapy, some symptoms tend to disappear, new symptoms arise, original symptoms transform, other symptoms relocate elsewhere, and so forth. All these symptomatic changes indicate whether the therapy is working against the disease, and the Eight Indicators provide the physician with a systematic code for diagnosing the patient's shifting symptomology.

The Eight Indicators form the basis for a method called

'differential diagnosis', whereby the physician carefully monitors the course of a disease and notes any symptomatic changes reflected by the Eight Indicators, then accordingly adjusts the herbal formulas, dietary advice, acupuncture, massage, and other therapies. Differential diagnosis enables the doctor to select 'the right tool for the job' during each progressive phase of the disease, so that therapies work in concert rather than conflict with the body's own natural healing mechanisms to facilitate the elimination of the disease from the system.

Western allopathic medicine regards symptoms of disease to be abnormal reactions to normal stimuli, as 'errors' to be 'corrected' with drugs and surgery. If the patient feels pain, the doctor prescribes painkillers. If there is swelling, drugs are prescribed to reduce it. The doctor gives sleeping pills for insomnia, stimulants for depression, antibiotics to kill germs, and recommends surgery to remove organs that fail to respond to drugs. None of these methods does anything to eliminate the root cause of the symptoms. On the contrary, they only contribute further to the patient's toxicity, weakening his or her system and eventually giving rise to even worse symptoms and more severe ailments.

By contrast, traditional medicine views symptoms of disease as normal responses to abnormal stimuli, as alarm signals indicating a defect in the environment or a mistake in lifestyle that must be corrected at the root source. Herbal medicine, diet, fasting, therapeutic exercise, acupuncture, massage, and other traditional healing methods eliminate the root causes of disease by removing the offending toxins from the body, purifying the vital fluids, restoring vital functions, and re-establishing optimum balance and harmony among the various organ energies of the human energy system. When this task has been completed, all abnormal symptoms naturally disappear and the patient is cured. If the patient then takes preventive measures to eliminate the environmental or lifestyle factors that caused the problem, the problem will not recur.

The Eight Indicators provide direct reflections of imbalances and aberrations in the vital organ-energy systems which regulate the human organism. These energy imbalances are closely associated with accumulations of toxic substances in the bodily tissues, vital fluids, organs, and glands. The blood and lymph, as well as the colon and liver, are particularly susceptible to pathological accumulations of toxic substances. Such toxins pollute the various vital essences which regulate the physical body, such as blood, lymph, bile, enzymes, hormones, and marrow, and impair the vital energy functions associated with those essences. Consequently, such vital functions as metabolism, digestion, respiration, excretion, immunity, and circulation are thrown off balance and fail to perform their tasks properly.

The herbs, dietary supplements, massage, and other methods used by traditional healers dissolve, dislodge, and help excrete toxic substances from the body, thereby eliminating obstructions to normal metabolism, circulation, immunity, and other vital functions and restoring natural balance among the body's energy systems. While the human energy system holds the ultimate key to successful diagnosis and therapy, detoxification and purification of vital essences and organ tissues are the primary methods employed to re-establish the energy balance upon which the vital functions of life depend.

As offending toxic substances are gradually driven out of the body during treatment, they usually cause a variety of additional symptoms that are clearly reflected by changes in the Eight Indicators. In alternative Western medical practice, these symptoms of detoxification are called 'cleansing reactions' or 'healing crisis', and they can be very unpleasant. Examples of common cleansing reactions are skin eruptions, headache, fever, dizziness, insomnia, swelling, aching joints, muscle pains, constipation, diarrhoea, flatulence, and fatigue. The appearance of such symptoms during therapy is a good sign because they indicate that the treatment is working successfully to purge, purify, and restore the body's vital fluids, organs, glands, and other tissues.

Conventional Western allopathic medicine views cleansing reactions as further symptoms of disease, rather than as normal responses to the body's elimination of disease, and therefore tries to suppress them by prescribing yet more allopathic drugs to counteract them, thereby halting the detoxification process and forcing the body not only to retain the original offending toxins but also to absorb the highly toxic by-products of the drugs themselves. A good example of this medical folly is the 'cold cures' sold in Western pharmacies, which do nothing at all to cure colds; instead, they provide a marginal measure of symptomatic relief by closing the ducts that excrete phlegm and mucus in the sinuses and throat, forcing these toxic discharges to back up in the lymph system. Although the patient may experience some temporary symptomatic relief from such drugs, sooner or later the retained toxins must be purged elsewhere, causing more virulent diseases, which are again treated symptomatically with more toxic drugs. Eventually such therapy leads to organ failures and surgery, and sometimes cancer, which is the final result of severe and prolonged tissue toxicity.

By contrast, traditional Chinese medicine deals with the symptomatic discomfort of cleansing reactions by periodically adjusting herbal formulas, diets, and other regimens in order to encourage and accelerate the detoxification and purification process, while simultaneously adding special herbs, foods, and other methods to help reduce the severity of cleansing reactions and minimize the patient's discomfort during the healing process. These adjustments are made according to progressive symptomatic changes revealed by the Eight Indicators. As soon as the offending toxic substances and aberrant energies are eliminated from the system, the cleansing reactions cease, purity of essence is restored, energy is rebalanced, and the patient is completely cured.

As the ancient proverb states, 'diagnosis is difficult' and requires many years of practical clinical experience, so there is no point in going into a deep and detailed discussion of the Eight Indicators of differential diagnosis here. Instead, we will review them briefly in order to establish a basic theoretical perspective on the subject and illuminate an alternative diagnostic approach to disease that contrasts sharply with the conventional Western method.

The Eight Indicators are called yin and yang, internal and external, cold and hot, empty and full.

Yin and yang

Yin and yang are by far the most important and fundamental indicators in the diagnosis and treatment of disease. In fact, the other six indicators are simply more specific manifestations of various aspects of yin and yang. In the final analysis, all diseases and their symptoms can be interpreted in terms of a loss of homeostatic balance in the yin and yang polarity of the body's various organ-energy systems. For example, high body temperature, constipation, flushed complexion, profuse perspiration, and hypertension are all signs of yang excess and indicate a 'yang disease'. Chills, diarrhoea, pale complexion, low vitality, weakness in the limbs, and aversion to cold are all examples of yin excess and indicate a 'yin disease'. Basically, yang diseases are treated with cooling yin herbs and other methods that boost yin and control yang energy, while yin diseases are treated with warming yang herbs and other methods that tonify yang and sedate yin energy. The *Internal Medicine Classic* states: 'If it's hot, cool it down; if it's cold, warm it up; if it's empty, fill it; if it's full, empty it.'

Yin and yang are known as the 'Commanders of the Eight Indicators' because all the other indicators 'belong' to either yin or yang. For example, the interior of the body is yin and the exterior is yang, and therefore 'external' symptoms indicate a yang disease while 'internal' symptoms indicate a yin problem. Similarly, 'cold' is a manifestation of yin and 'hot' manifests yang, 'empty' indicates a yin condition of energy deficiency and 'full' reflects a yang condition of energy excess. These indicators almost always appear in various combinations. Thus, if a 'hot' symptom appears on the surface of the body, it is called 'external-hot', which is also known as 'yang within yang'. If a 'cold' symptom appears externally, it is called 'external-cold', or 'yin within yang'. A 'full' symptom internally is 'yang within yin', and an 'empty-internal' condition is 'yin within yin'.

Each combination of indicators calls for a different therapeutic approach, and as various indicators move and transform, therapies are adjusted accordingly in order to ensure maximum efficacy. If an 'internal-hot' symptom moves to the surface and becomes 'external-hot', it means that the excess hot yang energy is successfully being driven from the internal organs outwards towards the skin for dissipation. The herb which moves evil hot energy from the inside to the outside will then be withdrawn, and herbs which dissipate excess heat from the body's surface will be added.

Internal and external

These indicators inform the physician where the disease is located and in which direction it is moving. They also reflect the extent and severity of the condition. As diseases get worse, they tend to move inwards from the surface of skin and muscles into the vital organs, glands, and bones. As conditions improve under therapy, they tend to move outwards towards the surface for elimination, so this is usually a sign that the treatment is working. Symptoms of internal disease include thirst, nausea, abdominal pains, aching joints, loose bowels, chest pains, and swelling. Symptoms of external disease include heat flushes, aversion to cold, stuffy nose, muscular pains, and headache.

Internal and external indicators always appear in conjunction with either hot and cold or empty and full symptoms. For example, hot flushes with no sweat and headache with muscular pain indicate 'external-full' conditions, whereas dizziness and fatigue, heart palpitations, cold sweat, cold hands and feet, shortness of breath, and sluggish speech indicate that the disease has developed into an 'external-empty' phase. Cold and hot, empty and full symptoms tend to shift rapidly between the surface and the interior during treatment, often indicating that toxic substances are being dislodged and propelled into excretory ducts, organs, and orifices for elimination. The physician must keep a careful watch on these movements in order to adjust the therapies so that they assist rather than interfere with the body's own natural healing mechanisms. At the same time, he or she must endeavour to alleviate the symptomatic discomforts of the patient's cleansing reactions.

Cold and hot

Cold and hot indicate the basic nature of the ailment by manifesting various types of aberrant energy, such as abnormally high or low body temperature, aversion to heat or cold, flushed or pale complexion, light or dark urine, hard or soft stools, and so forth. These symptoms can become quite complicated and unstable. For example, there are conditions known as 'hot on top, cold below', 'cold on top, hot below', 'hot stomach, cold intestines', 'hot intestines, cold stomach', and so forth. Bloodshot eyes and sore throat indicate hot symptoms in the Upper Burner, while accompanying abdominal bloating and diarrhoea indicate a simultaneous cold condition in the Lower Burner. Again, the physician must perform an extraordinary therapeutic balancing act to move and transform aberrant energies and to boost and balance the patient's own internal organ-energies with herbs, diet, massage, and other methods that work in harmony with the Great Principle of Yin and Yang and the Five Elemental Energies.

Empty and full

These indicators reflect the extent to which an ailment has depleted or inflamed the affected organ energies and the level of the patient's resistance to the ailment. Low resistance, physical weakness, and lack of vitality indicate a condition of 'empty energy', while hyperactivity, high blood pressure, and nervous energy indicate 'full energy'. Fullness of energy, however, is not necessarily a good sign, for it usually indicates an ongoing battle between the patient's protective 'pure energy' and the disease's intruding 'evil energy'. If the pure energy of resistance gains the upper hand, the evil energy of disease grows increasingly 'empty' and is finally driven out of the ven out of the system. If resistance is low, pure energy becomes increasingly 'empty', while evil energy grows 'full'. 'Full' conditions can also be caused by obstructions in one or more of the body's energy meridians, which cause the related organ energy to back up and spill over into other meridians, overstimulating and inflaming the affected organs.

'Empty' and 'full' are therefore primary indicators of relative energy levels and balances. Again, the related symptoms rarely manifest themselves singly but usually in combination with cold and hot, internal and external symptoms. They frequently transform, recombine, and relocate during the course of a disease's development and treatment, and these changes indicate how well the therapy is working and how it must be adjusted for maximum efficacy under changing symptomatic conditions.

Thus the physician establishes the root causes and basic nature of a disease by implementing the Four Diagnostics, then applies the Eight Indicators of symptomology to locate and differentiate the various symptoms of aberrant energy which the disease provokes. During the course of treatment, the differential diagnosis of symptoms becomes more important than the original cause and category of the disease, because the symptoms serve the physician as guiding signs for the therapies he or she employs to combat the disease, and indicate how those therapies must be adjusted as symptoms shift and transform while the disease runs its course. By monitoring the Eight Indicators, the physician is able to assist the body in the task of detoxification and purification and to align the therapies with the body's own natural healing mechanisms to effect a complete cure.

Depending upon the severity of the disease and the condition of the patient's essence and energy, the healing process can take a few days, a few weeks, several months, or a number of years, but when it is over, a complete cure has been achieved, without resorting to chemical drugs, radiation, radical surgery, or other debilitating allopathic methods, which often cause more diseases than they cure. As long as the patient follows up the treatment by adopting an effective programme of preventive health care, he or she can usually expect to live a long and healthy life.

PART II

The Branches:
Essence, Energy and Spirit

CHAPTER 9

Essence: Food

Essence refers to the vital fluids in the human organism.
All living things are born from fluid. The *Book of Change*
[*I Ching*] states: 'Heaven first produced water.' Taoists
say: 'Water is the mother of the Three Sources of Heaven,
Earth, and Humans, and essence is the root of primal
energy.'

Chang Ching-yueh, *The Book of Classifications*
(second century BC)

Essence is the fundamental material foundation of corporeal
human life and the primary element in Taoist internal alchemy.
Essence manifests its primordial prenatal aspect in the sperm and
ovum which form the human embryo upon conception and in the
primal procreative drive of sexual reproduction. The *Internal
Medicine Classic* states: 'Before a human body is formed, there must
first be prenatal essence.'

After birth, prenatal essence is stored in the 'kidney-organ
system', which in Chinese medical terminology refers to the
adrenal glands ('internal kidneys') and the testes or ovaries ('external kidneys'). The prenatal essence stored in the adrenals provides
the body's most potent internal source of life-supporting energy.
Every body is endowed with a limited supply of this primordial
energy (*yuan-chee*), and one's life span is determined by the rate at
which it is used up. The prenatal essence stored in the testes and
ovaries is activated at puberty and provides the sperm and ova
with which to procreate the next generation of human life.
Postnatal essence consists of the various vital fluids that sustain life
and is produced within the body in three basic forms. The first is
'blood essence', which includes all the elements that constitute
and are carried by the blood, such as red and white blood cells,
water, and the various nutrients assimilated from digested food.

The second is 'hormone essence', which takes two forms: 'life essence' includes all the various essential hormones secreted by the endocrine system, as well as neurochemicals, cerebrospinal fluids, and enzymes; 'sexual essence' refers to the various hormones and other secretions specifically associated with sexual functions, including sperm and ova. The third form of postnatal essence is called 'essential fluids' and includes all the body's heavier fluids, such as lymph and mucus, the synovial fluids that lubricate the joints, as well as tears, perspiration, and urine. All these fluids are synthesized from the essential nutrients extracted by digestion from food and water. The quality of these vital fluids, which constitute the 'essence of life', is therefore directly dependent upon the quality of nutrients in the diet and the efficiency of digestion and metabolism. The foundation of human life is rooted in nutrition: 'You are what you eat.'

In Taoist alchemy, postnatal essence 'resides' in the energy centre of the Lower Elixir Field, located slightly below and behind the navel, and is physiologically associated with the hypogastric plexus, a major nerve network in the abdomen which controls the digestive, excretory, and reproductive organs.

Diet and nutrition

The *Internal Medicine Classic* states: 'When essence is deficient, replenish it with food.' In other words, when any of the various essential fluids upon which all vital functions depend is deficient, the first place to seek replenishment is diet and nutrition. Hippocrates said precisely the same thing when he wrote, 'Your food shall be your medicine,' but ever since the turn of the twentieth century, Western medical practice has discarded this holistic healing principle in favour of drugs and surgery, with drastic results for human health.

Today nutritional therapy is once again gaining recognition in New Age Western medical circles as a safe and effective means of treating disease and degeneration in the human body, but in the East it has always remained a primary form of therapy. Traditional Eastern and modern Western concepts of what constitutes a healthy 'balanced diet' differ greatly, and so do their approaches to dietary supplements. In Western practice, refined nutritional supplements such as vitamins and minerals are prescribed to provide various nutrients that are missing or insufficient in one's diet. Such dietary deficiencies are often caused by modern farming and food-processing methods. The traditional Chinese approach to supplementation is to prescribe herbs such as ginseng and gentian, which enhance the power of the digestive system to extract and assimilate nutrients from whatever foods one consumes. Both methods work, and together their effects are synergistic.

The conventional Western notion of a balanced diet is to combine all major food groups at every meal, such as proteins and carbohydrates, fruits and vegetables. This approach violates the rules of trophology (the science of food combining) and can lead to digestive disaster, poor assimilation, and chronic constipation. Trophology is discussed in detail in *The Tao of HS&L*, to which interested readers may refer, and will therefore not be further discussed here. Instead, we will focus on traditional Taoist and holistic Western concepts of how to select and balance foods for optimum health according to the types of energy they release in the body.

In addition to their constituent biochemical nutrients, which is the only aspect of food that conventional Western nutrition recognizes, all foods have a basic bioenergetic nature which is imparted to the consuming organism. Traditional Taoist nutritional science categorizes foods according to these bioenergies, and Taoist diets are formulated in order to achieve an optimum balance between the various types of energy that foods release when digested and metabolized. Like all energies, food energies are polar, therefore they are categorized primarily in terms of yin and yang.

Yin foods have a cooling, calming effect on human energy, while yang foods are warming and stimulating. When selecting foods according to their yin and yang energies, you should seek balance not only among the foods selected, but also between the foods and the prevailing energy conditions inside and outside your body. For example, if your internal energy is in a state of extreme yin (tired, sluggish, depressed), you can balance and correct that condition by consuming yang foods, which will stimulate, warm, and elevate your energy. Similarly, if the external environment is extremely yin (cold, damp, overcast), you can resist the intrusion of these external 'evil energies' into your own system by consuming some warming, drying yang foods.

Until the recent advent of Western-style supermarkets and fast-food chains in the Far East, Chinese families routinely balanced their meals in this traditional manner. And even in the West, before the twentieth century people automatically ate more meat, butter, and other warming foods in the cold of winter, when fresh produce was scarce, and consumed more cooling fruits and vegetables in summer, when fresh produce was cheap and plentiful and livestock was still being fattened for winter. Thanks to refrigerators, super-markets, and long-distance transport, people now eat apples and oranges in midwinter and fatty meats in midsummer, thereby causing themselves all sorts of disease and distress and playing havoc with their internal energies. The following chart lists some basic foods and spices according to their warming (yang) and cooling (yin) properties:

	Cooling (Yin)	Warming (Yang)
Foods:	raw fruits	dried & stewed fruits
	raw vegetables	cooked vegetables
	summer squashes	winter squashes
	salad greens	cabbage
	tofu (bean curd)	tomato sauce
	seaweeds	avocado
	bulgur	root vegetables
	rice	lentils, kidney beans
	milk, yogurt	potatoes
	bean sprouts	oats, barley, kasha (buckwheat)
	raw fish (sashimi)	butter, cream, cheese
		nuts, seeds
		beef, lamb, chicken
		cooked fish
Spices:	curry powder	garlic
	parsley	ginger
	chilli peppers	basil, thyme, oregano
	coriander	black pepper
	tamari, soy sauce	bay leaf
	sugar	cloves
	salt	molasses
		miso
		chocolate, vanilla

From a modern scientific point of view, the most important aspect of yin and yang polarity in food is alkaline and acid balance, or pH. Yang foods are acid-forming and impart acidity to the bloodstream and cellular fluids, while yin foods are alkalizing to bodily fluids and tissues. Note that we're talking about the effects that foods have on the body's pH balance, not their own intrinsic pH values. Some foods that are acidic by nature, such as grapes and lemons, in fact have an alkalizing effect on bodily fluids when metabolized.

Biochemically, acids contain a high concentration of positively charged hydrogen (H+) ions, while alkalis contain a lot of negatively charged hydroxyl (OH-) ions. When a yang molecule of H+ meets a yin molecule of OH-, it's love at first sight: yin and yang unite, alkali and acid bond, positive and negative balance, and the resulting offspring is neutral water, the 'Mother of Life'. That's how the Great Principle of Yin and Yang operates on the molecular level of food chemistry in the body.

On a pH scale of 1–12, plain water is neutral at pH7. In order to function properly, blood plasma must remain slightly alkaline between 7.35 and 7.45. Even the slightest fluctuation in either direction can slow the heart beat and cause coma (acid) or race the heart and cause convulsions (alkaline), and if the imbalance is not immediately corrected, death is a certainty. Consequently, the body applies several internal mechanisms to maintain a constant homeostatic balance in blood pH, such as reducing excess acids into water and carbon dioxide and eliminating them through the kidneys and lungs, shunting excess acids into the stomach for digestive use, or transforming them into mineral salts.

Although it is also possible to overalkalize the blood, it is a rare occurrence. A far more common problem, especially on modern Western diets, is excess acidification of the blood, which results in a condition known as 'acidosis'. Acidosis is responsible for or contributes to a number of debilitating conditions, including demineralization of the bones (e.g. osteoporosis), nervous disorders, kidney stones, chronic fatigue, gout, arthritis, dental caries, and impaired immune function. By familiarizing yourself with the basic alkalizing (yin) and acidifying (yang) properties of various foods, you can easily maintain an optimum balance in the pH of your blood and other vital fluids and thereby protect your body from the ravages of acidosis.

The following chart lists major food groups according to their effect on body pH. Note that some foods, such as butter, are listed as 'neutral', which means that they neither alkalize nor acidify the system; instead, they diminish the acidity of acids and the alkalinity of alkalis and may therefore be consumed as buffers with either category.

acidifying	neutral	alkalizing
sugar, honey	butter	coffee, tea
alcohol, soft drinks	yogurt	fresh fruits
white flour & rice	cheese	fresh vegetables
meat, fish, fowl	tofu (beancurd)	seaweeds
eggs	soya sauce, miso	garlic
nuts, whole grains		salt
beans, legumes		

A quick glance at this chart reveals why modern Western diets are so highly acidifying. The standard American diet (SAD), for example, which derives over 90 per cent of its calories from acidifying foods, causes a state of chronic acidosis, the most obvious signs of which are a sour taste in the mouth in the morning and sour body odour. One reason so many Americans and Europeans rush to gulp down their first cup of coffee in the morning is because it has an immediate alkalizing effect on their perennial 'acid hangovers'.

Another aspect of food energetics is their associations with the Five Elemental Energies, which determine their 'natural affinities' (*gui-jing*) for various vital organ-energy systems in the body. Among the many properties and phases associated with the Five Elemental Energies, the Five Flavours are most obviously reflected in foods, and this is how Taoist alchemy categorizes this aspect of food energy. If, for example, your liver is weak, Chinese physicians might suggest that you eat more sour Wood-energy foods to boost your liver energy, but if your liver is overactive or inflamed, they would suggest that you abstain from sour foods. In this respect, it is interesting to note that Americans, who consume an enormous excess of sugary sweet Earth-energy foods, also have a very high incidence of chronic stomach ailments, such as hyperacidity, ulcers, and indigestion, and this might well be due to an overload in the stomach–Earth-energy system from sweets.

The chart below lists some common foods according to their Five Elemental Energy and Flavour associations, as well as their organ affinities:

Wood/sour/liver, gall bladder:

grains:	wheat, rye, oats, barley
beans:	lentils, green peas
vegetables:	bean sprouts, salad greens, green peppers, broccoli, string beans
fruits:	citrus fruits
meats:	chicken

water/salty/kidneys, bladder:

grains:	kasha (buckwheat)
beans:	kidney, black, pinto, adzuki
vegetables:	seaweeds
fruits:	blackberries, blueberries, black grapes, watermelon, cranberries
meats:	bluefish

metal/pungent/lungs, large intestine:

grains:	rice
beans:	soya beans & tofu, navy beans
vegetables:	white onions, cabbage, turnips, radish, cauliflower, celery
fruits:	pears
meats:	cod, flounder, beef, turkey

earth/sweet/stomach, spleen, pancreas:

grains:	millet
beans:	chickpeas
vegetables:	winter squash, yams
fruits:	sweet fruits
meats:	tuna, swordfish, wild birds

fire/bitter/heart, small intestine:

grains:	corn
beans:	red lentils
vegetables:	kale, mustard greens, endives, and other bitter greens, tomatoes, scallions
fruits:	apricots, strawberries
meats:	lamb, shrimp

As you can see, there is a lot more to food than meets the eye or tickles the palate. How well you feel, how clearly you think, and how successfully you adapt to your internal and external environments are all directly related to the sorts of energies you unleash in your system through your dietary habits. Massive advertising campaigns, clever junk-food packaging, huge supermarkets that stock everything under the sun all year round, fast-food outlets, and a widespread ignorance of nutritional science among the public as well as the medical establishment have misled most of the Western and much of the Eastern world down the debilitating path of obesity, malnutrition, immune deficiency, cancer, skin and dental problems, emotional imbalance, mental disturbances, and other diet-related ills.

Nevertheless, it's your mouth, your stomach, and your life. All you need to do is to familiarize yourself with the pharmaco-dynamics of food chemistry, learn how to combine foods properly at meals, and apply the Tao of Diet to eat your way to health and happiness.

Food alchemy: essence to energy

'Jing hwa chee,' states the first principle of Taoist internal alchemy. That means 'essence transforms into energy', which is precisely what Einstein said regarding the transmutable relationship between matter and energy, $E = mc^2$. In the alchemy of food, essential nutrients are transformed into energy by virtue of enzyme activity.

Enzymes are involved in every single biological function and physiological process in the body, including digestion and metabolism, immune response and cell division, muscular and cerebral activity, protein synthesis and antioxidant activity. About 5,000 different enzymes have so far been identified, each with a specific function and each requiring specific conditions of temperature and pH, and there are probably thousands more we don't know about yet. Without enzymes, the entire body would grind to a halt.

Enzymes are highly active biochemical agents produced by various organs and glands and within every cell in the body. Unlike ordinary chemical catalysts, enzymes are endowed with a spark of living energy, or *chee*, and it is this energy that gives them their remarkable bioactive powers. Enzyme energy can be detected by scientific instruments as a form of radiation that is emitted whenever enzymes are at work. No other type of biochemical essence displays such properties.

The enzymes required for digestion are produced primarily by the pancreas, as well as by thousands of tiny digestive ducts in the stomach and salivary glands in the mouth. Some enzymes, however, are present only in fresh unadulterated foods and are quickly destroyed when foods are subjected to chemical processing, irradiation, and prolonged cooking with high heat. Known as 'food enzymes', they are activated in the warmth and moisture of the mouth and stomach when food is chewed and swallowed. The more food enzymes you consume in your diet, the fewer enzymes your body needs to divert for digestive duty, and the more enzyme energy you save for other functions. And since your body must expend energy to produce enzymes, the more enzymes you consume with your food, the more energy you save and the longer you live.

Modern farming, food-processing, and cooking methods produce foods that are completely enzyme-dead, which means that diets based on cooked and processed foods require the body to direct a constant stream of enzymes into the digestive tract to break down these foods and extract their nutrients. This diversion of vital energy into enzyme production often exceeds the energy derived from the food itself, resulting in a net loss of energy. Obviously, such diets slowly but surely deplete vitality and therefore shorten life.

This situation is further aggravated by the overabundance of denatured foods in modern diets. Even the most potent metabolic enzymes cannot extract energy from food molecules whose electromagnetic valence has been altered or destroyed by chemical additives, gamma radiation, or microwave cooking, because damaged molecules do not react and combine normally with enzymes and other biochemicals and therefore do not yield much viable energy. Instead, they can cause faulty biochemical reactions that are suspected of being contributing causes of cancer. Only wholesome natural foods consumed in a relatively natural state produce wholesome natural energy for the body.

Perhaps this explains in part why the United States, despite its glut of food and high calorie intake, leads the world in the incidence of cancer. The SAD is virtually devoid of enzymes, and many of its constituent food elements have been abnormally damaged by chemicals and irradiation. Consequently, enzymes that under normal conditions would be performing the housecleaning and guardian duties of the immune system are all tied up trying to clear out the backlog of inert, denatured, partially digested foods in the digestive tract. What few viable nutrients are actually extracted from this mess often have faulty biochemical structures and fail to function properly when incorporated into the structural matrix of cells and tissues. The most glaring example of the carcinogenic properties of processed foods in modern diets is hydrogenated vegetable oil: when denatured fat molecules from margarine and other artificial fats are synthesized into the structure of cells owing to the absence of natural fats in the diet, those cells fail to respond properly under duress, paving the way for the growth of cancerous tumours. The fact is, in order for food alchemy to function properly, your body requires an abundant supply of active enzymes, some of which must enter the body as natural food enzymes via the diet, and processed foods simply cannot supply these vital elements. Instead, they burn up your own limited supplies of these vital metabolic elements.

In the following sections, we will discuss various food groups, diets, and supplements in order to determine what sort of eating habits sustain successful food alchemy and therefore promote health and longevity, and what sort of dietary factors inhibit proper food alchemy and therefore rob you of health and longevity.

Food profiles

The information presented below on various types of foods is meant to supplement and update the materials on diet and nutrition presented in *The Tao of HS&L*. For details on trophology and the therapeutic benefits of specific foods, readers may refer to the appropriate sections in that book and combine them with the new information below.

Sugar

Sugar is without question one of the most dangerous substances on the food market today. What we're talking about here is sucrose, the white crystalline sugar refined from cane or beet juice by stripping away all its vitamins, minerals, protein, fibre, water, and other synergists. White sugar is an industrially processed chemical not found in nature, and it is not fit for human consumption. Other sugars, such as fructose (in fruit and honey), lactose (in milk), and maltose (in grains) are natural substances with nutritional value. Raw sugar is a coarse, brown, sticky variety made by simply boiling down whole cane juice and it too is a wholesome food, but it is very difficult to find in the Western world. The so-called 'brown sugar' sold in supermarkets is nothing more than refined white sugar with some molasses spun back into it for colour and flavour. It is not a 'health food'.

Sugar suppresses the immune system by causing the pancreas to secrete abnormally large quantities of insulin, which is required to break it down. Insulin remains in circulation in the bloodstream long after sugar has been metabolized, and one of its main side effects is to suppress the release of growth hormone in the pituitary gland. Growth hormone is a primary regulator of the immune system, so anyone who eats a lot of sugar every day is going to experience a critical growth hormone deficiency and consequent immune deficiency caused by the constant presence of insulin in the bloodstream. Furthermore, refined white sugar is treated as a toxic foreign agent by the immune system owing to its unnatural chemical structure as well as the industrial contaminants it retains from the refining process. Sugar thus triggers an unnecessary immune response while simultaneously suppressing immune function, thereby debilitating the immune system with a double-edged sword.

Sugar is the chief culprit in many diseases and degenerative conditions. It can easily cause diabetes and is a major factor in candidiasis, both of which are epidemic in the industrialized Western world. Since sugar is 'nutritionally naked', the body must 'borrow' the missing vitamins, minerals, and other synergistic nutrients required to metabolize sugar from its own tissues. Heavy sugar consumption therefore causes a constant siphoning of nutrients from the body. Recent evidence suggests that sugar causes dental caries not so much by contact with the teeth but rather by leaching the teeth of calcium from within. Sugar depletes the body of potassium and magnesium, which are required for proper cardiac function, and is therefore a major factor in heart disease. The nutritional leaching caused by sugar can give rise to intense food cravings and eating binges, as the body seeks to replenish the nutrients 'stolen' from it by sugar.

Most people consume far more sugar than their bodies can possibly use for energy. When this happens, the liver converts the extra sugar into molecules called triglycerides and stores it as fat, or else produces cholesterol from the by-products of sugar and deposits it in veins and arteries. Sugar is thus a major factor in obesity and arteriosclerosis as well.

Sugar is an addictive substance. In *Sugar Blues*, William Dufty writes: 'The difference between sugar addiction and narcotic addiction is largely one of degree.' Abruptly giving up sugar invariably brings on the sort of withdrawal symptoms associated with narcotic drugs – fatigue, lassitude, depression, moodiness, headaches, aching limbs. Its addictive nature is also reflected in current per capita consumption in the USA – an average of 130 pounds of sugar per person per year, or about ⅓ pound daily. That qualifies as 'substance abuse'. Most people don't even realize how much sugar they're taking every day because much of it is hidden in other foods. A 12-ounce can of a typical soft drink, for example, contains about nine teaspoons of refined white sugar.

Sugar consumption in the USA is so high that is has also caused a social problem through its deleterious effects on behaviour, especially in children, who are displaying increasingly severe behavioural disorders and learning disabilities. In a recent study conducted by Dr C. Keith Connors of the Children's Hospital in Washington, DC, a 'deadly' link was established between the consumption of sugar with carbohydrates (such as breakfast cereal, cake, and biscuits) and violent behaviour, hypertension, and learning impediments. In other studies, chronic violence in prisons was remarkably reduced simply by eliminating refined sugar and starch from prison diets. Singapore in 1991 banned sugary soft-drink sales from all schools and youth centres, citing the danger that sugar poses to the mental and physical health of children.

If you or your children have a sweet tooth, you can easily satisfy it by concocting treats with honey, molasses, and barley malt, which are not only sweet but also nutritious and therapeutically beneficial.

Fat

Medical myths about fats have steered millions of Western people into self-destructive dietary folly in recent years. Natural unadulterated fats are not only highly nutritious, gram for gram they contain far more energy than any other type of food on earth, which makes them the most efficient fuel for essence-to-energy food alchemy. Natural fats contain nutrients which are absolutely essential for proper functioning of the brain, heart, and immune system, but despite this fact, the Western medical establishment, along with the media and processed-food industry, have condemned natural fats as killers and suggest instead that we all switch over to 'low-fat' or 'no-fat' products in which natural fats have been replaced by hydrogenated vegetable oils.

First, let's discuss why the body requires fats and how it uses them, then take a look at the artificial substitutes.

Natural fats such as butter, nut oils, and fish oils contain important nutrients called 'essential fatty acids', which are required for many metabolic processes and vital functions. That's why they are called 'essential' – because your body cannot function properly without them. Among other things, fatty acids are required to build and repair cellular membranes, especially in brain, nerve, and white blood cells, and to keep blood vessels clean and well lubricated. Two of them – linoleic and linolenic acid – cannot be synthesized in the body and must therefore be obtained from dietary sources. According to Dr Cass Igram, one of America's leading nutritional scientists, virtually all Americans are deficient in essential fatty acids.

Fats are about twice as efficient in producing energy as any other type of food, including complex carbohydrates and natural sugars. The essence-to-energy conversion of fats takes place in tiny power plants within each cell, called mitochondria, which prefer fat over all other fuels. But the fat must be natural and unadulterated in order to yield viable cellular energy. That means butter, meat, fish, nuts, seeds, and cold-pressed oils. The traditional Eskimo diet included mounds of raw fat from whales, seals, and fish, but

Eskimos never experienced problems with arteriosclerosis and heart disease until they switched from natural fats to processed American foods made with hydrogenated vegetable oils, sugar, and starch. The Japanese also eat a lot of natural raw fish oils in the form of sashimi and sushi, which contain abundant supplies of essential fatty acids. Cold-pressed olive oil has been a mainstay in Mediterranean diets for thousands of years, and these countries are known for their relatively low incidence of cancer and heart disease. In China, people traditionally used cold-pressed sesame and peanut oil for cooking and making condiments, and in India essential fatty acids are obtained by abundant use of clarified butter called ghee.

During World War II, when butter became scarce, American chemists fiddled around with vegetable oils to produce a butter substitute and came up with margarine and 'shortening'. They did this by heating various vegetable oils to over 500°F, then pumping hydrogen through it and adding nickel as a catalyst to harden it. The result of this chemical wizardry is a solid fat substitute with a molecular structure very similar to plastic.

When natural fats are eliminated from the diet in favour of hydrogenated-oil substitutes, the body is forced to use these denatured fat molecules in place of the natural fatty acids missing from the diet. White blood cells, which are pillars of the immune system, are particularly dependent on essential fatty acids. Here's how Dr Igram describes what happens to white cells when hydrogenated oils replace natural fats in the diet, excerpted from his book *Eat Right or Die Young*:

> These cells incorporate the hydrogenated fats you eat into their membranes. When this happens, the white cells become sluggish in function, and their membranes actually become stiff! Such white blood cells are poor defenders against infection. This leaves the body wide open to all sorts of derangements of the immune system. Cancer, or infections by yeasts, bacteria and viruses can more easily take a foothold . . . In fact, one of the quickest ways to paralyse your immune system is to eat, on a daily basis, significant quantities of deep-fried foods, or fats such as margarine . . . No wonder that a high consumption of margarine, shortening, and other hydrogenated fats is associated with a greater incidence of a variety of cancers.

Besides cancer, regular consumption of hydrogenated-oil products, including non-dairy creamers and toppings and virtually all processed and packaged foods, is closely associated with an increased risk of arteriosclerosis, heart disease, autoimmune diseases, candidiasis, and high blood pressure.

The heart is particularly fond of natural fats as fuel, and heart cells specialize in the conversion of fats into energy. In order to do this, however, a nutrient called 'carnitine' is required to deliver fats into the cells for combustion. 'Fats cannot be properly combusted without adequate amounts of carnitine,' writes Dr Igram.

Carnitine is an amino acid synthesized in the liver from two other amino acids – lysine and methionine – both of which must be obtained from dietary sources. If you have sufficient supplies of carnitine, you can eat all the natural fats you want, because carnitine helps burn fat, especially in the heart, which never rests.

Here we find a very interesting link with the traditional Taoist notion of the Five Elemental Energies and their associated organs, in which the liver is governed by Wood and the heart by Fire. According to the generative 'Mother-Son' relationship of Wood to Fire, the liver feeds the heart with energy, just as wood fuels fire. In terms of modern nutritional science, the liver provides the carnitine and the fat which the heart burns to produce energy.

The richest dietary sources of carnitine are lamb (especially the fatty parts), organ meats (especially liver and heart), fish, avocado, and wheat germ. The best sources of essential fatty acids are deep-water ocean fish such as tuna and salmon, as well as wild game, avocados, almonds, pecans, and pumpkin, pine, and sunflower seeds. The best choices in cooking oils are cold-pressed olive, corn, sunflower, sesame, and safflower oils. Clarified butter (ghee) is better than ordinary butter for cooking because it can withstand higher temperatures without damage. Avoid all products made with hydrogenated or partially hydrogenated vegetable oils, including commercial mayonnaise, bottled salad dressings, margarine, shortening, and virtually all processed foods.

Dairy

Cow's milk is meant for calves, and babies are meant to drink mother's milk until weaned from it. Nature has designed both types of milk and digestive systems accordingly. It is a scientifically documented fact that calves fed on pasteurized milk from their own mother cows usually die within six weeks, so it stands to reason that pasteurized cow's milk is not a wholesome, life-sustaining food for calves, much less for humans. Yet not only do adult humans feed this denatured animal secretion to their own infants, they also consume it themselves.

Cow's milk has four times the protein and only half the carbohydrate content of human milk; pasteurization destroys the natural enzyme in cow's milk required to digest its heavy protein content. This excess milk protein therefore putrefies in the human digestive tract, clogging the intestines with sticky sludge, some of which seeps into the bloodstream. As this putrid sludge accumulates from daily consumption of dairy products, the body forces some of it out through the skin (acne, blemishes) and lungs (catarrh), while the rest of it festers inside, forms mucus that breeds infections, causes allergic reactions, and stiffens joints with calcium deposits. Many cases of chronic asthma, allergies, ear infections, and acne have been totally cured simply by eliminating all dairy products from the diet.

Cow's milk products are particularly harmful to women. Milk is supposed to flow out of, not into, women's bodies. The debilitating effects of pasteurized cow's milk on women is further aggravated by the synthetic hormones cows are injected with to increase milk production. These chemicals play havoc with the delicately balanced female endocrine system. In *Food and Healing*, the food therapist Annemarie Colbin describes the dairy disaster for women as follows:

> The consumption of dairy products, including milk, cheese, yogurt, and ice cream, appears to be strongly linked to various disorders of the female reproductive system, including ovarian tumours and cysts, vaginal discharges, and infections. I see this link confirmed time and again by the countless women I know who report these problems diminishing or disappearing altogether after they've stopped consuming dairy food. I hear of fibroid tumours being passed or dissolved, cervical cancer arrested, menstrual irregularities straightened out ... Even infertility appears to have been reversed with this approach in several instances ...

Many women, as well as men, consume dairy products because their doctors tell them it's a good source of calcium. This is fallacious advice. True, cow's milk contains 118 mg of calcium in every 100 grams, compared to 33 mg/100 grams in human milk.

But cow's milk also contains 97 mg phosphorus/100 grams, compared to only 18 mg in human milk. Phosphorus combines with calcium in the digestive tract and actually blocks its assimilation. Dr Frank Oski, chairman of the Department of Pediatrics at the State University of New York's Medical Center, states: 'Only foods with a calcium-to-phosphorus-ratio of two-to-one or better should be used as a primary source of calcium.' The ratio in human milk is 2.35 to one, in cow's milk only 1.27 to one. Cow's milk also contains 50 mg sodium/100 grams, compared with only 16 mg in human milk, so dairy products are probably one of the most common sources of excess sodium in the modern Western diet.

Besides, cow's milk is not nearly as good a source of calcium as other far more digestible and wholesome foods. Compare the 118 mg calcium/100 grams cow's milk with 100 grams of the following foods: almonds (254 mg), broccoli (130 mg), kale (187 mg), sesame seeds (1,160 mg), kelp (1,093 mg), and sardines (400 mg).

As for osteoporosis, it is caused not so much by calcium deficiency in the diet as it is by dietary factors which leach calcium from bones and teeth, especially sugar. Sugar, meat, refined starch, and alcohol all cause a constant state of acidosis in the bloodstream, and acid blood is known to dissolve calcium from bones. The best way to correct osteoporosis is to consume the non-dairy calcium-rich foods mentioned above, while simultaneously cutting down or eliminating acidifying calcium robbers from the diet. A daily supplement of 3 mg of the mineral boron also seems to help bones assimilate and retain calcium.

From the traditional Chinese medical point of view, milk is a form of 'sexual essence'. For the human species to drink the sexual essence of another species can only lead to trouble, especially for females, because the hormones it contains will upset the sensitive balance of the human endocrine system.

If you insist on consuming dairy products, your best bet is goat's milk, which approximates the nutritional composition and balance of human milk. The only safe products made from cow's milk are fresh butter, which is a digestible fat, and fresh live-culture yogurt, which is predigested for you by lactobacteria, but even these should be consumed in moderation and preferably prepared from raw unpasteurized milk.

Meat

Westerners consume a far greater percentage of their calories from meat than Orientals do, and it shows in their complexion, body fat, and body odour. Meat is highly acidifying and warming (yang qualities), as well as putrefactive. According to the tenets of traditional Chinese medicine, elderly people require more meat than the young or middle-aged because of its warming yang properties and concentrated nutrients, but only if their digestive systems are in proper order.

The biggest problem with meat in the standard American diet is the pervasive contamination of US beef with antibiotics and steroid hormones. About 40 per cent of all the antibiotics produced in the USA are fed to cattle and other livestock, and this is passed on to the consumer in every hamburger, steak, and other food product made with US beef. This daily dietary intake of antibiotics depresses the human immune system and is an important contributing factor in acquired immune deficiency.

In addition to antibiotics, US cattle are fed synthetic hormones to accelerate growth, increase fat deposits, bring entire herds of cows into heat at the same time for breeding, increase milk production, and induce abortions in pregnant cows scheduled for slaughter. These hormones are suspected as a major cause of the high incidence of breast and ovarian cancer in American women, as well as premature puberty in American children. Since steroid hormones cause cattle to grow fat fast, it also stands to reason that they cause obesity in humans who consume the meat and milk of such contaminated animals. This is especially true for growing children, and is confirmed by the fact that whenever big American fast-food chains featuring beef and milk products set up operations in Asian countries, the once-healthy children there soon show all the signs of chronic ill health that plague American children: obesity, acne and pimples, respiratory infections, premature puberty, and behavioural abnormalities.

US cattle also absorb all the herbicides, pesticides, and chemical fertilizers used to grow the feed crops on which they are forced to gorge, and a high percentage of these hapless creatures arrive at the slaughterhouse riddled with cancerous tumours and tuberculosis. All this poison is passed directly on to the consumer, so if you like to eat beef, be sure it has been organically raised without drugs and hormones, and preferably range-fed rather than pen-fed.

For different reasons, pork is also a poor choice in meat. Owing to the pig's omnivorous diet, pork is even more acidifying than other meats. Pork is also very hard on the liver, largely because lard is difficult to digest. Researchers in Canada have established a close link between cirrhosis of the liver and pork consumption in sixteen countries studied. In countries where pork is consumed together with alcohol (beer and sausage, wine and schnitzel, etc.), the likelihood of liver cirrhosis rises by a factor of 1,000.

Commercially raised chickens are also kept confined in cages and fed on denatured feed contaminated with antibiotics, hormones, and pesticides. Chinese physicians have always recommended 'earth chickens' (tu-jee) as the only safe dietary source of chicken and eggs. Called 'free-range chickens' in the West, they run free around the farm, eating wild vegetation, insects, and worms, and getting plenty of fresh air and exercise.

The best choice in domestic meat is lamb. Sheep generally graze on open ranges, out in the sun and fresh air, and they are usually not contaminated with drugs. Lamb is the richest source of carnitine, which is required to deliver fat into cells for metabolism. Lamb has always been the meat of choice in the Middle East, Mediterranean, and Himalayan regions, where arteriosclerosis and heart disease have never been major problems. Even better than lamb is wild game, such as deer, elk, pheasant, and quail, although these products are hard to find these days.

Red meat should always be consumed as rare as possible, and preferably with horseradish or strong mustard, which stimulates the liver and gall bladder to secrete the juices required to break down the proteins and fats. Fresh ginger root aids the digestion of meat.

Eggs

Eating too many eggs can cause a highly acidifying and putrefactive excess of protein, especially when the diet already includes meat and seafood. The traditional Chinese dietary guideline stipulates that one or two eggs per week is sufficient for human nutritional needs. Women with ovarian cysts and other reproductive organ problems should abstain completely from eggs, because eggs are products of the hen's own sexual reproductive system and can therefore aggravate such problems in women.

Today, most commercially sold eggs come from chickens cooped up in small cages under bright lights and fed on dry feed laced with synthetic hormones and antibiotics. Such eggs do more damage than good to the human system and should be avoided. Try to buy free-range eggs, and don't eat them every day. The best way to cook eggs is soft-boiled or lightly poached, with the yolks remaining soft and intact for maximum nutritional value and digestibility. Raw egg yolks, without the whites, are an excellent source of protein such as lecithin, amino acids, and other nutrients.

Seafood

Fish

Deep-water ocean fish such as tuna and salmon are excellent sources of protein as well as fish oils that are rich in essential fatty acids called eicosapentaenoic acid (EPA) and docosaheyaenoic acid (DHA). EPA and DHA rank among nature's most effective blood thinners: they prevent sludging of blood platelets, dissolve clots, and dredge blood vessels of excess cholesterol and fatty deposits, thereby improving circulation and preventing heart attacks. Countries which consume a lot of deep-water fish, such as Japan and Pacific islands, have significantly lower rates of heart disease than non-fish-eating countries.

Like meat, fish is a warming and acidifying yang food. It is most easily digested and yields the most nutrients when eaten raw, such as sashimi in Japan and *poissons crux* in the South Pacific, or when lightly steamed or poached. Owing to the pollution of lakes, rivers, and streams throughout the world, freshwater fish is no longer such a good choice. Shellfish and reef fish should also be avoided because the shallow sea beds they inhabit are polluted.

Seaweed

Sea vegetables such as dulse, Irish moss, kelp, and *nori* are very good sources of iodine, calcium, phosphorus, iron, potassium, sodium, zinc, and manganese, as well as all the B vitamins, including B_{12}. Dried seaweeds such as dulse and *nori* also contain 20–30 per cent pure protein, more than some meats, which makes them valuable staples in vegetarian diets. Unlike fish, seaweeds are cooling, alkalizing yin foods, so they may be used to balance the excess acidification of meals based on meat, fish, or grains. Seaweeds also aid digestion, stimulate metabolism, lower blood cholesterol, and tonify sexual organs.

Another good reason to include sea vegetables in your diet is that they help neutralize and excrete radioactive toxins such as strontium-90 in the body. The sodium alginate they contain binds radioactive substances by a process called chelation; then they are harmlessly excreted through the kidneys.

Grains

The cultivation of cereal grains for food marked the transition from nomadic hunting and gathering to a sedentary lifestyle that permitted the rise of permanent cities and civilizations. Whole grains contain sufficient protein for most sedentary human requirements, plus the complex carbohydrates needed to provide the sort of sustained energy associated with mental rather than physical work. Meat-eating hunting societies have never been renowned for their intellectual prowess. Note, for example, the carnivorous Mongols, who conquered half the world on horseback, only to be seduced and absorbed by the elegant civilization of the grain-eating Chinese.

Due to their protein and carbohydrate content, grains are warming, acidifying yang foods, and like meat they should be balanced with cooling, alkalizing vegetables. Whole grains also contain fats, vitamins, minerals, and fibre, which makes them a truly 'whole' food. Most of the world's population depend on either rice or wheat for the bulk of their calories. But as a result of modern milling methods, which scrape away the nutrient-laden bran and germ and leave only the starchy white pith, most commercial grain foods are nutritionally naked. Only whole grains provide whole nutrition.

Grains can cause indigestion and flatulence if they are not thoroughly chewed and ensalivated in the mouth before swallowing. That's because all carbohydrates must begin their digestive journey in the mouth, where an alkaline enzyme called ptyalin is secreted from salivary glands to initiate the breakdown of starches. Another way to make grains more digestible is to roast them until golden brown before cooking. This process is called dextrinization, and it converts much of the hard-to-digest starch into easily digested simple sugars. For the same reason, it's always a good idea to toast bread well before eating it.

A serious problem with many grains on the market today is long-term storage in huge silos, which permits the growth of moulds that produce aflatoxin, one of the most potent carcinogens in the world. Corn is especially vulnerable to aflatoxin contamination, but so are wheat and other grains. Unless you have access to relatively freshly harvested grains, it's a good idea to take daily antioxidant supplements as a preventive measure against aflatoxin poisoning.

Beans

Beans complement whole grains as plant sources of essential amino acids, which is why they are often served together in meatless meals. Chick peas and millet, lentils and barley, rice and dhal, corn bread and black-eyed peas, rice and kidney beans are common examples of the grain-and-bean protein team. Together they provide the full spectrum of essential amino acids required for human nutrition, usually in a proportion of one part beans to two parts grain.

Except for soya beans, beans are warming, acidifying yang foods, like grains. Though much touted as a 'whole protein' food, soya beans and tofu are not very easy to digest, and they can also interfere with the absorption of zinc. Zinc deficiency is a common problem in vegetarian diets, and using tofu as a meat substitute only aggravates this deficiency. Furthermore, since zinc is vital for proper function of sexual glands, soya-bean products such as tofu can cool sexual energy, which is why tofu is a popular staple in Oriental monasteries, where celibacy is the rule. Unfortunately, when processed into tofu, soya beans lose most of their vitamin, mineral, and fibre content.

Beans may also be sprouted before consumption, in which case they may be eaten raw. Bean sprouts are rich in vitamins, enzymes, and amino acids, and are far easier to digest than whole beans.

Vegetables

Vegetables are the earth's most effective alkalizers, especially when consumed raw in salads or as freshly extracted juices. Cooling and cleansing, they are also high in fibre, which helps sweep post-digestive putrefactive debris from the intestinal tract. Their chlorophyll content protects the body against cancer, neutralizes toxins, and helps keep vital fluids pure. Easy to digest and non-putrefactive, fresh vegetables go well with meats as well as grains and help counteract the acidifying effects of both.

Crucifers

Cruciferous vegetables include broccoli, cauliflower, Brussels sprouts, mustard greens, and cabbage. These vegetables seem to have potent protective properties for mucous membranes, especially in the lungs and digestive tract, and they are therefore effective guardians against cancer, ulcers, and infections in these vital organs. Rich in antioxidant nutrients such as betacarotene, vitamin C, and selenium, crucifers guard your body against all sorts of toxins absorbed from polluted environments. Crucifers have always played important roles in traditional Asian diets, especially in China.

Roots

Root vegetables are rich in minerals and replete with the stabilizing energy of the earth in which they grow. A few roots, such as carrots and turnips, are commonly consumed as ordinary vegetables, but most of them are used as condiments, seasonings, and side dishes. Many, such as ginger, garlic, and burdock, also have potent medicinal properties.

Horseradish, a traditional condiment served with beef in England and with sashimi in Japan (where it's called *wasabi*), stimulates the liver and gall bladder, which are required to process proteins and fats assimilated from animal sources. Ginger has always been noted for its digestive properties in Chinese cuisine, and it is said that Confucius refused to eat a meal without it. Onions help clear congestion and cut through excess mucus in the digestive tract.

The most protective of all root foods is garlic, which has been used for millennia throughout the world for its well-known healing powers as well as its pungent flavour. In recent years, garlic has been shown to possess the following properties: inhibits growth of tumours; increases activity of white blood cells and macrophages; raises antibody production; destroys a wide range of harmful bacteria and viruses; provides a rich dietary source of the rare trace element selenium, which is a potent antioxidant; destroys fungus and yeasts such as candida. Not only is garlic one of nature's most powerful immune-system boosters, it is also prized in the Orient as a potent sexual tonic, which is why it is strictly prohibited in monastic kitchens throughout the Far East. Most practising Taoists include fresh garlic in their daily diets.

Leaves

Leafy greens contain abundant supplies of chlorophyll, one of nature's best cleansers and detoxifiers. Eating plenty of fresh leafy greens helps eliminate unpleasant body odour by neutralizing acidity and protein putrefaction. Fresh coriander is a particularly effective dietary deodorant.

Thanks to chlorophyll, green leaves have the capacity to convert the pure energy of sunlight into vegetable matter ($E = mc^2$ again), and when we consume and metabolize green vegetable matter, this solar energy is released into our own systems. Leafy greens thus serve as transformers and storehouses of revitalizing solar energy.

Nightshades

Among the most popular vegetables in Western diets today are certain members of the Solanaceae family, known 'nightshades', which includes twenty-two genera and over 2,000 species of plants. Among the nightshades are tobacco and many potent medicinal plants, some of them highly poisonous. Common foods from this shady family include potato, tomato, eggplant, and chilli peppers. The distinguishing feature of all nightshades is their rich alkaloid content. Alkaloids are potent plant chemicals, similar in molecular structure to proteins, with powerful physiological effects when consumed and metabolized. Caffeine, morphine, cocaine, nicotine, and belladonna are all alkaloids with well-known psychoactive effects and toxic properties. There is growing evidence that the alkaloids present in nightshade foods may have deleterious effects on human health, at least for some people.

It is interesting to note that, with the sole exception of eggplant, the traditional diet of China did not include nightshades, and that Taoist dietary guidelines have always strongly discouraged the consumption of nightshades, including eggplant. Tomatoes, for example, were brought to China from the New World by Spanish traders during the sixteenth century and were named 'foreign egg-plants' by the Chinese. Potatoes, which the Chinese call 'foreign yams', were also imported from the Western world, as were chilli peppers. Before this, the Chinese used nightshades only for medi-cine, not for food, and even in the West tomatoes and potatoes were once regarded as poisonous.

Today, nightshades such as tomato and potato have become ubiquitous in Western diets, particularly in fast food in the form of French fries and potato crisps, tomato sauce and ketchup. Potatoes and tomatoes are fast-growing, inexpensive and easy to store.

Recent research has implicated nightshades in the calcification of soft body tissues, a condition known as 'calciphylactic syndrome', which has become one of the most prevalent pathological condi-tions in all modern industrial societies. This syndrome, which occurs when nightshades remove calcium from teeth and bones and deposit it in tissues where it does not belong, is associated with arthritis, arteriosclerosis, cerebral sclerosis, kidney stones, gout, migraine, high blood pressure, bronchitis, osteoporosis, lupus, hypertension, and other common maladies. Many people have reported rapid recovery from these ailments when they completely eliminated nightshades from their diets. That includes smoking, because tobacco is also a nightshade, so smoking tobacco only com-pounds the severity of tissue calcification.

If you suffer from any of the above conditions, try abstaining entirely from all nightshades, including tobacco, for a period of six months. This cure works only if you eliminate *all* traces of nightshade alkaloids from your system, including those hidden in processed foods and condiments in the form of potato flour, tomato sauce, paprika, cayenne, tabasco, and so forth.

Fruit

Fruits are also alkalizing and cooling, except for certain tropical fruits such as mango and lichee, which are warming. Fruits are very easy to digest and metabolize, but only when eaten on an empty stomach. In fact, most fruits go straight through the stomach into the duodenum for digestion, which means if you put fresh fruit on top of a big meal, it has to sit and wait in the top of the stomach until the other food is digested, during which delay bacteria attack the fruit and ferment it, gobbling up all the nutrients and leaving you with gas and metabolic wastes. The best rule to follow with fruits is: 'Eat them alone, or leave them alone.' This is particularly true for melons and citrus fruits.

Fresh fruits are even more cleansing to the digestive tract than vegetables. A good way to detoxify and balance the pH of the entire alimentary canal is to eat nothing but fresh fruit for a period of one to seven days. It is best to select just one variety of fruit for cleansing purposes, top choices being grapefruit, lemon (as juice, diluted with water), watermelon, apple, or black grapes. You may eat the fruit whole or as a juice, the latter being somewhat more effective for cleansing purposes.

Nuts and seeds

Nuts and seeds are rich sources of amino acids and essential fatty acids, but you must eat them raw and as freshly harvested as possible to gain the full spectrum of their nutritional benefits. In the dry state, nuts and seeds can be quite difficult to digest due to their enzyme inhibitors, which enable them to be stored for a long time without going rancid. The best way to eat them is to cover them with water and let them soak overnight in the refrigerator. This inactivates their enzyme inhibitors, softens their fibres for easier digestion, and renders their nutrients easier to assimilate. Vegetarians can easily get all the essential amino and fatty acids which meat eaters get from animal protein simply by eating a handful or two of raw nuts and seeds every day. The best nuts for nutrition are almonds and pecans, and the best seeds are sunflower, pumpkin, and flax.

Fermented foods

Fermentation is at least as old a method of food preparation as cooking with heat. Yeast and other 'friendly' bacteria are added to raw ingredients and set aside to ferment, during which process the microbes break down complex carbohydrates and proteins into more easily digestible elements. Fermentation increases the vitamin and enzyme content of foods, aids digestion, and facilitates assimilation of nutrients. Fermented foods also colonize the intestinal tract with friendly flora, which control putrefactive bacteria, maintain proper pH balance in the colon, and increase the bulk and frequency of bowel movements. However, people with chronic yeast infections such as candida and those who are sensitive to salt should abstain from fermented foods.

Almost all culinary traditions include some form of fermented, food in the diet. Western cultures make yogurt, kumiss, and *kefir* (a yogurt-type drink) from milk, beer from barley and hops, and wine from grapes. In the East, Koreans eat fermented cabbage (*kimchee*) three times a day, China has its various fermented soya-bean products such as tofu and soya sauce, the Japanese make soups and sauces with fermented miso paste, Thai cuisine is laced with a pungent fermented fish sauce called *nam-pla*, and Indians drink a delicious beverage called *lassy* made with yogurt that is freshly fermented every day.

It is a good idea to include a moderate amount of fermented food in meals that are rich in animal protein and fat, in order to aid digestion. That's one reason why wine and beer are such popular accompaniments to the meat-heavy meals of classical Western cuisines. Even the Bible advises one to 'take a little wine for the stomach's sake'.

Processed food

If you wish to remain healthy and avoid ailments of the digestive organs, particularly cancer, you'd be well advised to eliminate all processed food completely from your diet. In the age of fast food, precooked frozen dinners, packaged snacks, and other 'convenience food', abstaining from processed food may seem difficult, but in fact it's not. It is just as quick to eat an apple as it is a package of potato crisps, just as convenient to have nuts and seeds and dried fruit for breakfast as packaged cereal with cow's milk, and just as easy to make an avocado sandwich as a hamburger. It's all a matter of habit.

Today, over 6,000 synthetic chemicals are officially condoned for use in the processed-food industry, including some that are known to have carcinogenic properties. Furthermore, processed foods also contain high levels of the debilitating, denatured ingredients we wish to avoid, such as white sugar, refined starch, pasteurized cow's milk, land-mined salt, and hydrogenated vegetable oils.

The human immune system correctly recognizes chemical food additives as toxic foreign agents and fights hard to rid the body of them, causing severe biochemical reactions and putting great stress on the immune system. After years of daily exposure to such inorganic chemicals, the immune system finally breaks down and burns out, leaving the body vulnerable to attack by microbes, toxins, and cancerous cells. Although the food industry has duped the public as well as government health agencies into believing that their products are safe for human consumption, there is abundant scientific evidence to the contrary, and this information is in the public domain, openly available to anyone who seeks it. Ignorance is therefore no longer a valid excuse for poisoning yourself with industrially adulterated foods. Only you control what goes into your mouth and down to your stomach.

Salt

Salt is absolutely essential to human health and nutritional balance. Salt alkalizes blood and other vital fluids, helps retain water, and is deeply involved in the biochemistry of metabolism. It's not salt per se that's so bad for human health, but rather the industrially refined, land-mined, mineral-deficient table salt sold on the market and hidden in packaged and processed foods. One to three grams of salt per day is a good measure for human nutritional requirements, but most Americans today consume 12–15 grams of salt daily.

In refining commercial table salt, manufacturers remove virtually all the minerals and trace elements, leaving a white crystal that is 98 per cent sodium chloride. Among the nutrients removed is magnesium, which is essential for proper immune function. Magnesium supports a process called phagocytosis, which enhances the assimilative power of scavenger cells that are responsible for controlling infectious bacteria and other unwanted microbes. Magnesium is also essential for proper function of nerve and brain cells, is involved in the metabolism of sugars and fats, and has been shown to lower mortality dramatically in heart-attack patients. A study in Canada showed a 66 per cent drop in the death rate of heart-attack patients who were given intravenous injections of magnesium, and Dr Cass Igram reports that magnesium injections resulted in a 90 per cent reduction in heart-attack mortality in a similar study in the USA.

Magnesium is essential to the internal alchemy of acid-alkaline balance in cellular fluids. Dr Jacques de Langre, director of the Grain and Salt Society, writes as follows about the importance of magnesium in maintaining proper body pH, in the 1992, Volume XVI, number 1 issue of the *Price-Pottenger Nutrition Foundation Journal*:

> The human organism functions at its peak only when the balance between acid and alkaline is maintained. All substances that nourish the body are either acid or alkaline. Magnesium possesses the remarkable ability to maintain the acid/alkaline balance within the organism. It also intervenes in the oxido-reduction mechanism. We know, for instance, that the human body is oxidized by the action of oxygen and becomes alkaline. Oppositely, an organism, under the action of hydrogen, is in reduction and becomes acid. This back and forth fluctuation passing from acid to alkaline and back again from basic to acid is a chemical phenomenon absolutely needed for keeping the body alive. This is where magnesium shines brightly.

Owing to modern farming and food-processing methods, magnesium is deficient in almost all foods today, including fresh vegetables and whole grains. Dr Igram reports that 76 per cent of all Americans are deficient in this vital mineral. The only viable dietary source of magnesium these days is whole, unrefined sea salt, especially the coarse grey variety harvested by hand along the Brittany coast of France, known as 'Celtic sea salt', which may be ordered from the Salt and Grain Society (see Appendix). The Epsom salts some people take as a magnesium supplement contains magnesium sulphate, which is rapidly excreted through the kidneys and therefore difficult to assimilate. Whole sea salt contains magnesium chloride and magnesium bromide, which are easily assimilated and metabolized in the human body.

The big ballyhoo in Western media and medical circles about avoiding salt to cut down on sodium and thus control high blood pressure is all based on the detrimental effects of industrially refined, land-mined table salt, which is 98 per cent sodium chloride. The health problems caused by this kind of salt is another typical example of how the processed-food industry has cornered the market on a vital food element, then refined and denatured it for 'convenience' (i.e. higher profits), duping the public into daily consumption of a product that undermines rather than supports health.

By contrast, Celtic sea salt contains only 82 per cent sodium chloride. Furthermore, the magnesium salts it contains naturally drain excess sodium from the body, thereby preventing the oedema, kidney malfunction, high blood pressure, and other ailments associated with excess sodium intake. Unrefined sea salt is the best, and sometimes the only, dietary source of bioavailable magnesium, an essential element that boosts immunity, prevents fatal heart attacks, and effectively maintains optimum yin-yang pH balance in vital bodily fluids.

Water

It does little good to spend a lot of time and money purchasing and preparing wholesome health foods if you continue drinking and cooking with contaminated water. All public-utility water these days is severely contaminated with toxic metals and other pollutants, as well as toxic chemicals deliberately added to 'purify' water. One reason that Taoist adepts used to retire to high mountains to cultivate advanced practices was the purity of the spring water available at high altitudes. Some adepts lived for months at a time on nothing but pure air and pure water ('sniffing air and sipping dew'), thereby purging their systems of toxins accumulated during the early years of their lives and purifying the primary ingredient in the human body's vital essence – water.

Tap water can contain any of over 1,000 toxic contaminants, including lead, aluminium, mercury, cadmium, asbestos, benzene, polychlorinated biphenyl, nitrates, pesticides, and radon. It also contains chlorine and fluoride, poisons supposedly added to 'kill germs'. If you drink such water long enough, it may kill you too.

Chlorine accumulates in your system and can cause, among other problems, heart and circulatory diseases. Chlorinated water also kills all the friendly intestinal flora in your digestive tract, such as acidophilus and bifidus. Fluoride is even worse. At a press conference held on 20 March 1990 in Washington, DC, Dr John Yiamouyiannis called for an immediate ban on the fluoridation of public drinking water, based on extensive studies of fluoride's damaging effects on human health. First of all, after examining the dental records of over 40,000 children in eighty-four different regions around the USA, his research concluded that fluoridation has had no significant impact on preventing tooth decay, and other studies have confirmed this finding. Worse yet, fluoride is closely associated with a significant rise in cancer in areas where it has been added to drinking water. Dr Yiamouyiannis reported:

> In 1988, researchers from Argonne National Laboratories, under contract by the United States Public Health Service, found that fluoride not only induces but promotes cancer. In a separate study, these Argonne researchers also confirmed the findings of scientists from the Nippon Dental University in Japan showing that the exposure of normal cells to fluoride transforms them into cancer cells.

Over fifty similar studies conducted on fluoridated water since 1952 have come to the same conclusion, and yet the practice continues throughout the world, because poisoning public drinking water with fluoride is more convenient and cheaper than properly purifying it for human consumption. When Philadelphia fluoridated its city water supply, the once famously healthy animals in the city's zoological gardens began to die off in great numbers from coronary diseases, which happens to be the greatest killer of humans in America. Even the US Food and Drug Administration has repeatedly warned that fluorine intake in excess of 2 mg per day can be toxic to humans, but you can easily ingest as much as 5 mg daily through the combination of drinking tap water, cooking with tap water, and eating processed foods and beverages manufactured with fluoridated tap water. Foods grown with phosphate fertilizers, such as most commercial produce, also contain lots of fluorides. It only requires three pints of fluoridated water per day to push your entire system into the toxic zone.

There's enough incriminating evidence against the safety of tap water to fill an entire book, but the gist is that long-term ingestion of such contaminated water is extremely hazardous to human health and should be strictly avoided. Drinking bottled water is not necessarily the answer, because studies have shown that many bottled waters are so carelessly produced that they often contain more bacteria and other contaminants than untreated tap water. Distilled water can be expensive, and in some people it causes a leaching of minerals from tissues. Your best bet is to filter your drinking and cooking water through activated carbon, one pound of which has the filtration capacity of 112 acres of surface topsoil. Be sure to purchase a good unit with the highest-quality activated-carbon filter and to change the carbon element regularly, depending on how much you use it. There are many such systems available today, including compact portable units for travelling.

CHAPTER 10

Essence: Diets and Supplements

What one eats, digests, and assimilates provides the energy-producing nutrients that the bloodstream carries to the brain . . . What you eat determines your state of mind and who you are.

Dr George Watson, *Nutrition and Your Mind* (1972)

Essential dietary guidelines

There are dozens of different diets being touted in health circles today – some of them useful, others downright dangerous – but the best guidelines of all are always your own knowledge and experience, based on study and personal practice. In formulating their personal diets, Taoists follow the principle of being firm in their goals (health and longevity) but flexible in their methods (diet and nutrition), frequently adjusting dietary and nutritional balance according to fluctuations in health, lifestyle, environmental conditions, seasonal cycles, residential locations, and so forth. Rather than trying strictly to follow arbitrary rules that stipulate which foods may or may not be eaten, as most fad diets require, the Taoist way is to follow firm principles of diet and nutrition and apply them flexibly from day to day, according to changing circumstances.

The general guidelines given below regarding various common diets should be combined with the information on food presented above as well as in *The Tao of HS&L*, in order to formulate your own personal dietary programme. By sticking to a few basic dietary principles rather than long lists of permitted and prohibited foods, you will be able to exercise culinary creativity in composing meals that satisfy your health requirements as well as your palate. As long as you follow a basically well-balanced programme, you need not worry about an occasional splurge or binge, especially if you practise periodic intestinal cleansing, such as fasting and colonic irrigation.

Standard American diet (SAD)

The standard fare served in coffee shops, diners, fast-food outlets, and most homes in America today constitutes a severe frontal assault on human health and defies almost all the principles of sound nutrition. If you wish to live a long and healthy life and guard your Three Treasures from disease and degeneration, you should avoid the SAD like a plague.

The SAD rejects the ancient premise that 'food is medicine' and denies that what you eat and how you eat it have direct effects on your health and vitality, physical as well as mental. It forbids nothing, ignores the scientific laws of food combining and food pharmacodynamics, and subordinates all health considerations to cost and convenience. It consists primarily of meat (especially hamburgers, hot dogs, bacon, ham, and cold cuts processed with toxic preservatives), pasteurized cow's milk products, refined white starch and sugar, artificial foods (such as margarine, synthetic sweeteners, non-dairy toppings and creamers), and all sorts of chemically preserved, industrially processed, canned, frozen, freeze-dried, sterilized, and cleverly wrapped junk foods.

According to a recent report prepared by the US Senate's Select Committee on Nutrition and Human Needs, average Americans obtain 42 per cent of their calories from fats (both animal and the carcinogenic hydrogenated-oil varieties), 12 per cent from proteins (mostly meat and milk), and 46 per cent from carbohydrates (of which more than half, or 24 per cent of the total diet, comes from sugar). In other words, 66 per cent of the calories in the SAD come from fats and sugars. Dr Cass Igram estimates that among those who follow the SAD, 100 per cent are deficient in chromium, manganese, and essential fatty acids, 79 per cent in folic acid, 76 per cent in magnesium, 75 per cent in selenium, and 65 per cent in calcium. Despite the glut of calories in the SAD, Americans rank among the most malnourished people in the world.

Besides the obvious degenerative diseases which such a deficient and imbalanced diet can cause, the SAD has also been linked to violent behaviour, learning disorders, aggression, and alienation, especially in children raised from infancy on this diet. Americans who wonder why their country suffers such a high and continuously growing incidence of heart disease, obesity, cancer, and AIDS, plus one of the highest murder and crime rates in the world, need look no further than their local supermarket shelves, fast-food outlets, and school lunch programmes for some of the most basic reasons.

Vegetarian diet

This is one of the oldest dietary systems in the world, both East and West. Plato and Pythagoras were strict vegetarians, and throughout the ages many Hindus and Buddhists have followed strict vegetarian diets. Properly practised, vegetarian diets can be very healthy, but they are not appropriate for all people in all circumstances.

Truly strict vegetarian diets that eliminate eggs and dairy products as well as all meat are called 'vegan'. Those that permit dairy products are called 'lacto-vegetarian', and those that also permit eggs are known as 'ovo-lacto-vegetarian'. Considering the ill effects of most of the pasteurized cow's-milk products and commercial chicken eggs on the market, the pure vegan diet is probably the best choice in vegetarianism.

However, those who follow this dietary system must be careful to avoid some common pitfalls. There is often a tendency to binge on sugar and starch to compensate for the absence of animal fat and protein. This can cause rapid weight gain, metabolic malfunctions, skin problems, and severe fluctuations in mood and energy. It is therefore important to ensure adequate intake of protein and essential fatty acids by consuming sufficient quantities of whole grains, beans, sprouts, nuts, seeds, and seaweeds, and to avoid refined sugar and starch.

Some people who follow vegetarian diets experience a critical deficiency of vitamin B_{12}, the richest dietary sources of which are meat, liver, and fish. However, if you eat plenty of whole grains, especially oats, as well as seaweeds, you should have no trouble getting sufficient supplies of B_{12} on a vegetarian diet, but *only* if you strictly limit your intake of sugar, which tends to rob your system of all B vitamins. Another good vegetarian source of B_{12} is fermented foods, such as *tempeh* (fermented soya bean), miso, sauerkraut, *kimchee*, and natural unpasteurized beer.

Climate is another important consideration. Most vegetarian diets originated in tropical and semitropical climates, where people don't require so many calories just to keep their bodies warm. In cold northern climates, however, people generally require some form of animal fat, such as butter, meat, or fish, in order to provide sufficient long-burning calories for warmth. Remember that gram for gram animal fat contains more than twice the potential energy of any carbohydrate, and that the heart, which has to work harder in winter, prefers fat over all other forms of dietary fuel.

Other factors include stress and sexual activity. If you are subject to chronic stress, you may need the more concentrated nutrients and energy contained in meat, fish, and fowl in order to compensate for the constant drain in energy reserves. And if you wish to maintain a sexually active lifestyle, which requires abundant supplies of 'sexual essence' (sexual secretions are composed largely of proteins and minerals), you may find that a purely vegetarian diet leaves you lagging and listless in bed, especially if your partner has the sexual appetite of a meat eater. One of the main reasons that Buddhist and Hindu monasteries in the East serve strictly vegetarian fare is to eliminate the sexually stimulating elements contained in animal foods from the diets of celibate monks and nuns, so that they may focus their energy and attention on spiritual practices.

Hospital diets

The food served to patients in most hospitals of Western medicine not only fails to contribute to their recovery but often creates new problems as well, especially in post-surgery and heart-attack patients. Items commonly found on hospital meal trays include spaghetti and meatballs, roast pork, fried chicken, scrambled eggs, canned and frozen vegetables, white bread, pasteurized cow's milk, pudding, cake, pie, and ice cream. Anyone who is sick enough to be hospitalized has no business eating this sort of food, which is not even good for healthy people. For one thing, hospital patients simply do not need all those calories. Secondly, digesting such heavy meals requires an enormous output of energy, especially enzyme energy, diverting vital essence and energy resources which the patient's body should be using for healing purposes. Third, such meals do not provide the nutrients which patients need to recover strength and rebuild tissues.

If you find yourself confined to a hospital for surgery or any other reason, insist on having your food brought in by a friend or relative who is knowledgable in the science of nutritional therapy, and send those hospital trays back to the kitchen. Select foods that are specifically beneficial to your condition, especially fresh fruit and vegetables, whole grains and bean sprouts, fresh fish and seaweeds, as well as plenty of vitamin and mineral supplements, and completely avoid anything canned, processed, preserved, and unnecessarily complicated in composition and cooking. If the hospital refuses to cooperate, go on a hunger strike. Fasting is an ancient cure for virtually all ills and will do you a lot more good than typical hospital food.

Raw food versus cooked food

Though some foods are most nutritionally potent when consumed raw, others require some form of cooking in order to render them digestible and/or easier to assimilate. You cannot digest raw rice or wheat, and even some vegetables which can be eaten raw, such as broccoli and cauliflower, become more digestible and nutritious when lightly steamed, poached, or sauteed.

Of all food groups, meat is the one that is most nutritionally depleted by cooking. Prolonged exposure to intense heat alters the protein molecules in meat, destroying much of its nutritional value. Overcooking meat (i.e. 'well done') completely destroys the natural proteolytic (protein-digesting) enzymes it contains, making it much more difficult to digest than raw or rare meat.

Meat eaters would therefore be well advised to eat their beef, lamb, and wild game as rare as possible, preferably bloody. Pork, which cannot safely be eaten bloody rare, should be avoided anyway, for reasons already explained. Raw deep-water fish, such as Japanese sashimi, is even more nutritious and easier to digest than rare meat.

As a general guideline, it's a good idea to consume about 40–50 per cent of your daily diet in the form of raw food. For one thing, following this guideline will induce you to include more fresh fruits and vegetables in your diet than you might otherwise be inclined to do. Raw fruits and vegetables are cooling, cleansing, and alkalizing to the system. Remember, though, that raw fruits are most nutritious, digestible, and cleansing when consumed alone on an empty stomach, either as a snack, a full meal, or a full day's fare. Raw vegetables, on the other hand, make great dietary adjuncts to meals based on either meats or grains, for they counteract the acidifying effects of such meals and provide abundant fresh fibre to help sweep digestive debris through the alimentary canal.

As for cooking methods, the best techniques for easy digestion and top nutrition are steaming, poaching, and stir-frying. All these methods are relatively quick, retain nutrients and moisture, and avoid scorching. Baking tends to dry food out and destroy all enzymes and most vitamins. It is best to avoid charcoal-grilled and smoked foods, because these methods of cooking produce polycyclic aromatic hydrocarbons, which are chemical carcinogens so powerful that they are commonly used to induce cancerous tumours in experimental laboratory animals. Scientists estimate that the hydrocarbons consumed in 50–100 charcoal-grilled hamburgers suffice to cause cancer in humans. Since these toxins are stored in the body and not easily excreted, the danger of consuming such foods grows greater over time.

Microwave ovens have become ubiquitous appliances in North American and many Western European kitchens, both at home and in restaurants, and their use is on the rise. Significantly, Russian safety standards for human exposure to microwaves are about one thousand times more stringent than American ones. The Russians should know: for years they used to beam microwaves at the American embassy in Moscow, resulting in several cases of cancer and numerous other debilitating health problems. Yet in the USA, microwave ovens are advertised as being perfectly safe.

Microwaves are very close to X-rays on the electromagnetic spectrum, and many studies, ignored by government health agencies, have indicated the serious health hazards of exposure to microwaves. Microwaves 'cook' food by alternating the magnetic polarity of its atoms thousands of times per second, causing changes in the molecular structure and producing heat by atomic friction, thereby giving food the appearance, texture, and taste of having been cooked. This artificial alteration of the electromagnetic polarity ruptures cell walls in food, releasing tremendous quantities of highly reactive free radicals, which are then consumed along with the food. So, not only does microwave cooking destroy the enzymes, nutrients, and energy potential of food, it also impregnates the food with free radicals, which are known to be carcinogenic, immunosuppressive, and major causes of aging and degeneration.

Food can also be prepared without heating, for example by fermentation and marination. In fermentation, friendly bacteria, such as certain yeasts and lactobacteria, perform the task of breaking down complex proteins and carbohydrates, in effect predigesting the food for human consumption. This process also produces many beneficial enzymes, vitamins, and other nutritional elements. Fermented foods promote and sustain the growth of friendly intestinal flora and help maintain proper pH balance in the digestive tract. They go especially well with meals that are rich in protein, fat, or starch, which their enzymes help digest. But if you have candida or any other chronic yeast infection, it's best to abstain from fermented foods until it has cleared up.

Meat and fish can be prepared by marinating them overnight in the refrigerator in strong vinegar or fresh lemon juice. This retains all constituent nutrients and makes meat and fish easy to digest as well.

Changing your diet: what to expect

Change and timely adaptation are the very essence of the Taoist way of life. Stubbornly clinging to outmoded and inappropriate habits is the first step on the path to stagnation and an early grave. This is especially true of dietary habits, because the food you eat must provide the building blocks from which your physical body is composed and also determines the quality and balance of energies your body derives from the nutritional essence in food. Reforming your eating habits is the first and foremost requirement for culti-vating the Taoist way of life in the modern world. Bear in mind, however, that dietary changes must always be made in a timely and flexible manner that accounts for the unique requirements of your individual lifestyle and metabolism, based on personal trial and error. Here are some hints on what to expect when you start to discipline your diet.

Quantity

First of all, the amount of food you ingest should not exceed the amount you require for your energy expenditure. The nutritional essence extracted from food produces energy, but the body con-verts only as much food into energy as it needs. The rest is stored as fat, calcium deposits, plaque, phlegm, impacted faeces, cysts, and other undesirable accumulations. An athlete or a construction worker requires a lot more protein and fat than a clerk or computer operator, while the latter need more complex carbohydrates than the former. You also need more warming fat and protein in winter and more cooling fruits and vegetables in summer. Just because everything is always available year round at your local super-market does not mean that you have to eat the same things throughout the year. Try to gauge the quantity and balance of the food you eat according to your energy requirements and environmental factors.

Detoxification

Switching abruptly over to a healthy diet usually triggers a detoxi-fication response called 'healing crisis'. You may experience frequent colds, flu, diarrhoea, profuse sweating, dark urine, skin eruptions, headaches, and other unpleasant symptoms, all of which are caused by the body's rapid elimination of toxic debris accumulated in organs and tissues by past eating habits. This is a natural, automatic cleansing response, but it only happens when the offending foods are totally eliminated from the diet. It is especially noticeable when you eliminate meat, milk, sugar, or drugs. The symptoms may last for a few days or a few weeks, depending on how toxic you are, but as soon as the toxic residues are thoroughly flushed out of your system, the symptoms will disappear.

For the brave and well-disciplined adept, three- to seven-day detoxification fasts are by far the most effective way to purge the system of toxins caused by past culinary crimes, in preparation for embarking on new dietary regimens. Fasting, especially in conjunction with colonic irrigation, triggers a powerful purging response throughout the entire body and all its tissues, usually with unpleasant but harmless side effects called 'cleansing reactions'. When it's over, your body is thoroughly cleansed and rejuvenated, and this is definitely the best condition in which to start a new dietary programme. One of the problems with intestinal tracts clogged and impacted with the detritus of many years of bad eating habits is severe impairment of the intestines' capacity to assimilate nutrients, regardless of how wholesome the food is. An intestinal tract swept clean of old impacted faeces and dried mucus will digest food far more efficiently and absorb nutrients much more completely than before, thereby enabling you to derive maximum benefits from improved eating habits. For those who cannot muster the self-discipline required for fasting, semi-fasts using fresh juices and cleansing supplements are also quite effective. Many of these methods are discussed in detail in the chapter on 'Fasting and Excretion' in *The Tao of HS&L*.

Withdrawal
When you quit using dangerous food substances such as sugar, starch, and pasteurized cow's milk, you are likely to experience withdrawal symptoms similar to those which occur when one abruptly gives up such drugs as alcohol, tobacco, and heroin. These symptoms of 'cold turkey' include headache, fatigue, irritability, insomnia, nervous tension, aching joints, sweating and chills, and intense craving for the substance withdrawn from the system. Taking only a small nibble of the offending substance -- the proverbial 'hair of the dog' – usually suffices to eliminate the withdrawal symptoms instantly, but then you have to start all over again.

Withdrawal symptoms are caused by the residues of toxic substances circulating in the bloodstream while the immune and excretory systems go to work flushing them out of tissues and cellular fluids for elimination via kidneys, lungs, colon, and skin. These symptoms occur because the body detoxifies its tissues faster than the excretory organs can eliminate them, resulting in a backlog of toxic residues floating around in the bloodstream. As soon as the last traces of the substance are eliminated, the symptoms cease, so it is important to persist in your cleansing programme until you are clean. After that, when your system is no longer biochemically addicted to the substance, an occasional nip now and then will not cause any problems.

Since fruits are more aggressively cleansing than vegetables, one way to decelerate the rate of detoxification and thereby lessen the severity of cleansing reactions is to add more vegetables and less fruit to your diet, especially during the first few months. Particularly good in this respect are carrot juice, cabbage, iceberg lettuce, and fresh sprouts. It also helps to take one to three daily doses of psyllium-husk powder (*Plantago ovato blond*) to push faeces and putrefactive debris through the colon. Chlorophyll powder or tablets is another good supplement to take when cleansing the system of past dietary follies.

Cravings and binges
One of the most common symptoms of withdrawal from substance abuse is an intense craving for the substance or something similar to it. These cravings can lead to binges. Cravings arise from two mechanisms: first, they are triggered by the familiar residues of the once-favourite substance as they circulate through the brain waiting for excretion during the cleansing process; second, they are provoked by sudden shifts in the yin-yang (alkaline-acid) balance of bodily fluids. For example, if you eliminate meat (an acidifying yang food) and adopt an alkalizing yin vegetarian diet, your body will shift over from its accustomed acidic state to an unfamiliar but far healthier alkaline condition. This might trigger a compensating craving for acidifying foods, but since you've given up meat, you might start binging on sugar instead, because sugar is highly and rapidly acidifying. In this case, the solution is to adjust yin-yang balance by eating plenty of whole grains and beans, which are acidifying, as a substitute for the meat, rather than turning to unwholesome sugar for dietary comfort. By familiarizing yourself with the pharmacodynamic alchemy of various types of foods, you can easily learn how to control your cravings and convert them into healthy habits, rather than binging on foods you wish to avoid.

Supplements

Debate continues to rage about the need for various forms of dietary supplements, especially nutritional supplements such as vitamins and minerals. For decades, conservative Western doctors have been ridiculing 'health nuts' for advocating the use of megadose vitamin and mineral supplements, insisting instead that people can easily obtain all the vital nutrients their bodies require from dietary sources. This deprives patients of quick and easy remedies for many common ailments. Nutritional supplements can prevent many common degenerative conditions from developing, are not expensive and do not require constant visits to the doctor's office.

Supplementing the human diet with food extracts, enzymes, and herbs is as old as the hills in the West as well as the East, and it has always been a primary method in traditional Taoist health programme. Today, dietary supplements are more important than ever in personal programmes of preventive health care. Below we'll discuss four important forms of supplements which can easily be incorporated into any healthy diet: nutrients, lactobacteria, food enzymes, and herbs.

Nutrients

In the cover story of the 6 April 1992 issue of *Time* magazine, recent research on 'The Real Power of Vitamins' revealed that daily supplementation of about a dozen essential vitamins and minerals has been shown to reduce significantly the incidence of heart disease, cancer, birth defects, and damage from environmental pollution. Despite the evidence in support of nutritional supplements, Dr Victor Herbert of New York City's Mount Sinai medical school was quoted as saying that taking vitamins 'doesn't do you any good. We get all the vitamins we need in our diets. Taking supplements just gives you expensive urine.' This is the sort of ill-informed nutritional advice most Western physicians still dispense along with their expensive and often debilitating pharmaceutical prescriptions.

There are three good reasons why everyone in the world who lives a mainstream modern lifestyle should take nutritional supplements in order to guard the Three Treasures against disease and degeneration.

1) Few people in the Western and much of the Eastern world today eat sufficient quantities of fresh vegetables and fruit to obtain the amounts of essential nutrients their bodies require. According to

the National Center for Health Statistics, a mere 9 per cent of adult Americans consume enough fresh produce to get the required daily doses of vitamins and minerals. Asians tend to eat more vitamin-rich fresh fruit and vegetables than most Westerners, but the invasion of Western fast-food chains and artificial food-processing methods into Asian countries is rapidly negating that former advantage. Furthermore, many people in modern societies simply do not have sufficient access to fresh produce, nor enough time to purchase and prepare them daily.

2) Even health-food fanatics who eat abundant amounts of fresh fruit and vegetables rarely get sufficient levels of many essential vitamins and minerals from their diets. That's because modern farming and marketing methods rob many crops of much of their nutritional value. Dr Michael Colgon of the Rockefeller Institute performed studies which showed that many of the oranges sold in American supermarkets today contain absolutely no vitamin C whatsoever, owing to the commercial practice of picking fruit long before it is mature for shipment to distant markets.

Another example of a vital nutrient missing in the food chain today is selenium, a trace element required by the body to synthesize the potent protective antioxidant enzyme glutathione peroxidase, which protects cells from cancer, toxic chemicals, heavy metals, radiation, and other free-radical damage. Selenium has been leached from the soil by chemical fertilizers and pesticides in about two-thirds of the arable land around the world, so that food grown in such soil is devoid of selenium. One of the most selenium-deficient regions in the world is the US Great Lakes area (including Wisconsin, Illinois, Indiana, Michigan, and Ohio), and these states also have one of the highest per capita cancer rates in the world.

Another practice which destroys nutrients is irradiation with gamma rays, a technique which extends the shelf life of fresh food but robs it of its nutritional value and shortens your life. Like so many other modern food-processing methods, it increases profits for purveyors at the expense of public health.

3) Highly reactive DNA-destroying, cell-killing, cancer-causing free radicals are present in our environments. Free-radical damage is caused by all sorts of environmental toxins, including pesticides, synthetic fertilizers, chemical food additives, heavy metals and toxic chemicals in water, air pollution, X-rays and other radiation, hydrogenated vegetable oils, artificial hormones in meat and poultry, chronic stress, and normal metabolic reactions.

The problem of free radicals and the protective powers of

antioxidants will be discussed in the chapter on 'The New Alchemy'. Suffice it to say here that certain vitamins and minerals, such as betacarotene, vitamins C, E, B_1, B_5, B_6, and the minerals selenium and zinc, have been conclusively proven to exert powerful antioxidant effects on free radicals in the human body, neutralizing free radicals before they can do any damage. Known as 'free-radical scavengers', antioxidant nutrients are quickly used up by the body's defence system in the presence of free radicals and must therefore be replenished daily. Even if you eat a well-balanced diet rich in fruit and vegetables, the fact that your body is constantly exposed to free radicals means that you are using up most of your essential vitamins and minerals as antioxidants, leaving insufficient levels for nutritional purposes.

The current RDA (recommended daily amount) levels for various vitamins and minerals set by the US Food and Drug Administration, which most of the world inexplicably follows, such as 60 mg of vitamin C, are absurd and useless guidelines that were established during World War II, when many foods were rationed. These figures indicate the minimum daily dosage required to prevent severe deficiency diseases such as scurvy and rickets, but they are not nearly enough to maintain optimum health and vitality, sustain immunity, and fight free radicals.

Take, for example, vitamin C, a potent antioxidant which boosts immunity, inhibits growth of cancerous tumours, prevents cataracts, and guards against heart attacks. Owing to the lack of a crucial enzyme in the liver, humans are one of only about half a dozen species on earth who cannot produce their own supplies of vitamin C from glucose and must therefore rely on external dietary sources for it. The FDA informs us that we require only 60 mg per day of this essential nutrient, but a 150-pound goat produces 13 grams (13,000 mg) of vitamin C *per day* for its normal nutritional requirements, and a lot more than that when distressed or diseased. Humans are subject to far more disease, distress, and free-radical damage than goats.

There are many good brands of vitamin and mineral supplements on the market today, as well as many well-informed books on how to use them. At the very least, you should be taking the following supplemental nutrients and dosages daily:

vitamin C	3–6 grams (in three doses)
vitamin E	800–1200 IU (international units)
vitamin B complex	50–100 mg
betacarotene	25,000–50,000 IU
selenium	250 mcg
zinc	50 mg

Lactobacteria

Lactobacteria such as acidophilus and bifidus are known as 'friendly' bacteria and inhabit the intestinal tract, especially the colon. They are extremely important for proper digestion and excretion and are responsible for maintaining proper pH balance in the colon. Lactobacteria increase the frequency, bulk, and ease of bowel movements, control flatulence, and reduce the putrefactive odour of faeces. They also suppress the growth of unfriendly putre-factive bacteria and keep infectious yeasts such as candida under control.

Lactobacteria are destroyed by chlorinated water, antibiotics, and diets high in animal protein, which support the putrefactive bacteria with which lactobacteria must compete for dominance in the gut. Since most people drink and cook with chlorinated water, take antibiotics, and eat a lot of animal proteins, their digestive tracts contain an average ratio of about 20 per cent lactobacteria to 80 per cent putrefactive bacteria. The correct ratio for optimum health is 80 per cent lacto to 20 per cent putrefactive.

People who eat a lot of yogurt think that they are getting plenty of lactobacteria into their systems, but that is not true, unless they make yogurt at home every day and consume it within twenty-four hours. After twenty-four hours, the lactobacteria in even the best yogurts begin to decline rapidly, leaving lactic acid, which is a waste product of lactobacteria metabolism. So yogurt is not a very viable dietary source of this important supplement. The same goes for freeze-dried acidophilus capsules: by the time they reach the consumer, most of the active bacteria are dead. However, yogurt is not the only or even the best source of friendly lactobacteria. The easiest and richest source of supplemental lactobacteria is cabbage. Cabbage feeds and promotes the growth of whatever friendly lactobacteria are already present in the digestive tract. It also sup-presses growth of putrefactive bacteria, controls gas, and reduces bowel odour. For therapeutic purposes, you must drink about half a cup of freshly fermented cabbage juice three times daily and also make cabbage a regular part of your bulk diet. Cabbage juice is also very good for healing stomach ulcers. Note that cabbage has always been a staple in the traditional diets of China, Japan, Korea, Thailand, and other Asian cultures, which are known for the digestibility and health-promoting properties of their traditional cuisines.

Another food that strongly promotes lactobacterial growth is Jerusalem artichokes (called 'sun chokes' in part of the USA). They contain a carbohydrate called inulin, which is neither digested nor absorbed by humans and therefore reaches the lower bowels intact. Lactobacteria love inulin, and they thrive on it; even moderate amounts of inulin can support abundant colonies of lactobacteria in the colon. Heavy-fibre foods such as bran, psyllium husk, carrots, and sprouts also help support lactobacteria by sweeping the colon clean of their enemies, the putrefactive bacteria.

One of the best supplemental sources for replenishing lactobacteria in the human digestive tract is Robert Gray's easy-to-prepare Cabbage Rejuvelac ferment. It is particularly important to replenish your intestinal lactobacteria colonies under the following conditions: after a course of antibiotics, which massacre all friendly intestinal flora; after a series of colonic irrigations, especially when using chlorinated water; after any prolonged fast or intestinal cleansing programme using cleansers such as psyllium and bentonite; if you have a weak digestive system and experience chronic constipation. To replenish your lactobacteria supply, take Rejuvelac daily for 30–45 days, longer if you wish, and repeat at least once each year. Here's how to make it at home:

In the morning, blend 1¾ cups (420 ml) of distilled or purified water with 3 cups (720 ml) of coarsely chopped, loosely packed fresh cabbage in a blender. Do not use chlorinated or fluoridated tap water, which kills lactobacteria. Start at low speed, then switch to high speed, for about thirty seconds. If you don't have a blender, use 2½ cups of very finely chopped, tightly packed cabbage with the same amount of water.

Pour the combined mixture into a jar, cover loosely, and let stand at room temperature for exactly three days. Then strain off the liquid Rejuvelac and discard the cabbage dregs.

Immediately measure out ¼ cup (60 ml) of fresh Rejuvelac and start your next batch by blending 3 cups coarsely chopped cabbage (or combining 2½ cups finely chopped cabbage) with 1½ cups (360 ml) of distilled or purified water, then pouring it back into the jar along with the ¼ cup of Rejuvelac from the first batch. Shake and let stand covered at room temperature for twenty-four hours. This and all subsequent batches require ¼ cup less water and take only one day to ferment owing to the ¼ cup of fermented Rejuvelac starter you now add each time.

Store the rest of the Rejuvelac in the refrigerator and take ½ cup (120 ml) three times per day, preferably with meals. Discard any leftover Rejuvelac after twenty-four hours. Continue making and taking Rejuvelac daily for one to three months, depending on how long it takes to establish regular bowel movements of bulky, well-lubricated stools. Resume supplementation whenever required, especially if chronic constipation recurs.

Good Rejuvelac should taste sour and slightly carbonated, a bit like yogurt or strong mineral water. If it tastes putrid, discard it and start over. Be sure the water you use is pure, and if you are living in an environment infested by airborne bacteria, try fermenting your Rejuvelac in a room with a negative-ion generator, which removes harmful bacteria from the air and thus prevents your ferment from contaminating.

Replenishing your colonies of friendly intestinal bacteria takes some time, but it is well worth the effort, because it prevents all sorts of digestive disorders and degenerative conditions. A good way to get started is first to detoxify the entire digestive tract with a three- to seven-day fast, using intestinal cleansers and colonic irrigations, or any combination of these methods. Follow up by replenishing your lactobacteria colonies with one to three months of Rejuvelac, then help support their growth by including plenty of cabbage and other fresh vegetables and fruits in your diet and eliminating or cutting down on dairy products, meat, and refined sugar and starch. You'll be astonished at how much better you feel after doing this.

Food enzymes

Enzymes are probably the least understood and most important forms of essence in the human body. Over 5,000 different enzymes have so far been identified, and they are involved in each and every vital function in the body. Without adequate supplies of enzymes, the body soon gets sick, degenerates, and dies. Here's what the late Dr Edward Howell, one of America's foremost authorities on enzymes, wrote about these vital biochemicals in his book *Enzyme Nutrition*:

> Enzymes are substances that make life possible. They are needed for every chemical reaction that takes place in the human body. No mineral, vitamin, or hormone can do any work without enzymes. Our bodies, all of our organs, tissues, and cells, are run by metabolic enzymes. They are the manual workers that build our bodies from proteins, carbohydrates, and fats, just as construction workers build our home. You may have all the raw

materials with which to build, but without the workers (enzymes) you cannot even begin.

There are three basic types of enzymes: food, digestive, and antioxidant. Antioxidant enzymes are produced by the body to neutralize free radicals before they cause damage to cells and tissues. You need plenty of selenium and zinc in your diet to produce the most important antioxidant enzymes, which are superoxide dismutase and glutathione peroxidase. Digestive enzymes, of which there are twenty-two, are also produced by the body, in the pancreas, which secretes them as needed into the duodenum to handle the final stages of digestion. Pancreatic enzymes, however, only work in the duodenum, not in the stomach, and then only if the pH balance in the duodenum is precisely correct (slightly alkaline), which is not the case for most people on highly acidifying modern diets.

Food enzymes, of which there are four major varieties, occur only in fresh raw foods, and they are responsible for handling the initial stages of protein, fat, and carbohydrate digestion in the acidic medium of the stomach. You cannot produce these enzymes yourself, and they are totally destroyed in food by cooking, pasteurization, canning, chemical additives, microwaves, and exposure to heat over 118° F. No vitamin, mineral, or any other supplement can substitute for the work they do, and without them cooked and processed foods can be only partially digested in the stomach, a condition which permits ever-present bacteria to ferment carbohydrates and putrefy proteins, causing digestive distress and other health problems. So unless you are eating a diet that consists of well over 50 per cent raw food, you should supplement your diet with food enzymes at meal times. Even if you do eat a lot of raw foods, taking food-enzyme supplements is still a good idea because they greatly enhance your immune system's capacity to digest dead or diseased cells, dissolve tumours and cysts, remove excess cholesterol deposits, kill bacteria and viruses, and eliminate any other undesirable elements composed of proteins, fats, and carbohydrates.

In Taoist alchemy, enzymes are the elements which trigger the conversion of nutritional essence into energy in every cell of the body. Traditionally, the Chinese obtained their food enzymes not only from raw foods, but also from various soya-bean products fermented with aspergillus-fungus enzymes. In addition to fruit, vegetables, and fermented soya-bean products, the Japanese also derive food enzymes from raw fish and raw beef. There is no better way to fortify the potency of your body's essence and enhance the energy you derive from it than by consuming plenty of enzyme-rich raw food and taking food-enzyme supplements daily. Bear in mind that only high-calorie raw foods are rich in enzymes, which means that bananas and mangoes contain far more food enzymes than apples or oranges, and raw fish and beef contain much more than lettuce or tomatoes.

The four essential food enzymes contained in unadulterated raw foods are the following:

Protease
This digests proteins in food, as well as unfriendly bacteria, damaged cells, the protein film surrounding some viruses, and inflammatory substances such as pus in injured tissues. Of all properly digested protein, 56 per cent is converted into glucose upon metabolic demand, which means that protease enzyme supplements ensure an adequate backup supply of glycogen (the precursor to glucose) in the liver, thereby preventing hypoglycaemia and chronic fatigue and increasing stamina and energy reserves.

Amylase
This digests carbohydrates in food, as well as pus and phlegm. In combination with lipase, it can digest many types of virus, including herpes, and remove hard, encrusted mucus from the lungs and bronchial tract. Try amylase and lipase together next time you or someone in your family has an asthma attack or some other chronic lung or bronchial condition.

Lipase
This digests fats, as well as the fatty walls surrounding some viruses. Also helps dissolve and digest fatty accumulations, such as cholesterol in the arteries.

Cellulase
This digests cellulose, so that it can easily pass through the system as bulk. Cellulose contains no essential nutrients, but it is a good source of fibrous bulk for the bowels.

There are many good food-enzyme supplements on the market, including Dr Howell's 'N-Zime' formula, made entirely from vegetable sources. Do not confuse food-enzyme supplements with digestive-enzyme supplements made from extracts of animal pancreas. The latter are similar to the digestive enzymes produced by your own pancreas and work only in the alkaline medium of the duodenum during the final stages of digestion. Food enzymes, which your body cannot produce, work in the acidic medium of the stomach and insure that the crucial first stages of digestion are properly performed.

Herbs

Medicinal herbs are the world's most ancient form of dietary supplement, and nowhere has this tradition been more studiously researched and practised than in China. Taoist recluses in the remote mountains of ancient China were responsible for the early evolution of Chinese herbal medicine, and today virtually all practising Taoists still use and experiment with herbal supplements.

The subject of herbal supplements could fill several large volumes by itself, so we will only briefly discuss a few of the most basic varieties here. First and foremost in Taoist herbal tradition are the tonic supplements. Tonic formulas fortify the body's essence by stimulating secretions of vital hormones throughout the endocrine system and by building strong blood. They boost immunity, enhance sexual vitality, improve circulation, and increase available energy. However, they are strictly preventive formulas designed to guard good health and should not be used when ill. The chapter on 'Tonic Herbal Formulas' discusses this topic in further detail and provides some tried-and-true formulas for the reader's reference.

Most Taoists, especially after the age of forty, use ginseng supplements regularly. In addition to its tonic properties, ginseng also enhances digestion and assimilation of nutrients, nourishes vital fluids, and regulates blood pressure and blood sugar. In China, ginseng has always been highly regarded as the 'King of the Myriad Medicines'.

All herbs are classified according to the Five Flavours, an aspect of the Five Elemental Energies. The flavour with the most potent benefits in preventive medicine is bitter, a flavour that is generally disliked and avoided in contemporary sugar-loving Western cultures, but which Oriental cultures still recognize and value for its therapeutic properties. Bitter herbs such as gentian root, burdock root, wormwood, and goldenseal have the following properties:
- Detoxify blood and lymph
- Stimulate liver and gall bladder
- Clear cholesterol from veins and arteries
- Alkalize blood and other bodily fluids

- Are antibiotic, antiviral, and antiparasitic
- Stimulate digestive secretions, improve appetite, and enhance assimilation of nutrients.

Clearly, modern Western societies could use a strong dose of bitter brew as a daily supplement to compensate for all the highly acidifying, cholesterol-promoting, difficult-to-digest foods they consume. In fact, during medieval times, Western cultures were quite familiar with the benefits of bitter herbs, as evidenced by the bitter liqueurs and digestives brewed by monks in monasteries to aid digestion, control flatulence, and prevent disease. Today, many of these bitter remedies, such as Benedictine, Fernet Branca, and vermouth, are still widely available, though few people seem to be aware of their health benefits. Angostura bitters, a popular cocktail ingredient made from gentian root, is a great digestive aid that is available in any bar or grocery shop. Just dilute about half a teaspoon in an ounce or two of water, soda, or ginger ale, and take it about half an hour before meals as a digestive stimulant.

Bitter herbs not only aid digestion and balance the pH of the body's vital fluids, they also aggressively remove toxic substances from the blood, lymph, and tissues, and accelerate their excretion from the body. These detoxifying properties are particularly important today, when everything from air and water to food and drugs is contaminated with dangerous toxins. For lymph detoxification, blood purification, and general disease prevention, the herbal supplements most highly favoured by Taoists include garlic, burdock, scullcap, liquorice, Mishmi bitter, wormwood, and dandelion.

CHAPTER 11

Guarding Your Essence

It is the toxic filth in our systems which kills us. That is why people age so rapidly today – they are actually rotting and decaying from the inside out.

V. E. Irons (1981)

In the Taoist system of preventive health care, diet and nutrition, including supplements, form the first line of defence. Our bodily essences are derived directly from the food and water we consume, and they may be further strengthened, balanced, and protected by the judicial use of the various types of supplements discussed above.

In addition to diet and nutrition, there are a few other preventive measures you can implement in order to guard health on the fundamental level of essence. Perhaps the most important of these in today's toxic world is internal tissue cleansing and the purification of vital bodily fluids, such as blood and lymph. This and other methods are briefly discussed below.

Bowel and tissue cleansing

Most natural-therapy healers agree that chronic constipation and toxic colons are the root causes of many of the diseases and most of the degenerative conditions that plague the modern world, especially people on Western diets. 'Purging the bowels eliminates the source of poisons, thereby permitting blood [essence] and energy to regenerate naturally,' wrote the Chinese physician Chai Yu-hua over three hundred years ago. Today this is truer than ever.

Even if your bowels move every day, it is likely that you are nevertheless constipated. The word 'constipate' comes from the Latin root *constipare* which means 'to press together'. This agrees well with the traditional Chinese term for constipation, *bien-mee*, which means 'compressed faeces'. In other words, constipation is a condition characterized by compressed, tightly packed faeces.

Constipation is caused by the long time that food in modern diets requires to transit through the digestive tract from mouth to anus. Contributing factors include improper food-combining, insufficient fibre, highly mucus-forming foods, protein putrefaction, enzyme-deficient food, and stress, all of which delay digestion and slow down excretion. The longer faeces remain in the bowels, the drier and more densely compressed they become. Healthy stools should be bulky and mushy and break up when the toilet is flushed. If you'd like to know what healthy stools are like, simply try taking an intestinal cleansing supplement made with powdered psyllium-seed husk twice a day for a week or two, or try a month or two of daily doses of fermented cabbage juice, or both, and you will experience what may well be your first normal bowel movement in memory.

Constipated stools not only move slowly through the bowels, they also deposit layer upon layer of slimy mucoid matter on the walls of the colon, where they gradually become impacted and form tough, rubbery adhesions that obstruct the bowels and thereby further delay excretion. These foul deposits continue to accumulate layer upon layer, year after year, throughout your life, and the toxins they contain continuously seep into the bloodstream by osmosis through the colon wall, which is laced with miles of capillaries. The blood picks up these toxins and circulates them throughout the body, thereby poisoning tissues, weakening organs, impairing immunity, and causing various degenerative conditions. The fact of the matter is that your tissues are only as clean as your blood, and your blood is only as clean as your bowels. Therefore, by cleansing the bowels you purify the blood, and the blood then detoxifies the tissues.

Normal healthy bowels manifest a natural response called the 'gastrocolic reflex', whereby the bowels are automatically stimulated to move every time the stomach is filled. The combination of poor eating habits and modern notions of 'toilet training' has virtually destroyed our inherent gastrocolic reflex. In primitive societies, children run around naked and are encouraged to squat down and defecate whenever the urge strikes, but in modern 'civilized' societies children are taught to override the gastrocolic reflex by restraining their bowels until the urge becomes overwhelming. The modern sit-down toilet, which inhibits complete bowel movements, has further aggravated the situation. Therefore, the only way to recover normal bowel functions is to cleanse your bowels thoroughly of accumulated toxic debris, completely reform your eating habits, and retrain yourself to use the toilet properly and frequently. 'Properly' means squatting instead of sitting on the toilet, and 'frequently' means heading for the loo whenever you feel even the slightest urge to move your bowels.

A variety of methods and materials for cleansing the bowels, detoxifying the tissues, and purifying the blood, including a seven-day fast with daily colonic irrigations, are discussed in detail in the chapter on 'Fasting and Excretion' in *The Tao of HS&L*. After completing a bowel- and tissue-cleansing programme you will notice a refreshing feeling of physical lightness, a higher level of energy, and an elevated spirit. That's because energy is derived from essence and in turn fuels spirit, so by cleansing and purifying your bodily essences, you naturally harvest more potent and abundant energy, which in turn sustains a more elevated, luminous spirit. This is basic Taoist alchemy at its best.

Women readers please note that if you undertake a seven-day fast for bowel cleansing and tissue detoxification, you may experience alterations in your menstrual and ovulation cycles, especially the first time you try it. This is a perfectly natural result of purifying your body's essences, rebalancing your body's energies, and harmonizing vital functions. Therefore, if you are using some version of the rhythm method for birth control, such as the one discussed in *The Tao of HS&L*, you should wait until your cycles have re-established a predictable pattern before again relying on this method. This usually takes only two months, and as your bowels and tissues get cleaner, subsequent fasts will have little or no effect on your menstrual cycles.

Exercise and physical therapy

'Flowing water never stagnates, active hinges never rust,' wrote the great Chinese physician and Tao master Sun Ssu-mo 1,300 years ago. By remaining active throughout his life, Dr Sun lived to the age of 101. The human body was designed to move on its own two legs, not to sit in cars and stand in lifts while machines do all the work. Dr Sun's use of 'water' and 'hinges' as metaphors is significant: not only must we keep our 'hinges' (joints) active, we must also keep our 'water' (blood, lymph, and other bodily fluids) flowing. 'Rusty hinges' such as arthritis, rheumatism, and lower-back pains and 'stagnant water' such as circulatory, excretory, and lymphatic problems have reached epidemic proportions in this age of ambulatory machinery and sedentary lifestyles. Physical exercise is an absolute prerequisite for maintaining the health and vitality of our physical bodies. Without sufficient exercise, the body atrophies; so, as they say, 'use it before you lose it'.

By far the best form of exercise is traditional Chinese *chee-gung*, which is discussed in a later chapter, as well as in the chapters on 'Breathing' and 'Exercise' in *The Tao of HS&L*. Besides *chee-gung*, any form of physical exercise with an aerobic aspect to it is helpful in preventive health care, as long as you do not overexert yourself. The problem with so many athletic exercises, such as jogging and field sports, is that people do not practise them regularly enough to stay in shape for the considerable demands such sports make on the body. Consequently, many people hurt rather than help themselves with their athletic endeavours. One of the advantages of *chee-gung* is that it may be safely practised by young and old, male and female, weak and strong, all with equal benefit.

Short of *chee-gung*, the best form of therapeutic exercise is swimming, which gently exercises all joints, muscles, and tendons in conjunction with rhythmic breathing. Golf is good if you walk rather than ride a motorized cart, because it makes you exercise and breathe in the open, freshly ionized air of the greens. Walking in the woods and fields and doing dance aerobics are also effective methods for keeping hinges active and fluids flowing.

Another good form of physical therapy is massage, particularly traditional Thai massage, which combines Indian yoga with Chinese acupressure in a highly effective technique that tones muscles, stretches tendons, loosens joints, stimulates circulation, drains lymph, and balances energy. Other good therapeutic massage systems are Chinese *tui-na* ('push and rub'), which focuses on joints and energy points, and its Japanese cousin, *shiatsu*. In fact, almost all forms of massage are good physical therapy, as long as the therapist is properly trained.

The same goes for chiropractic, which is an excellent way to align and limber your body's 'hinges' and balance its energies: performed by well-trained hands, chiropractic therapy can cure and prevent myriad ailments, but unqualified hands can leave your body completely 'unhinged'.

Skin brushing

One of the best ways to cleanse the entire lymphatic system is by brushing the surface of the body with a soft dry brush made of natural vegetable bristles. The traditional Chinese version of this method uses the dried fibres of a gourd fruit called 'silk squash', known as a loofah in the West, but natural-bristle brushes have proven to be far more effective. The brush should have a long handle, soft natural bristles, and always be kept dry.

Dry skin brushing stimulates the lymph canals to drain toxic mucoid matter into the colon, thereby purifying the entire lymphatic system. This enables lymph to perform its house-cleaning duties by keeping the blood and other vital tissues detoxified. Most people today have chronically toxic lymph fluids and swollen lymph nodes, a condition which promotes toxicity throughout the system by robbing lymph of its power to clean the blood and cellular fluids. In addition, skin brushing is highly stimulating to surface circulation of blood and leaves you feeling invigorated.

Skin brushing need be performed only once a day, preferably first thing in the morning, and it takes only a couple of minutes. If you're feeling sluggish, toxic, or ill, you may want to do it twice a day. The body should be dry and naked, and the brush should be swept once or twice in the same direction across every surface of the body except the face. Do not scrub, massage, or rotate the brush on the body; just sweep it across the skin in long smooth strokes in the general direction of the colon. Brush up the arms from the hands to the shoulders, up the legs from feet to hips, down the back and torso, up the buttocks, down the neck, and across the shoulders. After a few days, you may notice a gelatinous mucoid material in your stools: that's toxic lymph which has drained into your colon owing to skin brushing.

For a thorough lymphatic cleansing, perform skin brushing daily for about three months. Thereafter, twice a week is sufficient to keep your lymph quite clean, but you should resume daily brushing whenever you're feeling ill.

Acute illness

When acute illness strikes, such as fever, flu, bronchitis, or diarrhoea, it is often a sign that your blood, lymph, lungs, and/or colon have become so toxic that the body must take emergency measures to purge toxins from your tissues and restore a healthy homeostasis. As your tissues become more toxic, your system becomes ever more vulnerable to abnormal environmental energies (Six Evils), emotional stress (Seven Emotions), and the ever-present germs inside and outside the body.

A fever, for example, is nothing more than the body's way of burning off bacteria and other microbes, and it has been scientifically proven that most microbes associated with human disease perish in the heat of fever conditions. Taking drugs to lower fever is, in most cases, self-defeating and only prolongs your misery by permitting offensive bacteria to survive in your system. The same goes for runny noses, hacking coughs, profuse sweating, and diarrhoea, all of which are the body's safety valves for forcefully purging the system of toxic debris.

The best way to guard your essence and recover your health during most acute illnesses is, first, immediately to stop eating all acidifying, mucus-forming foods, particularly meat, dairy products, starch, and sugar. Instead, either fast on distilled or filtered water, or else consume only fresh fruits and vegetables, preferably as freshly extracted juice.

Second, perform skin brushing twice daily to purify your lymph so that it is able to detoxify your blood and tissues. If possible, take one or two enemas or colonic irrigations each day as well, immediately after skin brushing, to flush accumulated wastes from your colon and trigger the cleansing response throughout your body.

Third, take appropriate herbal remedies, particularly of the bitter variety, to accelerate the detoxification and purification process further. You'll find some excellent Chinese patent herbal medicines for various common ailments listed in the chapter on 'Remarkable Remedies'. For detailed guidance in the use of Chinese medicinal herbs, you may also refer to the author's book *Chinese Herbal Medicine*.

Last but not least, remain relaxed and get plenty of rest until the disease has run its course, the toxins are purged from your system, and your energy has recovered its strength and balance.

Dual sexual cultivation

Predictably, the 'Tao of Sex' section in *The Tao of HS&L* aroused strong interest among readers, particularly males. For most Western readers, the idea of prolonging sexual intercourse for up to an hour or more by restraining male ejaculation is an exotic novelty and a far cry from the syrupy romance and debauchery with which most Western sexual lore is associated. The taboos and titters surrounding sex in Judeo-Christian tradition have prevented Western societies from exploring the therapeutic benefits of sexual activity, so this is one area where the Western world stands to learn a lot from the traditional cultures of East Asia and India.

Like a strong appetite for food, strong sexual drive has always been regarded as a fundamental sign of good health and flourishing vitality in Taoist tradition. How this drive is expressed in practice can make all the difference between health and disease, regeneration and degeneration, even life and death. The same principle applies to food: how we satisfy our appetites for food determines whether our eating habits help or hinder our quest for health and longevity. Like nutritional needs, there are right ways and wrong ways to manage sexual needs, and the choice has nothing whatsoever to do with morality.

According to the Taoist view, overt sexual drive stems from the expansive Wood energy of the liver, an energy associated with the spring season, while sexual essence comes from the potent condensed Water energy of the kidneys. While sexual activity releases and relaxes the tension caused by the pent-up Liver/Wood energy of sexual drive, it can also exhaust or stagnate the Kidney/Water energy that supplies the hormones for such activity. For men, the problem is depletion of kidney energy due to excessive ejaculation. For women, the problem can be stagnation of kidney energy due to insufficient or incomplete orgasm. For both men and women, kidney energy and sexual potency can also be easily exhausted by chronic stress. Since sexual satisfaction is a good antidote for stress in both men and women, a way of sexual intercourse must be found that prevents sexual depletion in men while providing complete satisfaction to women. That way is the 'Tao of Yin and Yang', whereby yin is fully released and satisfied through orgasm, while yang is carefully controlled and conserved by regulating ejaculation in order to prevent exhaustion, all according to age, health, season, and other relevant factors. The reasons and traditional methods for practising the Tao of Yin and Yang are presented in detail in *The Tao of HS&L*.

Taoists regard sexual activity as being good for health if it leaves you feeling relaxed, refreshed, and elated, but bad if it leaves you feeling exhausted, weak, or frustrated. That means 'different strokes for different folks'. Despite its enlightened attitude and scientific rationale, Taoist sexual yoga has over the ages often been accused of being a mere excuse for unbridled debauchery. And in fact there have always been, and still are, charlatans and deviants who invoke the Tao as a smokescreen for lechery. We should not be fooled by popular myths about sex, nor should we suppress this natural drive because of prudery or unpleasant experiences in the past. Instead, we should familiarize ourselves with the real facts of sex, ignore all the nonsense, then find a loving and understanding partner.

Properly practised, sex can be one of the fastest, most effective, and most enjoyable ways to build up abundant supplies of potent hormone essence, boost energy, enhance immunity, and prolong life. Far from conflicting with spiritual values, sex can forge a strong foundation of essence and generate potent reserves of energy as a basis for progress on the higher paths of spiritual cultivation.

After reforming your eating habits, learning how to use supplements, disciplining your sexual activities, and taking other measures to protect and nourish your essence, it's time to take another step on the path of Taoist alchemy by starting to work directly with energy.

CHAPTER 12

Energy: Human and Artificial

> Science tells us that everything is energy and that matter
> is nothing more than energy in a different form. The chair
> we sit on is simply energy vibrating at a much slower
> rate. Our bodies are a composite of many different energy
> patterns and vibrations. In fact, the universe and every-
> thing in it is made up of different levels of vibration.
>
> Dr John Veltheim, *reiki* energy therapist (1992)

Vital energy is the most fundamental element in the medical,
meditative, and martial-arts traditions of all Oriental cultures.
Called *chee* in Chinese and *prana* in Sanskrit, vital energy is the
immaterial but highly functional force that drives the universe and
animates humans and all other living things. According to Taoist
internal alchemy, energy is derived from essence and in turn commands essence, which means that energy and matter are mutually
dependent. Similarly, energy fuels spirit and is in turn commanded
by spirit, which means that mind controls matter via its command
over energy.

The primary forms of energy permeating the universe are light,
heat, electricity, magnetism, and nuclear forces. Just as light and
heat are closely related and often manifest themselves together, as
in a flame, so electricity and magnetism are inseparably connected.
All these forces are directly involved in the human energy system.

The primary attributes of all universal energies are movement
and transformation, and the prerequisite for the movement of energy is a polar field. Electromagnetic energy moves and transforms
by virtue of the dynamic tension established by electromagnetic
fields with opposite poles, referred to as 'positive' (yang) and
'negative' (yin).

The surface of the earth (negative pole) and the ionosphere
(positive pole) act as charged plates which create a powerful

electric field that envelops the entire planet, with polarity ranging up to thousands of volts per foot. The earth's electromagnetic field continuously ionizes air molecules in the atmosphere, and when we breathe, we absorb the electrical energy they carry. Breathing plugs us into the earth's electromagnetic field and tunes our energy systems into the frequency of the earth's energy pulse. Human health and vitality depend largely on the degree to which we are able to absorb the atmospheric energy of the earth through breathing, and this in turn depends on three factors:

- our breathing method
- the quality of the air we breathe
- the strength of the electromagnetic field in which we breathe.

Shallow erratic breathing impedes the assimilation of energy from the atmosphere and thus impairs vitality. Pollution radically reduces the atmospheric energy we absorb from air even with the best breathing methods, because polluted air contains an abnormally high concentration of heavy, sluggish, positive ions, which counteract the energizing influence of negative ions. Abnormal electromagnetic fields generated in our immediate environments by electric power lines and transformers, microwave radiation, radio and television broadcasts, home appliances, and other modern technology interfere with our bodies' access to the energy of the earth's normal electromagnetic field and can have devastating effects on human energy systems. Furthermore, high rise buildings and steel-reinforced concrete structures can reduce electromagnetic fields in living and working environments to virtually zero, which means that the air in such environments is devoid of the vitalizing electromagnetic energy of the earth. That's why sitting for hours at a desk in a high-rise office building can leave you feeling more exhausted that spending a whole day doing hard labour out in an open field.

Human energy: the Taoist view

Taoists have known about the earth's electromagnetic field for at least 5,000 years. *Chee-gung* ('energy work') tunes the frequency of human energy with that of the earth, thereby establishing energy resonance among the Three Powers of heaven (sky), earth (ground), and humans (practitioners). The early Taoists called the positive pole of the sky 'yang' and the negative pole of the earth 'yin' and referred to the electromagnetic energy this field generates as *chee*.

In Chinese, 'weather' is *tien-chee* ('celestial energy'), terrestrial energy is *dee-chee* ('earth energy'), and 'electric energy' is *dien-chee*.

As we discussed earlier, human energy has two basic aspects, known as 'prenatal' or 'primordial' and 'postnatal' or 'temporal'. Postnatal energy is of two types: 'celestial', which humans derive from air by breathing; and 'terrestrial', which is obtained from food and water by digestion and metabolism. Together these postnatal human energies are referred to as Fire or yang energy. Primordial energy is derived from the prenatal original essence (*yüan-jing*) we receive upon conception from the sperm and ovum of our parents, and it is stored in the glands of our bodies in the form of highly potent hormones, especially in the adrenal glands. The energy we derive from our prenatal essence is called Water or yin energy. In his book *The Root of Chinese Chi Kung*, Dr Yang Jwing-ming, a Taoist master teaching *chee-gung* and martial arts in Massachusetts, writes:

> Generally, the Chi is generated or converted naturally and automatically from the Essences within your body. These Essences include the inherited Original Essence which goes to make Water Chi, and the Essence from food and air which is transformed into Fire Chi. This natural Chi generation is the major source of your lifeforce.

Chee takes many different forms in the human energy system. Besides the basic Water and Fire energies derived from prenatal and postnatal essences, human energy differentiates itself into the Five Elemental Energies associated with the paired yin-yang organ systems, the energies of the Seven Emotions generated by the temporal postnatal mind, the nourishing *ying-chee* that flows within the energy meridians, the protective *wei-chee* that forms an aura of guardian energy around the surface of the body, and other types. But ultimately it's all derived from the same basic sources: food, air, and the 'original essence' of hormones.

External environmental energies, such as the Six Evils of adverse climate and weather and their even more malevolent modern cousins – microwave radiation and abnormal electromagnetic fields – can easily invade and distort human energy systems, especially when the protective shield of guardian energy is weak or defective. Chinese *chee-gung* restores normal pulse in the human electromagnetic field, thereby permitting the adept to tune in to the earth's soothing energy field and receive a revitalizing boost of natural energy that clears the system of damaging abnormal energies.

On the postnatal level, *chee-gung* improves digestion, metabolism, respiration, and other vital bodily functions, but its greatest benefit is an elevation in the soothing, rejuvenating Water *chee* derived from original essence. Because of the abnormal nature of modern life, with all its overeating, constant excitement, chronic stress, drugs, and electromagnetic pollution, almost everyone has a morbid excess of deviant Fire energy coursing through their systems, and *chee-gung* practice can counteract this excess by suffusing the body with restorative Water *chee*. However, in order for this to work, not only must *chee-gung* be properly practised every day, but the practitioner must also endeavour to reduce to an absolute minimum those aspects of his or her temporal lifestyle that generate deviant Fire energy and undermine vitality.

The rejuvenating vital energy upon which human health depends is called 'True Energy' (*jeng-chee*), and it is this type of energy that *chee-gung* cultivates. As we have seen, spirit commands energy, which means that whatever is going on in your mind and brain directly affects the quality and circulation of energy in your system. Therefore, when practising *chee-gung*, it is important to do so with a quiet and 'empty' mind, which means that the chronically overactive cerebral cortex, the source of our ongoing internal dialogue with ourselves, must be stilled during practice. The *Internal Medicine Classic* states: 'When the mind is quiet and empty, true *chee* will rise to its command, and the danger of disease will turn to safety.' In modern medical parlance, this means that the cerebral cortex, which operates at high frequency, must be inhibited so that the entire autonomous nervous system may switch over to the calming, restorative parasympathetic mode, which operates at the low frequencies of the earth's own electromagnetic pulse. This is why the practice of 'sitting still, doing nothing' (meditation) is such an effective adjunct to *chee-gung* or any other restorative health regimen.

The human energy network

The electromagnetic nature of human energy has been recognized by traditional Chinese medicine and Taoist alchemy for at least 5,000 years and was recorded in the *Internal Medicine Classic* over 2,000 years ago. This energy was found to flow through the human body via a complex network of channels (*mai*), meridians (*jing*), and capillaries (*luo*) interlacing the entire human system. Along the major meridians were found particularly sensitive energy points called *hsüeh*, which function as energy relay terminals, much as transformers along power lines do. The meridians and their power points are the basis of acupuncture and acupressure healing techniques, for they can be used directly to manipulate the magnitude, balance, and flow of vital human energies.

Dr Robert Becker of the Upstate Medical Center in New York has confirmed this view of the human energy network by demonstrating that the major points used in acupuncture have significantly lower electrical impedance and therefore higher conductivity than other surface areas of the body. Tests at the Veterans' General Hospital in Taipei showed that whenever an organ associated with a particular acupuncture point is ailing, the electrical impedance of that point changes acutely. The energy points and meridians not only feed vital energy to their related organs, they also reflect any pathological disturbance in those organs, thus providing physicians with a convenient and highly accurate tool for diagnosis as well as therapy.

Each of the twelve major meridians is connected to a specific organ-energy system and its vital functions (Fig. 8). In addition, each organ meridian is also associated with other physiological functions that may appear unrelated to that organ, but in fact are connected to it via the invisible meridian network. For example, it is well known in Chinese medicine that eye problems are often related to liver malfunction and that tinnitus (ringing ears) reflects kidney problems. Consequently, when a Chinese physician talks about the 'liver' or the 'kidneys', he is referring to more than conventional Western doctors do when they mention those organs. The Chinese physician is taking into account that particular organ's ordinary biological functions, other peripheral activities governed by the organ's energy, related emotional and psychic phenomena, and any symptoms occurring along areas of the body through which that organ's meridian runs.

In addition to the major organ meridians, each of which controls one of the twelve organ-energy systems, there is also a network called the 'Eight Extraordinary Channels' (chee-jing ba-mai) (Fig. 9). While the twelve major meridians function as 'rivers' of energy to irrigate the organs and tissues with vitality, the eight extraordinary channels function as 'reservoirs', storing and feeding energy into the twelve organ meridians as required, or taking up the overflow when they get overloaded. It is these eight channels that are primarily influenced by the practice of chee-gung, which fills them up with True Human Energy to be distributed as needed into the twelve organ meridians. Among the eight reservoir channels, the two most vital are the Governing Channel that runs up the spine from perineum to head and the Conception Channel that runs down the front of the body from head to perineum. These are the

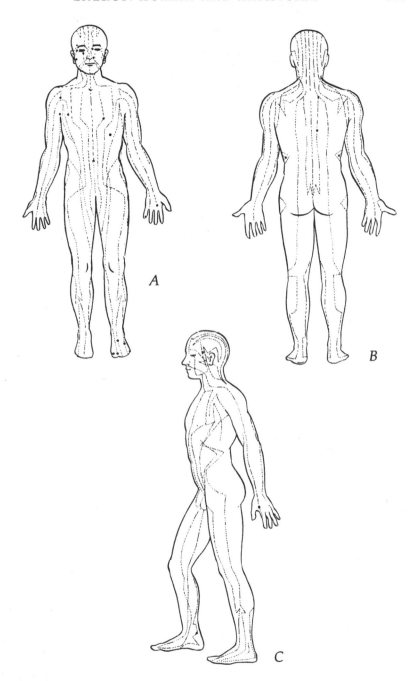

Fig. 8 **The twelve major meridians: each meridian is related to a specific organ-energy
system and regulates that system's vital functions.**
A. Front: yin-organ meridians
B. Back: yang-organ meridians
C. Side: side view of major meridians

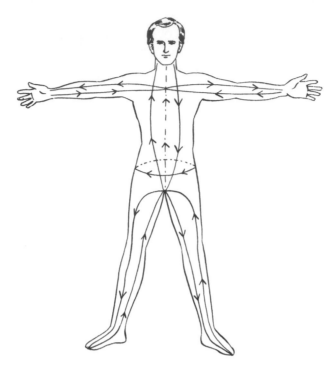

Fig. 9 **The Eight Extraordinary Channels.**

two primary channels activated by Taoist internal alchemy and the two major reservoirs for True Human Energy. Among the eight channels, only the Governing and Conception channels have their own vital points; the other six have their terminals located along the major organ meridians.

Branching out from the twelve major meridians and eight extra-ordinary channels are fifteen subnetworks of finer energy capil-laries (*luo*) and countless 'grandchild' webs which spring from those networks to cover every tissue and cell in the body. For the purposes of *chee-gung* and medical therapy, attention is usually confined to the twelve organ meridians, the eight reservoir channels, and various vital energy points along them. More advanced *chee-gung* practices, such as meditation, also work with the Central or 'Thrusting' Channel, which together with the Governing and Conception channels controls the movement and distribution of energy from the root sexual centres below to the higher cerebral centres above.

As you can see from the illustrations, the meridians and channels are very logically distributed. Six of the organ meridians run through the arms and upper torso, and six run through the legs and lower torso. The six running along the front and interior surfaces of the body control the yin organs, while the six running along the back and exterior surfaces are connected to the yang organs. Similarly, the Governing Channel that runs up the spine controls the six major yang meridians, while the Conception Channel in front regulates the six major yin meridians. Together, these fourteen energy vessels and their subsidiary networks form a third circulatory system, in addition to the blood and nervous systems. In terms of function, the energy channels are more closely related to the circulation of blood than to the nervous system, as evidenced by the ancient Taoist maxim that 'blood follows where energy leads'. One cause of 'tired blood', or anaemia, is insufficient circulation of vital energy, which deprives blood of vitality.

The human energy network has many vital health functions. It regulates blood circulation, sends protective *wei-chee* to the surface to guard against external attack, and carries nourishing *ying-chee* to the organs, glands, marrow, brain, and other internal tissues to fuel their vital functions. The internal circulation of nourishing energy

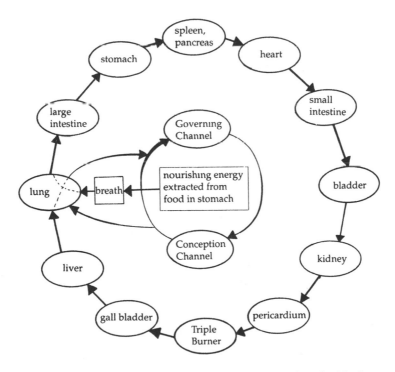

Fig. 10 **The internal circulation of nourishing energy extracted from food in the stomach is driven by breath through the twelve organ-energy meridians and regulated by the Governing and Conception channels, which also serve as reservoirs for storing surplus energy and distributing it as required.**

follows a set pattern, as illustrated in Fig. 10. The distribution of internal energy revolves around the Governing and Conception channels and is driven by the organ energy of the lungs, hence the importance of correct breathing in human health.

In the pathology of disease, all ailments and their symptoms are reflected in the meridians and vital points and are attributed to some sort of imbalance or functional failure in the flow and distribution of protective and nourishing energy. An experienced Chinese diagnostician can pinpoint the problem by applying pressure to a related energy point, which will feel painful when the related organ is diseased or dysfunctional. To cure the disease, the physician prescribes herbal remedies that correct the imbalance by releasing the energies required for healing and conducting them to the ailing organ by the 'natural affinity' (*gui-jing*) of the herbs' specific energies for the related organ-energy system. He might also treat the ailing organ by applying acupuncture or acupressure to the related meridians and points. Advanced adepts of internal alchemy can perform many healing functions for themselves as well as for others simply by channelling energy into ailing organs via the meridian system.

Western medicine has much to learn from traditional Chinese energy-healing techniques.

Electromagnetic fields

The Western scientific view

Electric currents always generate magnetic fields around the conducting material. In *The Root of Chinese Chi Kung*, Dr Yang quotes Dr Richard Broeringmeyer, publisher of the *Bio-Energy Health Newsletter*, as follows: 'Life is not possible without electromagnetic fields, and optimum health is not possible if the electromagnetic fields are out of balance for long periods of time. Magnetic energy is nature's energy in perfect balance.'

The entire earth is surrounded by its own geomagnetic field, which is influenced and sometimes distorted by solar winds, especially by solar flares, which can cause magnetic storms within the earth's field. A lesser-known fact is that by the direct currents flowing through the human brain, our heads generate their own magnetic fields, which extend outwards several feet. The nature and configuration of this magnetic field is directly influenced by cerebral activity. This is the aura often depicted around the heads of saints and holy persons in Eastern as well as Western religious paintings. The entire body also has its own electromagnetic field, complete with positive yang and negative yin poles (Fig. 11). As Dr Yang points out:

> When a piece of steel is placed inside a magnetic field, it becomes a magnet. Since our bodies are made up of conductive material, and we are in the magnetic field of the Earth, it is reasonable to assume that our bodies are like magnets. Since a magnet has two poles which must be located on the centerline of the magnet, we can easily guess that the poles of our bodies must be somewhere on the head and the bottom of the abdomen.

Human energy fields have been scientifically proven to be directly affected by electromagnetic activity in the earth's field, and this influence is the source of what are known as 'biorhythms' or 'biocycles'. Typical examples of human biorhythms affected by the earth's electromagnetic field are the twenty-eight-day female menstrual cycle, which follows the cyclic influence of the moon on the earth's field, and sleep/wake cycles, which are easily disrupted by lunar phases and solar flares. It therefore stands to reason that

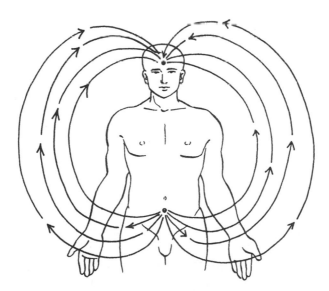

Fig. 11 **The human electromagnetic field is a microcosm of the earth's electromagnetic field, to which it must stay tuned for optimum health. Earthly energies gather in lower abdomen (negative pole) and move up to head (positive pole), where heavenly energies focus.**

human biorhythms can also be adversely affected by electromagnetic fields generated by power lines, microwave transmissions, and other artificial sources.

Homing pigeons find their way home by tuning into the earth's
field by crystals of the magnetic mineral magnetite located on the
surface of their brains. This magnetic organ enables them to navi-
gate their way home through darkness and fog. When small bar
magnets are attached to their heads to negate their sensitivity to the
earth's field, they lose their sense of direction and their way.

Dr Robin Baker of the University of Manchester in England has
located a similar mass of magnetite crystals high up behind the
nasal passages in humans, slightly in front of the pituitary gland.
This is precisely the point which Taoist adepts and Hindu yogis cite
as the Upper Elixir Field or 'Celestial Eye'. It is one of the most
powerful energy centres in the human system, and when 'opened'
through the practice of *chee-gung* and meditation, it provides perceptions and insights that are inaccessible to the uninitiated.

Once regarded as the body's master gland, the pituitary has in
recent years been overshadowed in importance by the mysterious
little pineal gland, located in the exact centre of the brain, just above
the pituitary. The pineal secretes a wide range of vital neurohormones, such as melatonin and serotonin, which influence virtually
all human functions, including moods, sleep/wake cycles, appetite
and sexual drive. The pineal has been found to be highly sensitive
to the slightest fluctuation in the earth's magnetic field, and these
fluctuations directly influence its secretions of 'vital essence'. The
pineal is therefore likely to be even more sensitive to the far more
radical electromagnetic fluctuations caused by power lines, broadcasting stations, computer terminals, and other electronic technology. The earth's magnetic field has a strength of 0.5 milligauss;
the power lines running through your neighbourhood, home, and
office, generate a 100-milligauss field.

Besides the magnitude of magnetic fields, human energy is also
influenced by the frequency at which they pulsate. The earth's field
pulsates in a range of 1–30 hertz (Hz), or cycles per second, with the
greatest field strength occurring between 7 and 10 Hz. This is precisely the frequency at which the human brain operates under
normal conditions. It is also the frequency that *chee-gung* practice
restores throughout the human energy system.

Thus the human body has a dual sensory system: the ordinary
nervous system, which controls the limbs, motor functions, and
ordinary sensory organs, such as eyes and ears; and the electromagnetic control system, which is sensitive to the normal

micropulsations of the earth's field as well as the high-frequency pulsations produced by human technology. The latter system regulates the vital energies of the organs (Five Elemental Energies), senses injuries on the surface and interior of the body, triggers repair and healing responses, mediates the essential secretions of the pituitary and pineal glands, manages the immune system, and operates through the invisible network of energy channels and their vital points. This electromagnetic system can be directly regulated and balanced by the practice of *chee-gung*.

Human bioenergy fields have been photographed in Russia by a technique called 'Kirlian photography'. Dr Thelma Moss of the University of California at Los Angeles has conducted extensive studies on human and plant bioenergy fields, and has come to the intriguing conclusion that the 'green fingers' displayed by talented gardeners is due to the strength and healthy balance of their energy auras, which they transmit to plants through contact with their fingers. It has long been known in the Orient, and recently confirmed by Western science, that the hand is a very powerful conductor of human energy, and this is the basis of the 'laying on of hands' healing method.

Electromagnetic pollution

The impact of electromagnetic fields and microwave radiation, whether natural or abnormal, on human health and energy is now becoming established in Western science. The implications of this fact for modern human lifestyles are enormous.

First, let's take a look at the effects of natural aberrations in the earth's electromagnetic field – the magnetic storms caused by solar flares. Solar flares have been known to cause blowouts in electric power and telephone lines and to disrupt radio and television transmissions. Dr Robert Becker has produced evidence that major magnetic storms coincide closely with a significant rise in admissions to mental hospitals and with outbursts of extremely aberrant behaviour in patients already confined in such institutions. It would be interesting to see what sort of influence magnetic storms have on summit meetings, political campaigns, and other events that determine the course of human affairs.

The course of evolution itself may have been changed by the periodic reversal of the earth's northern and southern magnetic poles. This occurred, for example, during the Cretaceous period, coinciding with the disappearance of the dinosaurs. Reversals in the earth's polarity happen three or four times in every million years. But this pattern predates the advent of artificial magnetic fields, so no one can accurately predict when the next one will be.

Since humans learned to harness electric power, we have created vast networks of electromagnetic fields across the entire length and breadth of the planet, forces with more than enough strength to override the earth's own gentle subsonic pulse. The frequencies at which electric power systems, radio and television signals, and microwave transmissions operate do not exist in nature and can cause severe disturbances in human energy systems, which in turn give rise to physical and mental health problems.

Take for example Vernon, New Jersey, a small town of 25,000 which happens to rank fifth in the USA in the number of microwave transmitters. The incidence of Down's syndrome, a birth defect caused by genetic damage to the foetus and/or parents, in Vernon is 1,000 per cent above the national average. Other studies have found this birth defect in children whose fathers were military radar operators. You can well imagine how reluctant government authorities are to acknowledge this scientifically established evidence, for it would require them to dismantle most of the huge radar stations and other microwave transmitters upon which modern military forces depend. It would also unleash an avalanche of litigation against the government for condoning such public health hazards.

Brain tumours and other cancers have also been linked to the abnormal frequencies produced by radar and other microwave transmitters, including cellular telephones. Dr Robert Becker, one of America's leading authorities in the field of electromagnetic pollution, writes as follows in his book *Cross Currents*:

> The scientific data at this time indicate that microwaves have major biological effects at power levels *far below* those required to cause heating [such as microwave ovens]. The majority of these effects are productive of various disease states, primarily cancer and genetic defects, in those exposed and in their unexposed offspring . . . The hazard comes from the fact that exposure to microwaves, like exposure to any abnormal electromagnetic field, produces stress, a decline in immune-system competency, and changes in the genetic apparatus. Thus, the levels of exposure that the government says are 'safe' are in fact not safe at all.

Anyone who keeps a microwave oven or cellular phone at home is risking injury to the health of the entire family, including foetal damage. Is it really worth the 'convenience'?

Ordinary electric power lines and transformers operate at 60 Hz in the USA and 50 Hz in Europe. In 1980, the Public Service Commission of the New York State Department of Health commissioned Dr David Savitz of the University of North Carolina to conduct a thorough study on the effects of the field emitted by ordinary electric power lines on people living near those lines. Five years and $500,000 later, Dr Savitz concluded that at least 20 per cent of childhood cancers in the areas he studied were produced by exposure to electric power-line magnetic fields as weak as 3 milligauss. The study showed that such fields not only promote cancer, they also inhibit the production of vital neurohormones in the brain, resulting in severe behavioural disorders and learning disabilities. The field generated within 50 feet of standard power lines in the USA is 100 milligauss, which is over thirty times higher than the 3-milligauss magnitude that Dr Savitz's research linked to cancer and brain damage.

Embarrassed by the results of its own study, the NY Public Service Commission ignored its conclusions and promptly set a 'safe' power-line electromagnetic-field level of 100 milligauss, claiming that the public had already 'accepted' such a health risk. The public has of course never been informed of this risk.

In 1988, Dr Marjorie Speers of the Department of Preventive Medicine at the University of Texas Medical Branch in Galveston reported results of a study on brain tumours in workers whose jobs expose them to a field of 60 Hz. The incidence of brain tumours in such workers was thirteen times higher than in those in an unexposed control group. Dr Becker writes in Cross Currents: 'At this time, the scientific evidence is absolutely conclusive: 60-Hz magnetic fields cause human cancer cells to permanently increase their rate of growth by as much as 1,600 per cent and to develop more malignant characteristics.'

These and other studies show that the magnetic fields of electric power lines and transformers, as well as microwave radiation, primarily damage two types of tissue: brain tissue and rapidly growing tissues, such as developing foetuses, young children, and cancerous tumours. Brain tissue and rapidly growing tissues are the two types of human tissue which normally display the greatest electrical activity, and this is what renders them particularly sensitive to electromagnetic fields. This agrees well with the traditional Taoist view, which cites children as having far more active energy auras than adults and identifies the brain as the main centre of the refined electromagnetic energy associated with True Human Energy.

In June 1989, the *New Yorker* magazine ran a three-part series on the health hazards of exposure to electric power lines and computer terminals, based on several exhaustive scientific studies. These studies found that leukaemia and other cancers in children are closely linked to exposure to electric power fields, and that pregnant women who work long hours at computer terminals suffer a significantly higher rate of miscarriage than others. If you or your children sleep in a room within 50–100 feet of electric power lines or transformers, you'd be well advised either to switch rooms or, if necessary, move elsewhere. The same goes for your places of work, recreation, and other activities.

A growing number of people whose work exposes them to artificial electromagnetic fields, as in the computer and electronics industries in California's Silicon Valley, have been reporting the full range of symptoms associated with immune deficiency syndrome, including chronic fatigue, hypersensitivity, allergies, headaches, chronic depression, and the inevitable cover-all of 'flu-like symptoms'. The medical establishment's claims that HIV causes AIDS is based on the observation that HIV kills or impairs the function of some T-cells in a culture dish in the laboratory. Recently, Dr Daniel Lyle of the Veterans' Hospital in Loma Linda, California, exposed human T-cells in a culture dish in the laboratory to a 60-Hz electric field (similar to ordinary power lines) for forty-eight hours. He reported a significant impairment of the T-cells' capacity to fight foreign cells and microbes. This implicates abnormal electromagnetic fields as a causative factor in AIDS, yet today the entire population is chronically exposed to immunosuppressive electromagnetism in homes, offices, and schools, as well as in hospitals and clinics. In fact, one of the most hazardous of all such environments is the modern operating room, with all its various electronic and microwave gadgets.

Besides the growing incidence of Down's syndrome, sudden infant death syndrome (SIDS) is also on the rise throughout the industrially developed world. It has already been established that abnormal electromagnetic fields have a suppressive influence on the pineal gland, which secretes melatonin and other vital neurochemicals. Recent studies have revealed that victims of SIDS have significantly lower levels of melatonin in their brain plasma than ordinary infants, so it is reasonable to conclude that melatonin deficiency is associated with SIDS and that some environmental factor is suppressing melatonin secretions in SIDS victims. In England, Dr Cornelia O'Leary of the Royal College of Surgeons reported eight SIDS deaths in one weekend within a seven-mile radius of a high-security military base where a powerful new radar system was being tested that weekend. Indeed, military radar facilities have been implicated time and again in unexplained outbreaks of cancer, birth defects, and autoimmune diseases among otherwise healthy people living nearby, but government authorities consistently cite 'national security' as an excuse not to acknowledge and investigate this issue. What good are elaborate defence facilities built against alleged foreign threats if they kill and disable our own children?

The medical establishment is fond of citing a minor reduction in the mortality rate of a few types of cancer as evidence that they are 'winning the war on cancer'. In fact, there has recently been such a rapid increase in the incidence and mortality rate of other, formerly negligible cancers, such as brain, spinal, and colon cancer, that the overall incidence and mortality rate for all cancers has risen significantly. Another formerly rare cancer that has increased in incidence in the USA by a whopping 80 per cent between 1973 and 1980 is melanoma skin cancer. Ozone depletion is usually cited as the cause. However, one place where the incidence of melanoma is four times greater than the already rapidly rising national average is among the staff at the Lawrence Livermore National Laboratory in California. This institute is deeply involved in developing exotic new weapons systems using high-intensity magnetic fields and high-frequency microwaves.

Studies in Sweden and England have observed significant rises in suicide rates among young people living and going to school in close proximity to electric power lines or radar stations. Manic depression and suicide are often related to low levels of serotonin, also secreted by the pineal gland. The record shows that between 1950 and 1977 in the USA, the suicide rate among 15–19-year-olds rose fourfold for males and twofold for females. This time frame coincides with a manifold increase in the exposure of children to television sets, electric appliances, electronic toys, fluorescent lighting, power lines, and so on.

While there is nothing much you can do about electromagnetic pollution from power lines, radar stations, broadcasting towers, and other public sources condoned by the government, short of moving to a less exposed location, there is no need to spend hours irradiating yourself with television, electric blankets, and other home appliances. Bearing in mind that fields of only 3 milligauss have been conclusively linked to greatly increased risks of brain cancer, genetic damage, and birth defects, let's take a quick look at the fields generated by common household appliances.

Television
In addition to the electromagnetic field generated by the power source, television sets also emit X-rays that can penetrate 2–3 inches into the human body. With most sets, you must sit at least 42 inches away from the screen in order to avoid exposure to dangerous fields. Those fields emit in all directions and can easily penetrate wood and other solid materials, so be sure that no one has a bed or desk placed against the opposite side of a wall where a television set is located.

Electric blankets
These devices produce fields in the 50–100-milligauss range, far above safe levels. Dr Nancy Wertheimer of the University of Colorado studied the effects of electric blankets on pregnant women and found a far higher rate of miscarriage among women who use them. They are more dangerous than other electric appliances because they are so close to the body and there is a long period of continuous exposure during sleep.

Electric razors
When operated from a plug-in power line, electric razors generate highly intense fields ranging from 200 to 400 milligauss. Men who use electric razors would be well advised to discard them in favour of safety razors.

PCs and VDTs
Personal computers and video display terminals have been linked to a doubling in the rate in miscarriages and a much higher than average rate of birth defects in women who operate them during pregnancy. Non-pregnant women also report a variety of disorders, including menstrual irregularities, headaches, chronic fatigue, and depression.

Fluorescent lights
The detrimental effects of abnormal light waves emitted by fluorescent tubes, especially on children, are discussed in detail in *The Tao of HS&L*. In addition to abnormal light, these devices also produce abnormal electromagnetic fields. A 10-watt fluorescent tube produces a twenty times stronger field than an ordinary 60-watt

light bulb. In offices and school rooms lit by multiple banks of fluorescent tubes in the ceilings, everyone in the room is irradiated.

Electric clocks
Ordinary plug-in electric clocks produce fields of 5–10 milligauss at a distance of two feet. Since alarm clocks are usually placed within this distance from the head for up to eight hours every night, it would be a good idea to use an ordinary wind-up or a battery-operated alarm clock instead.

Hair dryers
These produce a field of 50 milligauss at six inches, which is more than enough to increase the risk of brain tumours and other cancers, as well as genetic damage. It has long been noted that female beauticians have abnormally high rates of breast cancer, which may well be due to the occupational hazard of operating hair dryers within six inches of their breasts.

Electric stoves
A 12-inch burner on an electric stove produces a field of 50 milligauss at a distance of 18 inches. If you do a lot of cooking at home, it's much safer to use gas.

Telephones
Cordless and cellular telephones, as well as wireless intercoms and all radio-controlled toys and household appliances, create electromagnetic fields when in use, and in the case of phones, which are held against the head, the abnormal field goes straight through the brain. Exposure to radio-generated electromagnetism has been linked to increased risks of leukaemia in amateur radio operators, so you might want to think twice about buying your children toys that are operated by remote radio control.

In summary, it has become abundantly clear that the simple chemical-mechanistic view of human health upon which orthodox Western medicine is based fails to account for vital factors: energy and energy fields. The human organism and the various energies that animate it evolved within the energy band of the earth's own natural electromagnetic field, a field which modern technology distorts and overrides by power lines, broadcasting stations, microwave transmitters, household appliances, and military installations. When government agencies assure you that 'everything is all right' and your doctor tells you there's 'nothing to worry about', it does not mean there's no risk. Only a few decades ago, the same agencies and doctors denied that smoking cigarettes posed any significant health risk, and they still deny that white sugar, hydrogenated vegetable oils, and food additives can cause cancer and immune deficiency. It is up to individuals to familiarize themselves with the facts and demand corrective measures by exercising the powers of collective dissent and the ballot box, for the evidence is in, and it is conclusive: electromagnetic fields exert decisive influences on human health through the medium of energy. As Dr Robert Becker writes in *Cross Currents*:

> The data obtained in the past few years indicate very clearly that we must now include the Earth's normal geomagnetic field as an environmental variable of great consequence when we deal with the basic functions of living things. In my opinion, this knowledge is probably the single most important discovery of the century. It provides us with a key to the mechanisms by which all electromagnetic fields produce biological effects, and it may enable us to determine more accurately the risks involved in our technological uses of such fields.

CHAPTER 13

Chee-gung:
The Skill of Energy Control

Chi Kung [*chee-gung*] is the science of working with the
body's energy field.
Dr Yang Jwing-ming, *The Root of Chinese Chi Kung* (1989)

Chee means 'breath' and 'air' as well as 'energy', indicating the vital
role breathing plays in transmitting the atmospheric energy of air
into the human system. *Gung* means 'work', 'skill', and achievement' and refers to any skill that requires a lot of time and effort to
achieve. *Chee-gung*, which enables the practitioner to cultivate
and control his or her own energy, may therefore be translated as
'energy work' or 'energy skill'.

Chee-gung has four basic applications: health, longevity, martial
power, and spiritual enlightenment. In this book, we are concerned
mainly with the first two goals – promoting health and prolonging
life – which are prerequisites for achieving any other goals that
require a lot of time and energy. Whether you use the enhanced
health and longevity which *chee-gung* provides for purposes of
power or enlightenment, hedonism or mysticism, is entirely up
to you.

Chee-gung dates back to prehistoric times in ancient China and is
mentioned in the earliest written records of Chinese history.
Originally practised as a form of therapeutic dance to cure rheumatism and ward off other symptoms of excess Damp Evil in the
flood-prone Yellow River basin where Chinese civilization first
evolved, *chee-gung* gradually developed into a complete system of
human energy management with medical and martial, as well as
meditative, applications. In a second-century AD text entitled *Dance
Verse*, the scholar Fu Yi wrote: '*Chee-gung* is an art that pleases the
spirit, slows the aging process, and prolongs life.' In the *Collective
Commentaries on Chuang Tzu*, dating from the same period, Cheng
Yuan-lin wrote: 'Breathing practised together with movements

resembling a bear, bird, and other animals helps move our *chee*, nourishes our bodies, and builds our spirits.' In those days, *chee-gung* was based primarily on movements learned by observing animals in nature. Arm exercises, for example, were drawn from the manner in which birds flap their wings, leg exercises imitated a tiger's gait, shoulder postures were learned from watching bears, and so forth. This early form of *chee-gung* was called *wu chin hsi*, or the 'Play of the Five Beasts'.

From the earliest times, the importance of soft, flowing exercise in cultivating the essence and energy that lie at the root of human health was clearly recognized by the Chinese. In the fourth-century BC Confucian classic entitled *Spring and Autumn Annals*, we find the following statement: 'Flowing water never stagnates, and the hinges of an active door never rust. This is due to movement. The same principle applies to essence and energy. If the body does not move, essence does not flow. When essence does not flow, energy stagnates.'

The renowned physician Hua Tuo, a centenarian who flourished during the Eastern Han dynasty (AD 25–220), prescribed a series of energy exercises called *dao-yin* ('induce and guide') for various common ailments, including arthritis, rheumatism, digestive disorders, nervous afflictions, and circulatory problems. He wrote: 'The body requires exercise, but exercise must not be excessive . . . When the blood pulses unobstructed through the veins, illness cannot take root. This is like a door hinge that cannot rust owing to frequent use.' Ko Hung, a great alchemist and one of China's most prolific Taoist writers, who lived in the century after Hua To, wrote in his monumental Taoist compendium *Bao Pu Tzu* ('Embracing the Uncarved Block'): 'The onset of illness is a sign that *chee* is not flowing. One must exercise in order to unblock the myriad meridians and facilitate the free flow of *chee*.' *Chee-gung* has been practised as a form of preventive as well as curative health care ever since ancient times in China.

During the fifth century AD, Chinese *chee-gung* took a giant evolutionary step forward under the influence of the eccentric, ragged old monk from India named Bodhidharma, whom the Chinese called Ta Mo. Formerly the prince of a minor kingdom in southern India, Bodhidharma gave up his wealth and title in order to practise an ascetic, esoteric form of Buddhism called 'tantra', which stressed the importance of personal practice and spontaneous in-sight. Following a visionary impulse, Bodhidharma crossed the barren plateaus of Tibet on foot and suddenly appeared on the scene in southern China during a period of political disunity and intellectual ferment known as the Six Dynasties Era.

Many legends enshroud the mysterious figure of Bodhidharma in Chinese history. He was renowned for his ability to sit in silent meditation for days on end without stirring. What is known for certain is that he brought *pranayama* breathing exercises from India, combined them with Chinese *dao-yin* and 'Play of the Five Beasts' forms, and taught this new system to monks and martial artists in Chinese monasteries, such as the famous Shao Lin monastery. Ever since that time, Bodhidharma has been revered as the patron saint of all schools of Chinese martial arts, including offshoots in Korea and Japan, and also as the founder of Chan Buddhism, better known in the West by its Japanese name, Zen. The unique system of breathing and exercise which he devised is the source of all subsequent schools of *chee-gung* in China.

Bodhidharma is credited as the author of two remarkable classics which have become the bibles of *chee-gung* for martial artists, meditators, and medical therapists alike. One is called the *Tendon Changing Classic* (*Yi Jin Jing*) and the other the *Marrow Cleansing Classic* (*Hsi Sui Jing*). These two manuals go hand in hand, and together they lead the adept from the most basic stretching exercises up to the most advanced techniques of internal energy alchemy. Dr Yang Jwing-ming has written a good English translation and commentary on both classics under the title *Muscle/Tendon Changing and Marrow/Brain Washing Chi Kung,* listed in the appendix 'Recommended Reading'.

The forms of *chee-gung* taught in the *Tendon Changing Classic* and *Marrow Cleansing Classic* are different but complementary. The *Tendon Classic* focuses mainly on toning and energizing the muscles, tendons, and fasciae, on circulating energy through the twelve major organ meridians, on moving energy to the surface to enhance the guardian shield of *wei-chee,* and on cultivating post-natal Fire energy. The marrow-cleansing exercises direct energy inwards into the bones and marrow and upwards into the spinal fluids and brain, build up reservoirs of energy in the eight extraordinary channels, and cultivate prenatal Water energy by transforming the original essence of hormones.

Students of *chee-gung* usually begin their training with exercises derived from the *Tendon Changing Classic,* which builds physical strength, enhances health and vitality, increases energy resources, and forms a firm foundation for the more advanced practices derived from the *Marrow Cleansing Classic.* The term 'tendon changing' refers to the significant increase in the power, flexibility, and resilience of muscles and tendons brought about by these exercises, which pack and store energy into a condensed form of connective tissue called 'fasciae'. Fasciae are flat, slippery, flexible tissues which envelop and lubricate all muscles, tendons, and ligaments. Thanks to their concentrated content of electrolytes – mineralized fluids which conduct electric energy in ionic form – fasciae have the capacity to absorb and store the electrically charged ion energy of *chee*.

The term 'marrow cleansing' refers to the rejuvenation of marrow effected by the practice of exercises from the classic of that name. In *The Root of Chinese Chi Kung*, Dr Yang explains the importance of marrow-cleansing exercises as follows:

> According to Chinese medicine, your body deteriorates mainly because your blood loses its ability to feed and protect your body. Your bone marrow produces the red blood cells and one type of the white blood cells, but as you grow older, the marrow becomes 'dirty', and produces fewer and fewer useful blood cells. However, if you know how to 'wash' the marrow, it will start once again to produce fresh, healthy blood. Your body will begin to rejuvenate itself, and restore itself to the glowing health of youth . . . To keep the marrow fresh and alive and functioning properly, Chi must be plentiful and continuously supplied. Whenever there is a shortage of Chi, the marrow will not function properly.

In traditional Chinese medicine as well as Taoist alchemy, the brain is regarded as a form of marrow, since it too is a soft, secreting tissue encased in bone. Therefore, the marrow-cleansing exercises are also designed to guide and sublimate energy upwards through the spinal fluid into the brain, thereby stimulating the secretion of neurohormones and enhancing all cerebral functions. Marrow-cleansing exercises also stimulate the entire endocrine system to produce abundant supplies of vital hormone essence as fuel for internal energy alchemy.

Of all forms of vital essence, by far the most potent is the 'sexual essence' of male and female hormones, semen, and other sexual secretions. One of the unique hallmarks of the *Marrow Cleansing Classic* is a series of solo sexual exercises – or 'sexercises' – for male and for female adepts. These exercises, which sometimes strike newcomers to the Tao as rather bizarre, are designed to be practised alone, not with sexual partners, and they specifically stimulate the body to secrete extra supplies of sexual hormones, semen, lubricants, and related sexual fluids. The enhanced sexual vitality obtained thereby was not meant to be used for sexual intercourse, for these exercises were practised by celibate monks and recluses as well as by lay persons, but rather to provide adepts of internal alchemy with extra supplies of sexual essence. This essence is then transformed into energy and sublimated upwards into the spine and brain to accelerate spiritual development. A set of basic 'sexercises' for men and women is presented below in the illustrated section on exercises.

Since the time of Bodhidharma, *chee-gung* practice has been categorized into various degrees of internal and external forms called *nei-dan* ('Internal Elixir') and *wai-dan* ('External Elixir'). *Nei-dan* and *wai-dan* are opposite poles of practice on a scale calibrated according to the degree of stillness and motion in any particular form of exercise. On the extreme end of the Internal Elixir scale is still-sitting meditation, while examples of extreme External Elixir exercises are such 'hard' moving forms as weight lifting, fighting techniques, and field sports. While exercises from the *Tendon Changing Classic* are somewhat more externally oriented than those from the *Marrow Cleansing Classic*, both are balanced forms which include elements of *nei-dan* and *wai-dan* harmoniously combined, and most of the traditional Chinese *chee-gung* exercises which evolved from these two classics stand in the middle of the Internal/External Elixir scale (Fig. 12).

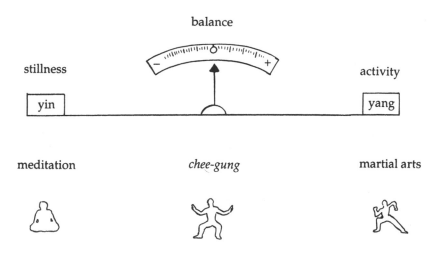

Fig. 12 Internal (*nei-dan*) and External (*wai-dan*) scale in Taoist practice: *chee-gung* balances the internal stillness of meditation with the external activity of martial arts.

The key to achieving balance between *nei-dan* and *wai-dan* forms is to establish a state of calm awareness in which the high-frequency activity of the cerebral cortex is put to rest in order to permit the restorative low-frequency oscillation of the parasympathetic nervous system to take over control of the body's organs and functions. In this state, the soothing low-frequency pulse of the earth's electromagnetic field harmonizes and boosts the human energy system. As the *Tendon Changing Classic* states: 'Of paramount importance is to seek movement within quiescence and to seek quiescence within movement, moving softly and continuously until one enters the sublime state.' Internal energy is induced to flow by virtue of soft, continuous external movements harmonized with deep, diaphragmic breathing, under conditions of mental calm and quietude. Because of this *chee-gung* is sometimes referred to as 'moving meditation'.

Benefits of chee-gung practice

The benefits of *chee-gung* practice may be summarized in two words which crop up again and again in the literature and lore of esoteric Taoist alchemy: balance and harmony. Balance includes equilibrium between yin and yang, Fire and Water, body and mind, and harmony refers to synchrony among the Five Elemental Energies of the internal organ systems, the Three Treasures of essence, energy, and spirit, the Three Powers of heaven, earth, and humans, and the various electromagnetic frequencies of our internal and external environments. Let's take a brief look at what this means in concrete terms of physiology and bioenergetics.

Central nervous system

Beginners often ask why *chee-gung* exercises must always be performed like a slow-motion movie. 'Why not just speed up and get on with it?' they ask. Speed is the scourge of modern life and the enemy of rest and relaxation. In the mad rush to 'save time', people today subject their central nervous systems to such extreme and chronic states of hypertension that they undermine their own health and shorten their own lives, wasting precious reserves of energy in a self-defeating battle against time.

The psychophysiological effect of performing soft, slow movements in conjunction with deep diaphragmic breathing is to switch the autonomous nervous system over from the chronically overactive sympathetic mode to the calming, restorative parasympathetic mode, in which the body's various vital functions and energies are balanced and harmonized and secretions of vital essence such as hormones and neurochemicals are stimulated. In order to initiate this switch-over in our circuitry, we must perform the exercises slowly, softly, and smoothly with a calm and quiet mind. Once the parasympathetic system has taken over control of the central nervous system, its calming influence helps to promote and maintain mental tranquillity. In this way, *chee-gung* counteracts the chronic stress and strain of daily life on the body as well as the mind, which in Chinese medicine are inseparable, and restores optimum equilibrium to essence, energy, and spirit. In Taoist parlance, *chee-gung* balances the depleting yang Fire energy of temporal life by cultivating the soothing, restorative yin Water energy derived from hormones and neurochemicals.

Bio feedback of the endocrine and nervous systems

When asked to summarize the essential mechanism of *chee-gung*, Master Luo Teh-hsiou of Taiwan put it this way:

> When properly practised, *chee-gung* activates the parasympathetic circuit of the central nervous system, thereby stimulating the production of neurochemicals which cause the endocrine system to secrete hormones that enhance vitality and boost immunity. Those hormones also help sustain further production of calming parasympathetic neurochemicals. This mutual interaction continues until perfect equilibrium is established between the nervous and endocrine systems, and when that happens, the true energy of human health and longevity is generated.

In other words, *chee-gung* orchestrates perfect balance between body and brain by establishing a condition of beneficial biofeedback between the nervous and endocrine systems. This fosters a form of energy called 'True Energy' (*jeng-chee*), which is the basis of human health and longevity.

In an article entitled 'Mental Muscle' in the May 1992 issue of *Omni* magazine, Kathy Keeton describes this same mechanism in modern medical terms:

> Over the past ten years, there's been an explosion of evidence linking the power of the mind to the health of the

body, and experts in the new field of *psychoneuroimmunology*, or PNI, are gaining a greater understanding of how the brain and the body can cooperate to fight off illness. It's been discovered, for one thing, that there are nerve fibers in the thymus, the immune system's master gland, as well as in the spleen, the lymph nodes, and the bone marrow – all vital parts of the immune system. Some immune system cells have receptors for neuropeptides, chemicals that are produced within the brain itself. In other words, there's a growing body of evidence to suggest that the brain talks directly to the immune system via this electrochemical version of AT&T.

Over the past 5,000 years in China, Taoist science has accumulated a vast reservoir of evidence linking the powers of body and mind, neurology and immunology, and has developed specific techniques for activating that link, but only recently have Western investigators taken a serious look at this remarkably effective system of human health care.

Acid/alkaline balance

Another aspect of yin and yang which *chee-gung* effectively regulates is the acid/alkaline balance in the bloodstream. Physical exercise acidifies the blood with lactic acid, while deep breathing has the opposite effect of alkalizing the blood. Therefore, excess physical exercise or deep breathing, when performed alone, can lead to imbalances in blood pH. *Chee-gung*, which combines gentle rhythmic movements of the body with deep diaphragmic breathing, maintains optimum balance between acidity and alkalinity in the blood and other bodily fluids.

Harmonizing the human electromagnetic field with the earth

Research at Jiao Tong University in Shanghai, China, has shown that the energy emitted by *chee-gung* masters during practice pulses at a frequency of 2–10 Hz, which falls within the normal subsonic range of the earth's own natural electromagnetic field. *Chee-gung* thus tunes the human energy system into the natural frequency of the earth, thereby 'plugging' the practitioner directly into the earth's energy field. This has a soothing, rejuvenating effect on the human energy system and helps correct energy imbalances and biochemical disorders caused by exposure to artificially generated electromagnetic fields.

Circulation

Chee-gung practice is perhaps the most effective of all ways to improve circulation of blood and energy. 'Stagnant blood' and 'stagnant energy' have for thousands of years been recognized by Chinese physicians as primary causes of human disease, degeneration, and death. Since 'blood follows where energy leads', promoting circulation of energy through the meridian network automatically enhances circulation of blood through veins, arteries, and capillaries. Deep diaphragmic breathing acts as a pump or 'second heart' to drive energy and blood through their respective vessels, while slow rhythmic movements of limbs and torso draw blood and energy into every nook and cranny of the body. This particularly benefits the brain by irrigating it with abundant supplies of freshly oxygenated blood, glucose, and other nutrients. The pineal and pituitary glands, which secrete vital neurochemicals such as serotonin, melatonin, dopamine, and growth hormone, are stimulated and balanced by enhanced cerebral circulation of blood and energy and by restoration of natural electromagnetic frequencies in the brain. Enhanced circulation also nourishes and energizes all the other vital organs and glands and helps detoxify tissues by carrying away metabolic wastes and delivering white blood cells, enzymes, and other immune factors to dissolve accumulated toxins, damaged cells, and undesirable microbes and parasites.

Immunity and resistance

Chee-gung expands and strengthens the radiant shield of protective *wei-chee* around the body, thereby guarding against invasion by adverse environmental energies (The Six Evils) as well as abnormal electromagnetic and microwave radiation. People often remark on the 'glow of health' which radiates from practitioners of *chee-gung* and Taoist meditation. If you stand next to such a person and close your eyes you can actually feel the aura of guardian energy emanating from his or her body. People who have developed so-called 'astral vision', an innate ability shared by all humans but dormant in most, can 'see' such auric energies as waves of coloured light.

The internal immune system also receives a strong boost from the regular practice of *chee-gung*, which stimulates secretions of vital hormones throughout the endocrine system, especially in the all-important adrenal cortex. Being strategically placed on top of the kidneys, the adrenal glands receive a stimulating massage from the descending diaphragm with every inhalation. The thymus gland, which produces T-cells and is located near the heart, benefits from the rhythmic expansion and contraction of the chest during deep breathing exercises. Bone marrow, which produces red and white blood cells, is cleansed and energized by *chee-gung* practice, which drives energy into the fasciae, tendons, and bones. The rhythmic movement of limbs in conjunction with deep diaphragmic breathing also stimulates the flow of lymph, keeping it fresh and clean so that it may properly perform its blood- and tissue-purifying duties. It has long been observed in China, and more recently in the West, that people who practice *chee-gung* suffer a far lower incidence of colds, flu, infections, and other common maladies, even when directly exposed to infected people.

Energy balance

Chee-gung is without question the most effective guardian and regulator of human energy. Among other things, it immediately corrects any imbalances in yin and yang, Water and Fire, and Five Elemental Energies in the human system. Since the stress and toxicity of modern living inevitably leads to a state of extreme yang and Fire excess, *chee-gung* provides a simple and effective method for correcting this imbalance on a daily basis. Dr Yang Jwing-ming describes this aspect of *chee-gung* as follows:

> Chi Kung practitioners believe theoretically that your body is always too Yang unless you are sick or have not eaten for a long time, in which case your body may be more Yin. When your body is always Yang, it is degenerating and burning out. It is believed that this is the cause of aging. If you are able to use 'Water' to cool down your body, you will be able to slow down the degeneration process and thereby lengthen your life. This is the main reason why Chinese Chi Kung practitioners have been studying ways of improving the quality of Water in their bodies, and of reducing the quantity of Fire.

Chee-gung has six basic effects on human energy which, over time, greatly improve the quality, balance, and availability of energy, and enhance the efficiency of digestion, metabolism, circulation, excretion, sex, cellular division, and other vital functions which depend upon steady supplies of energy:

Movement
Chee-gung keeps energy circulating through the body's vast network of energy channels, thereby preventing stagnation.

Transformation
Chee-gung activates internal alchemy, transforming and refining sexual and nutrient energy into cerebral and spiritual forms, which in turn expand awareness and improve cerebral functions. It promotes the efficient conversion of nutrient and hormone essence into energy and tames Fire by cultivating Water.

Exchange
Chee-gung expels stagnant and polluted energy from the system by dredging the energy channels with pure potent energy derived from food, air, and conversion of hormone essence. It also enhances the body's exchange of energy with the environment and with sexual partners.

Balance
Chee-gung keeps the vital energies properly balanced and harmonized at all levels, including yin and yang, Fire and Water, Five Elemental Energies, sacral and cranial, heaven and earth, nourishing and protective.

Storage
Chee-gung generates, collects, and stores energy in various vital energy centres, especially the three Elixir Fields in the lower abdomen, solar plexus, and brain. It fills the reservoirs of the Eight Extraordinary Channels with fresh energy, which is then distributed as required into the twelve major organ meridians. It also stores energy in the electrolytes of the body's vital fluids, particularly the brain, spine, marrow, fasciae, and endocrine glands.

Control
Energy commands essence, and spirit commands energy, hence the practice of *chee-gung* trains the mind to take conscious command of energy. This is an extremely useful skill which may be effectively used to control emotions, direct healing energy to ailing or weak organs, prevent 'rebellious' organ energy from

rising into the head, and improve the efficiency of internal alchemy during *chee-gung* and meditation practice. When highly developed, energy control may be applied to project healing energy to others.

Points of practice

When practising *chee-gung*, it helps to bear in mind a few basic points, foremost of which are the Taoist themes of balance and harmony. When we speak of balancing Fire and Water, for example, you should be aware that Fire energy springs from the heart, belongs to yang, and runs through the heart meridians along the arms, while Water comes from the kidneys, belongs to yin, and is conducted by the kidney channels in the legs. Synchronized movements of arms and legs combined with deep diaphragmic breathing bring these two basic energies into harmony.

Similarly, the Three Powers of heaven, earth, and humanity each has its own locus on the body. The energy of heaven is drawn down through the crown of the head, the energy of earth comes up from the soles of the feet, and they meet and mix with human energy in the pelvic region, particularly in the Lower Elixir Field below the navel and in the coccyx. A 2,000-year-old text on *chee-gung* inscribed on jade tablets states: 'Celestial energy is activated above, and terrestial energy below.'

'Externally, practise the form; internally, practise the meaning,' advises an ancient Taoist maxim. This means that you should practise the forms properly with your body, while contemplating the inner meaning and purpose of those forms with your mind. Here again we see why *chee-gung* is regarded as a form of moving meditation.

Breathing

Correct breathing is the most important aspect of *chee-gung* practice, for breath is the key to energy control as well as the bridge between body and mind. The longest chapter in *The Tao of HS&L* is the one on breathing, so readers may refer to that for detailed information on the subject. Here we'll briefly review a few basic points on the role of breathing in *chee-gung* practice.

The major difference between the way most adults ordinarily breathe and the way *chee-gung* adepts breathe is in the use of the diaphragm and abdomen as breathing pumps. This is what is meant by 'deep' breathing: the breath is drawn deep down into the bottom of the lungs by virtue of diaphragmic flex, which causes the abdomen to expand on inhalation and contract on exhalation. Inhalation is the yin stage of breathing: it condenses air into the lungs and draws energy down into the lower abdomen, driving it through the meridians and into the marrow and brain. Exhalation is yang: it expands breath outwards and causes energy to spread externally towards skin and muscles, enhancing the radiant shield of protective *chee* around the body.

Not only does the diaphragm act as a pump to circulate blood and energy, it also massages the internal organs. Dr Yang Jwing-ming writes in *The Root of Chinese Chi Kung*:

> Deep and calm breathing relaxes you, keeps your mind clear, and fills your lungs with plenty of air so that your brain and entire body have an adequate supply of oxygen. In addition, deep and complete breathing enables the diaphragm to move up and down, which massages and stimulates the internal organs. For this reason, deep breathing exercises are also called 'internal organ exercises'.

Deep abdominal breathing is also the key to tapping the potent resouces of 'original essence' and converting it into pure Water energy. In his book on the *Tendon Changing Classic*, Dr Yang explains:

> In order to increase the quantity of Chi, you must find its source. It was discovered that Chi has two major sources. One is the food and air you take in. The Chi which comes from this source is considered Fire Chi. The second source is the Original Essence you inherited from your parents. The Chi converted from this source is considered Water Chi . . . Since it is relatively easy to control the quality of food and air, most of the research has been directed at increasing the quantity and improving the quality of Water Chi.
>
> After long years of study and research, it was concluded that in order to increase the quantity of Water Chi, you must imitate the way a baby breathes. When a baby breathes, its abdomen naturally moves in and out. Finally, the Chi Kung practitioners discovered that there is a spot in the lower abdomen which can store an unlimited amount of Chi, once it has been converted

from the Original Essence which resides in the Kidneys. The trick of increasing the efficiency of the conversion of Original Essence to Chi is through abdominal exercises.

There are many different breathing techniques used in *chee-gung* and meditation, nine of which are briefly described below:

Natural breathing
This is the beginner's breath. Rather than trying actively to control your breathing, you simply observe and feel its rhythmic rise and fall in the abdomen. Emotional calm and mental quietude are pre-requisites for this and all other types of regulated breathing, because emotions and thoughts have a disruptive impact on rhythmic breathing patterns.

Chest breathing
This is the way most people ordinarily breathe, by expanding and contracting the ribcage rather than the diaphragm and abdomen. It is most suitable for bursts of intense exercise and fast motion, such as 'hard' forms of martial arts, but it is an impediment to *chee-gung* and meditation practice.

Normal abdominal breathing
This is the primary breath in *chee-gung* and meditation, performed slowly, deeply, and deliberately with the diaphragm, letting the abdomen expand on inhalation and contract on exhalation. It massages the internal organs and glands, tones the abdominal muscles, draws energy into the Lower Elixir Field, and promotes the conversion of original hormone essence into cool, restorative Water energy.

Reverse abdominal breathing
This is an advanced version of abdominal breathing used for some exercises by experienced *chee-gung* adepts. The diaphragm expands downwards on inhalation as in normal abdominal breathing, but instead of letting the abdomen expand outwards, you contract the abdominal muscles to draw the abdominal wall inwards. On exhalation, you relax the muscles and let the abdomen expand outwards as the diaphragm rises. Internal abdominal pressure is greatly increased with this breath, enhancing the diaphragmic massage of the vital organs, giving an extra boost to circulation of blood and energy, and driving *chee* into the marrow and up to the brain.

Breath retention
Breath retention is a popular technique in Indian *pranayama* breathing, but is not used much in *chee-gung* practice. It is, however, employed by some Taoist adepts for advanced meditation. The method is discussed in detail in *The Tao of HS&L*, and readers should not go beyond the instructions given therein without personal guidance from an experienced master. Many strange things can happen as a result of prolonged breath retention when improperly practised, including deviations which Taoists refer to as 'playing with fire, possessed by demons' (*dzou huo ru muo*). Don't play with fire!

Long breathing
This method works with full, deep, long inhalations and exhalations. Abdominal and natural breathing use only 70–80 per cent of lung capacity, whereas long breathing works with full capacity. This type of breath increases the amount of oxygen absorbed and carbon dioxide expelled, drives more energy out to the skin on exhalation, and packs more energy into the marrow on inhalation. It is usually practised in sitting-meditation *chee-gung* rather than with moving exercises.

Body breathing
With this breath, you focus on the feeling of expansion and contraction in the abdominal region and visualize the radiant bubble of energy around your body expanding and contracting at the same time, like a big balloon. As you progress with this breath, you may actually start 'breathing' through your skin, exchanging energy directly with the external environment. This can be practised standing still or sitting still.

Palm and sole breathing
In this mode of breathing, you feel and visualize *chee* entering and exiting from the vital energy points located in the middle of the palms or soles as you breathe. The palm point is called the 'Labour Palace' and the sole point is the 'Bubbling Spring'. These are powerful points, and it usually does not take long for beginners to be able to feel *chee* flowing through them. The feeling is somewhat akin to a valve or flap opening and closing at the beginning of inhalation and the end of exhalation. This is a good way to expel excess heat from the body and to absorb fresh *chee* from the environment. It may be practised standing or sitting still, as well as during moving exercises.

Transport breathing
This breath requires a lot of concentration and a basic familiarity with the feeling of *chee* moving within the meridians and channels. Using the mind to lead energy and the breath to drive it, you transport *chee* to any organ, limb, or tissue you wish to energize. It's an excellent self-healing technique and can be used to dissolve tumours and cysts, stimulate sluggish organs and glands, and deliver blood and energy to stagnant tissues. This method requires extensive practice and is most effective during still sitting. Beginners may wish to try it in conjunction with natural or normal abdominal breathing, because it's a good way to start cultivating mental control over the flow of internal energy.

Most of the time you'll be using the normal abdominal mode of breathing in your *chee-gung* practice. In order properly to regulate your breathing patterns during practice, it's helpful to keep the following eight qualities in mind:

Silent
Make your breathing as silent as possible. This requires that you breathe slowly and smoothly and keep your mind focused on your breath.

Fine
The stream of air flowing in and out of your nose and throat should be very fine, like a gentle breeze, not coarse and choppy like a rustling wind.

Slow
Each and every inhalation and exhalation should be performed slowly and deliberately, without rushing on to the next breath. To do this, your mind must also be completely calm and unhurried. Instead of watching the clock, watch your breath.

Deep
Draw each breath deep down into the abdomen by letting the lungs push the diaphragm downwards. This does not mean filling the lungs 100 per cent full, for that would cause the chest, shoulder, and neck muscles to tense up. Inhale to about 70–80 per cent capacity, remaining as relaxed as possible while the abdomen expands, then switch slowly and smoothly over to exhalation and draw the abdomen inwards as the diaphragm rises.

Long
Make your inhalations and exhalations as long as possible without straining or tensing the chest and abdomen. This requires that you breathe deeply and slowly and keep your mind focused on your breath.

Soft
Cultivate a feeling of softness and smoothness while you breathe by keeping your muscles relaxed, your breath slow, and your mind calm.

Continuous
Each inhalation should flow smoothly into the next exhalation, followed by another inhalation, and so forth, without pausing or retaining the breath in between. Let inhalation and exhalation follow one another naturally and continuously, like the pendulum of a clock.

Even
Try to make your inhalations and exhalations even in length and duration. This requires emotional equilibrium and mental quietude. It also provides the mind with something to focus on during practice.

General rules of practice

When adapting *chee-gung* as an integral part of your daily routine, you should follow the traditional guidelines formulated by the ancient Chinese masters, based on thousands of years of experience. Observing these rules will accelerate your progress and help avoid common pitfalls along the way:

● Do not take up the practice of *chee-gung* with any preconceived notions or grand expectations regarding results. Simply follow instructions and practise diligently, keeping your mind open and aware.

● Do not permit your mind to get distracted by external phenomena or peculiar sensations while practising *chee-gung*. Remain peripherally aware of your surroundings and sensations, but focus attention primarily on the form and content of the exercises you're practising.

● Try to keep your mind clear of discursive thoughts and avoid the mental rambling of internal dialogue.

● Keep the Five Thieves of sensory distractions under control during practice: sight, sound, smell, taste, feel. Instead of letting the senses reach outwards turn them inwards and focus their attention on breath, energy, pulse, and vital organs.

● Regulate your sexual activities, especially during periods of intensive *chee-gung* practice. Men should either practise 'Dual Cultivation' methods, retaining semen and regulating ejaculation according to Taoist precepts, or else reduce frequency of intercourse. Men should not practise *chee-gung* immediately after ejaculation or ejaculate immediately after practice.

● Avoid exposure to excess heat or cold during practice. In hot weather, practice in the shade, not out in the sun. When it's cold, dress warmly.

● When feeling ill or fatigued, practise gently and slowly, without excessive exertion, and stop to rest when you get tired.

● Avoid exposure to winds when practising. *Chee-gung* opens the pores and energy channels, so it's easy to contract 'wind injury' in strong cold, dry, damp, or other conditions of Wind Evil. Wind also has a tendency to scatter *chee* during *chee-gung* practice. For the same reason, it's best not to bathe for at least twenty minutes after practice, until the pores close.

● Remove watches, bracelets, and any other binding objects from the limbs, and loosen belts and buttons, especially around the waist. Even the slightest pressure against the skin can inhibit abdominal breathing and obstruct energy flow.

● Regulate your diet properly in order to provide the best possible fuel for the essence-to-energy conversion of internal alchemy. Especially avoid refined sugar and starch, deep-fried foods, dairy products, and pork. Eat plenty of fresh fruit, vegetables, and wholegrain products.

● Empty your bladder before practice, if it feels full, but do not urinate immediately after *chee-gung*. The fluids in the bladder help to collect and store energy in the Lower Elixir Field, so you should not drain the bladder for at least twenty minutes after a practice session, in order to give the energy you've collected a chance to enter and circulate in the Governing and Conception channels.

● Do not commence practice if you are emotionally upset, and do not get emotionally upset during or immediately after practice. Emotional outbursts scatter energy, and if this happens during *chee-gung* practice, it can be quite harmful.

● Do not practise on a full stomach. It's best to wait about two hours after a full meal and at least one hour after a light meal before commencing a practice session.

● Do not practise *chee-gung* or meditation during heavy thunder-storms, lightning, hurricanes, typhoons, and so forth. Violent, unstable *chee* can enter your energy system in such weather conditions and severely upset your energy balance.

● Do not try to rush ahead of your own level in practice. Be patient and advance step by step along the path. Practise all exercises as correctly as possible, and do not proceed to a higher level until you feel you have mastered the techniques you're working with first.

● Always commence practice with a calm mind. Do not bring problems at work, home, or school into a practice session. It is impossible to relax the body and regulate the breath unless your mind is clear and calm.

● Always swallow the clear sweet saliva secreted from the glands below the tongue during practice. Known as 'medicinal brew' or 'sweet dew', this secretion is highly beneficial to the stomach and is also regarded as an immune factor in traditional Chinese medicine. Spit out any phlegm coughed up from the lungs or drawn down from the sinuses, but do so gently. Hard, forced spitting during practice scatters *chee*.

● Remain confident in your practice, and do not permit doubts and impatience to undermine your determination to persist in your practice. 'Practice makes perfect' applies to *chee-gung* as well as to any other skill.

Silence is golden

In some Asian traditions, such as the Tibetan, energy is often referred to as 'speech'. That's because speech expends a tremendous amount of breath and energy, and unless it comes out in the form of mantras, chants, or prayers, speech is usually undisciplined, uneven, and often unnecessary. The 'motor mouth' syndrome which seems to infect many people in crowded urban environments exhausts energy reserves and can actually lower resistance and impair immunity. As the Tao master and martial artist Chang San-feng said 600 years ago: 'Forget about words and your energy won't scatter.' The Taoist adept and writer Liu I-ming agrees: 'When the mouth speaks, energy scatters.' Unless you have something important to say, it's always best to keep your lips buttoned, because idle gossip and marathon monologues are like leaking tyres: they permit your energy to escape and leave you flat. Silence is an effective way to conserve energy for more important internal uses.

An ancient Chinese adage says: 'Disease comes in through the mouth; disaster comes out through the mouth.' The first is obvious: open mouths invite germs, dust, and airborne toxins to enter our systems. The second clause refers to the fact that we often create our own personal disasters by talking too much and too carelessly, thereby offending others, revealing things about ourselves that would be better kept secret, making bad impressions on people, and so forth.

So choose your words carefully, speak softly, and don't say any more than necessary.

Signs of progress

Beginning practitioners of *chee-gung* usually experience a variety of sensations which may at first alarm or confuse them but which in fact are quite harmless and may usually be taken as signs of progress. These sensations indicate that energy channels are opening up and that energy and blood are circulating freely in tissues formerly deprived of sufficient circulation. As soon as your body and energy system grow accustomed to enhanced circulation of blood and energy, these symptoms will gradually disappear. Sometimes, however, they may also indicate incorrect posture, improper breathing, or inappropriate environmental conditions for practice, in which case you must take corrective measures to eliminate them. These sensations should serve you as guidelines without alarming or distracting your practice.

Hot or cold sensations, especially in hands, feet, and head
Hot flushes in various parts of the body indicate that energy and blood are flowing abundantly into tissues normally deprived of sufficient circulation, while cold feelings may be caused by practising in cold weather without sufficiently warm clothing, by exposure to wind, or by mental and emotional tension, which blocks circulation.

Numbness and tingling
Beginners often experience numbness in the legs, knees, or ankles, because their muscles and tendons are not accustomed to maintaining the Horse posture for prolonged periods of time. Tingling in the hands and feet is also quite common, owing to enhanced circulation of blood and energy in the extremities. These symptoms usually disappear after a few weeks or months of regular practice.

Soreness and pain
Soreness is generally felt in the thighs and lower back, because these muscles are not accustomed to supporting body weight in the Horse stance for prolonged periods. When the muscles and tendons become properly toned and energized, soreness will disappear. Sometimes aches and pains are the result of incorrect posture, which should promptly be corrected.

Headache and eye ache
These aches are commonly experienced by beginners, who tend to get *chee* stuck in their heads from strained breathing or incomplete circulation of energy. As channels open and breathing grows smoother, these symptoms gradually subside. Headache can also be caused by tensing the shoulders and neck during practice, which causes energy to congest in the head. Therefore, it is important to conclude each practice session by performing a short series of cooling-down exercises to draw excess energy down from the head and store it where it belongs in the lower abdomen.

Trembling
This is a very common sign in the beginning stages of practice. Trembling usually occurs in the limbs and abdomen and is generally caused by the sudden infusion of blood and energy into the muscles. It can also be caused by muscular tension, which obstructs energy flow, in which case you must perform some loosening exercises and focus on physical relaxation during practice. Practising beyond your capacity can also result in tremors. Sometimes your entire body will begin to tremble spontaneously, even though you are practising correctly and within your capacity. This is a good sign of progress, for it indicates that energy is flowing strongly through the Eight Extraordinary Channels. Whenever this happens, you should neither encourage nor discourage it. Just let it follow its course naturally, and it will gradually fade away.

Warm sweat
Sweating is very common in *chee-gung* practice, especially in the beginning stage. It indicates that energy is flowing to the surface of the body and opening the pores. If there is any excess Fire energy inside your system, it will be driven to the surface and expelled through the pores as warm sweat. Even though *chee-gung* exercises appear to be very calm and gentle from the outside, they generate and circulate high levels of energy on the inside. You must be careful to protect your skin from exposure to wind and cold during

practice, and if you sweat a lot, dry yourself off immediately after practice and do not take a shower for at least twenty minutes.

Insomnia
The enhanced vitality of essence, energy, and spirit which *chee-gung* generates can cause changes in sleeping patterns, resulting in a period of insomnia as the entire system readjusts to higher levels of hormones, energy, and awareness. When this happens, focus your mind on your breath while lying in bed waiting to fall asleep. Eventually, when your system has adjusted itself to enhanced energy circulation, you will find it easier than ever to fall asleep, you'll sleep more soundly, and you'll require less sleep each night.

Dry throat
This is caused by the increased flow of air through the throat during practice. It can be alleviated by keeping the tongue pressed to the palate, which stimulates the secretion of clear 'sweet dew' from the salivary glands beneath the tongue. Swallowing this saliva from time to time will keep the throat lubricated.

Sexual Stimulation
This a common sign of progress, caused by the enhancement of hormone production in the sacral region, particularly the testicles and ovaries, and by the strengthening of kidney energy, which governs sexual potency. It is important not to waste this enhanced sexual essence and energy on reckless sexual activity, which will only undermine your practice. Enhanced sexual vitality should be used as a foundation for raising and refining energy to nourish the brain and cultivate the spirit. It may also be used to practice Dual Cultivation sexual yoga with an experienced partner.

Deviations and corrections

Sometimes, owing to incorrect posture, strained breathing, or absent-mindedness, energy will get stuck in a particular spot and cause discomfort. This is called 'deviant energy', and it should be corrected immediately, otherwise it can obstruct the nervous and circulatory systems. The six most common deviations and their corrections are as follows:

Dizziness
Dizziness can be caused by accumulating too much blood and energy in the head, breathing too hard, or holding the breath. It can

be corrected by massaging the temples, stroking the palms of the hands briskly down the back of the head and neck, rolling the eyes around in circles, and massaging the neck and shoulder muscles with the thumbs.

Pressure in the Upper Elixir Field
Sometimes a dull throb will be felt at the energy centre between the eyebrows, as energy accumulates there during practice. This pressure can grow and become uncomfortable unless you pause to correct it by gently massaging the spot with the tips of your middle and forefingers, then stroking the fingertips sideways from that point across the eyebrows to the temples and down the jawbone.

Pressure in the Middle Elixir Field
Pressure below the heart and around the ribcage can be caused by breathing too forcefully, breathing with tensed chest muscles, or breathing more deeply than your diaphragm's flexibility permits. Two ways to correct this are by placing the palms on top of each other over the heart and rubbing firmly but slowly in circles, or by massaging the ribcage from the sternum out towards the sides with the palms.

Pressure in the Lower Elixir Field
This deviation usually manifests as tremors in the abdominal muscles, a dull throb behind the navel, or discomfort in the gut. It is readily corrected by placing one palm over the other on the navel and rubbing firmly but slowly in circles, while breathing naturally and relaxing the body.

Sexual pressure
When energy gets stuck in the sacrum, or when enhanced secretions of sexual hormones are not sublimated into energy, it can cause a buildup of sexual pressure that manifests itself as nocturnal emissions and frequent erections in men, pressure in the nipples and vagina in women, and sexual fantasies in both. In this case, excess sexual energy must be redistributed from the sacrum upwards to the brain and outwards to the limbs. One of the quickest ways to do this is by flexing the anus and perineum in order to draw excess sacral energy up through the coccyx and spinal channels into the head. You may also practise the yoga posture known as the 'Candle', or 'shoulder stand', which drains excess fluids from the sacrum and draws them towards the head. Another way to correct this deviation is to engage in a prolonged

session of Dual Cultivation sexual intercourse, without male ejaculation, in order to circulate and sublimate excess sexual essence and energy.

Modes of chee-gung practice

There are seven basic modes of *chee-gung* practice, each of which has its own specific purposes and parameters, as follows:

Preparation
This is the warm-up stage of practice performed at the beginning of every session in order to stretch tendons and ligaments, tone muscles, open energy channels, stimulate circulation, and generate a strong polar field.

Mobilization
This is the main part of *chee-gung* practice, in which deep abdominal breathing is combined with slow rhythmic movements of the limbs and torso in order to generate and mobilize the flow of energy through the meridians and distribute blood and *chee* to the brain, organs, glands, muscles, marrow, and every other tissue in the body.

Collection
This is the cool-down stage of practice performed at the end of every session in order to collect and store energy in the Lower Elixir Field below and behind the navel. Failure to practise this stage may cause energy to scatter and be lost, or else to get stuck in the head or chest as deviant energy. Many masters believe that collection exercises direct energy down into the bladder, where electrolytes in the urinary fluid hold and store it until it enters into general circulation in the Governing and Conception channels, or 'Microcosmic Orbit'. That's why most masters advise adepts not to urinate for fifteen to twenty minutes after a session.

Stillness
This is what is known as 'meditation' in the West. Adepts usually begin to practise still-sitting meditation after they have achieved a certain degree of proficiency in the moving meditation of *chee-gung* exercises. Sitting *chee-gung* focuses on circulating energy internally, opening vital points called 'passes', and sublimating energy upwards from sacrum to head in order to cultivate spiritual power.

Healing
This mode of practice is meant to be used specifically for healing purposes, either self-healing or healing others. It is an advanced method which requires substantial experience and a firm command of mind over energy. Practised alone, it involves using the mind to lead energy to ailing parts of the body. Practised on others, it requires that the healer focus and project his or her internal energy outwards through the hands and into the patient's body, where it balances and fortifies the patient's own energy. This type of healing has become very popular today in China, where it is currently under intensive scientific investigation.

Spontaneous motion
This mode usually occurs spontaneously during still-sitting or standing practice, at the intermediate or advanced stage, and is marked by sudden, involuntary tremors or rocking motions in the head, limbs, torso, or entire body. Such motions should neither be resisted nor encouraged, but rather permitted naturally to run their course. They usually indicate a transition from a lower to a higher level of practice.

Extraordinary power
This mode may only be practised by highly advanced adepts, for it involves the restoration of primordial powers inherent in all humans but long lost to virtually everyone. These powers, such as clairvoyance, extrasensory perception, healing, moving objects at a distance without touching them, and other so-called 'miraculous' powers, can be reawakened and brought under voluntary control with *chee-gung*, but only after many years of diligent practice.

The exercises introduced below, as well as in *The Tao of HS&L*, involve only the first three modes of practice – preparation, mobilization, and collection – which should always be performed in that order. In other words, you should begin every practice session with a series of preparatory warm-up exercises, then perform the main energy-circulation exercises, and conclude each session with a few cool-down exercises to collect and store energy in the lower abdomen. For warm-up, you may select any combination of the warm-up exercises given in *The Tao of HS&L*, or else some simple yoga stretches, or any other form of slow, gentle calisthenics. For the main practice, select a set of exercises from those given below and those in the previous book, depending on what you wish to accomplish. For cool-down, use the set of collection and storage manoeuvres presented at the end of the exercise section below.

Chee-gung exercises

Three types of *chee-gung* exercises are presented below: exercises to boost the immunity and vital-organ functions; solo 'sexercises' for men and women to stimulate secretions of sexual essence and generate sexual energy; and a set of cool-down exercises for collecting and storing energy in the lower abdomen. These may all be practised in combination with the exercises introduced in the breathing and exercise chapters of *The Tao of HS&L*, which readers should review for additional background information and practical pointers. By way of quick review, here's a list of tips on *chee-gung* practice, most of which is performed in the standard 'Horse' stance (Fig. 13).

Feet
Place your feet shoulder-width apart; parallel for men, splayed outward at 45 degrees for women. Weight should be evenly distributed between both feet and centred on the front pads rather than the heels.

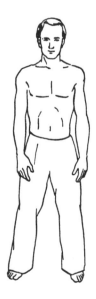

Fig. 13 **The Horse stance, standard beginning posture for most chee-gung practice.**

Knees
The joints of the knees should be relaxed and slightly bent in order to ensure free flow of blood and energy between feet and hips and place the bulk of your body weight on the thighs.

Hips and pelvis
The hips should be relaxed and body weight supported by the thighs. Tuck the pelvis forward a bit in order to keep the lower spine straight and evenly aligned with the upper spine and neck.

Anal lock
Slightly contract and lift the anus and perineum during the inhalation stage, and relax them on exhalation. This helps open up the 'pass' at the coccyx and encourages energy to enter circulation in the Microcosmic Orbit.

Abdominal lock
Slightly pull in the abdominal wall at the end of inhalation in order to enhance internal abdominal pressure. This stimulates circulation of energy and provides invigorating pressure on the internal organs.

Chest
Keep the chest as loose as possible by slightly rounding the shoulders and relaxing the thoracic cavity. Tension in chest and rib muscles inhibits diaphragmic breathing and blocks circulation of energy.

Spine
Keep the spine straight and stretch the vertebrae upwards by raising the back of the neck up and tilting the pelvis forwards to tuck in the butt. This is a prerequisite for inducing energy to flow from the sacrum up the Governing Channel along the spine into the head.

Shoulders
Keep the shoulder muscles relaxed and let the shoulders droop. This helps relax the chest and stretch the spine.

Elbows
Keep your elbows slightly bent and your arms hanging loosely down the sides, with the hollows of the elbows facing the ribs and palms facing towards the rear. This facilitates a free flow of energy through the arm channels.

Wrist and hands
The wrists should be totally relaxed, and the hands should hang loosely down without any tension in the fingers. Keep your fingers slightly bent and palms hollowed. An old *chee-gung* adage, 'The hands are the flags of *chee*,' means that the hands are sensitive to the 'winds' of energy, projecting internal energy outwards and drawing external energy inwards through palms and fingertips.

Head and neck
Keep the head suspended as though it were hanging by a string attached to the crown. Do not tilt the head forwards or backwards, right or left. Apply the neck lock to keep the back of the neck straight and aligned with the spine so that energy flows freely into the head.

Chin and throat
Tuck the chin slightly in towards the throat, but without tilting the head forwards. This keeps the back of the neck straight and gives a slight stretch to the upper vertebrae.

Eyes
Keep the eyelids relaxed, eyes partly closed but not shut tight, and eliminate all tension in the eye muscles. Do not focus your eyes on any particular object; just let them gaze unfocused on the ground or straight ahead.

Lips and teeth
Keep your lips closed without tensing the mouth, and let the upper and lower teeth touch without clenching the jaw muscles.

Tongue
Keep the tip of the tongue lightly pressed against the upper palate, behind the front upper teeth. This forms a bridge for energy to descend from the point between the brows down into the throat and chest. It also stimulates secretion of saliva from the glands beneath the tongue. This saliva should be swallowed from time to time as it collects in the mouth.

Exercises for boosting immunity

All *chee-gung* exercises boost immunity by enhancing and harmonizing the Three Treasures. However, some exercises were specifically designed to stimulate the glands, organs, and other mechanisms directly involved in immune functions. It is a good idea to include some of these exercises in your daily *chee-gung* programme.

According to the tenets of Chinese medicine and Taoist alchemy, the human immune system has three primary centres: the thymus gland, located in the centre of the chest over the heart at a vital energy point midway between the nipples, called *tan-jung*; the adrenal glands, located on top of the kidneys and regulated by a point along the spine, called *ming-men*; and the spine. If we draw a schematic diagram of the thymus, adrenals, and spine, lo and behold, we see a familiar image: the 'Supreme Ultimate' symbol of the Tao itself! (Fig. 14) Note that the thymus is associated with the heart, which is governed by Fire, while the adrenals are associated with the kidneys, governed by Water. The spine and its potent cerebrospinal fluids regulate the circuitry of the sympathetic and parasympathetic branches of the autonomous nervous system, govern the biofeedback between the endocrine and nervous systems, and maintain the brain's control over organs, limbs, and other tissues throughout the body.

Another line of defence is managed by the kidneys and the liver, which are responsible for filtering and purifying the blood. Blood boosts immunity by carrying metabolic wastes, toxins, and microbes out of cells and tissues for excretion, and by delivering nutrients, oxygen, enzymes, and immune factors into the cells and tissues. The blood's defence functions depend entirely on its purity and pH balance, which in turn depend on proper kidney and liver functions.

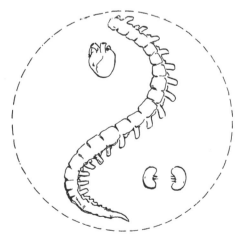

Fig. 14 **Schematic depiction of three pillars of the human immune system: thymus, adrenals, and spine.**

According to Taoist alchemy, the sweet clear saliva secreted from the glands under the tongue also has potent immunological properties. Master Chang San-feng said:

> The key is to let the mouth fill with salvia as energy rises and circulates during periods of stillness. You should visualize this saliva as sweet dew, like honey. Buddhists refer to it as the elixir of enlightenment. Swallow it, and use your mind to drive it down into the cauldron of the lower abdomen, where it crystallizes and nourishes primordial energy.

Keeping the tongue pressed against the palate during *chee-gung* and meditation practice stimulates these beneficial secretions. Two tongue exercises specifically designed to increase these secretions are given below.

The pituitary gland and bone marrow also play important roles in human immunity by secreting vital hormones and producing red and white blood cells. In Chinese medicine, the brain is regarded as a form of marrow and all exercises which energize marrow also draw energy into the brain. In order to draw energy into the brain and marrow, *chee-gung* exercises must be performed slowly, smoothly, and softly. Meditation is even more effective in energizing these innermost tissues.

Thymus tap (Fig. 15)
Technique: Stand in the Horse stance, completely relaxed. Make a fist with the right or left hand and raise it up to the middle of your chest. Start tapping the spot midway between the nipples with a rhythm of one hard followed by two softer taps: *one*, two, three; *one*, two, three; etc. Tap hard enough to vibrate the sternum and create a deep drumming sound in the chest. Continue for three to five minutes, breathing naturally and keeping your mind focused on the vibrations in the chest. You may practise this in the morning as part of your warm-up, or just before bedtime, or both. Practising at night before going to sleep is particularly beneficial because the thymus gland becomes most active approximately ninety minutes after you fall asleep. Since the thymus shrinks in adults during the late teens or early twenties, it's a good idea to make this exercise a regular part of your practice, in order to stimulate this gland's immune functions.

Benefits: Stimulates the thymus to produce T-cells, which are primary immune factors. Draws blood and energy into the thymus,

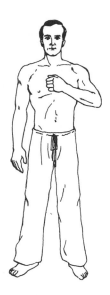

Fig. 15 **Thymus tap.**

thereby energizing and nourishing it. With regular daily practice, this exercise will increase the size of the thymus and improve its immune functions. The rhythmic vibrations not only stimulate the thymus, they also vibrate throughout the chest, gently massaging and energizing the lungs, heart, bronchial tubes, and throat.

Kidney rub and tap (Fig. 16)
Technique: Stand in the Horse and relax. Raise the hands behind the back at kidney level and start rubbing briskly up and down over the kidneys, using the backs of the hands. Continue until the kidneys start to feel warm, which usually takes only two or three minutes. This is a great way to warm up the entire body on cold winter mornings. After rubbing, you may also tap the kidneys gently with the backs of the hands, alternating left and right. Do not tap any harder than is comfortable, and if your kidneys are sore or sensitive, then skip this phase of the exercise until you have developed more strength in this area.

Benefits: Stimulates secretions of the adrenal glands and draws blood and energy to the kidneys, thereby warming up and energizing the entire system. Tapping also helps dissolve crystals before they form kidney stones and stimulates the kidneys' filtering and excretory functions.

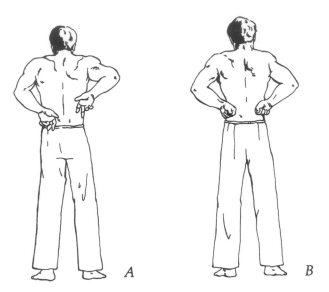

Fig. 16 **Kidney rub (A) and tap (B).**

Spinal stretch (Fig. 17)
Technique: This exercise may be performed standing, but it's easier and just as effective when done sitting on a low stool or chair. Sit with feet wider than shoulder width apart, hands placed firmly on knees, spine erect. Inhale, then extend the chin and lean forwards, stretching the entire spine as you follow your chin forwards and down between your knees. At that point, tuck your chin in against your chest, arch your spine upwards and start lifting your torso back up by pushing the hands against the knees. Keep your chin tucked in until the spine is once again erect, and inhale slowly as you rise. Then raise the head, look straight ahead, and commence another cycle on exhalation. The key is alternately to bow and arch the spine and stretch the vertebrae in conjunction with deep diaphragmic breathing.

Benefits: Stretches the entire spinal column and aligns the vertebrae. Stimulates all nerves along the spine and promotes free flow of cerebrospinal fluids and energy. The alternate bowing and arching of the spine also provides direct stimulation to the thymus and adrenals and encourages energy to rise up along the spinal channels into the brain.

Tongue roll
Technique: First, extend the tongue and stretch it out as far as possible, then roll it back into the mouth and curl it up until the tip

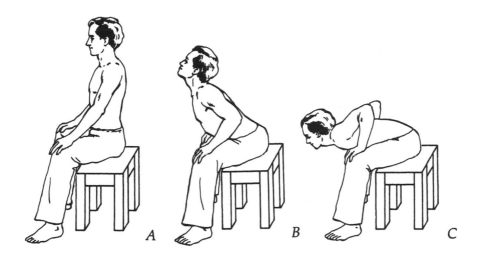

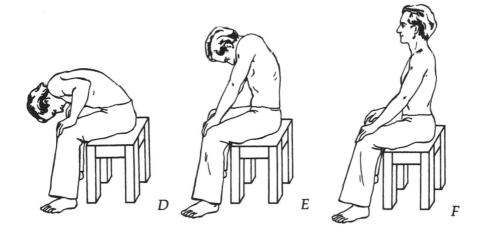

Fig. 17 Spinal stretch
A. Starting posture; inhale.
B. Extend chin and stretch forwards; start exhalation.
C. Full stretch forwards; complete exhalation.
D. Tuck chin in and arch spine up; breath pause.
E. Straighten back up; start inhalation.
F. Return to start; complete inhalation.

touches the soft palate at the top of the throat. Repeat about a dozen times. Second, roll the tongue rapidly in circles either clockwise or counterclockwise, whichever is more comfortable, along the upper and lower gum lines between teeth and lips. Continue rolling circles until the tongue muscle feels tired or numb. Swallow any saliva secreted from beneath the tongue.

Benefits: Stimulates secretion of beneficial saliva from glands beneath the tongue. Not only is this beneficial to the immune system when swallowed, it also helps to eliminate bad breath by digesting offensive bacteria in the mouth. Stretching the tongue also tonifies the heart, because the tongue and heart muscles are connected.

Palms raised to heaven to regulate the Triple Burners (Fig. 18)
Technique: This is the first exercise in a series called 'Eight Pieces of Brocade', a classical *chee-gung* set derived from the *Tendon Changing Classic* and specifically designed to promote healing and boost immunity. Stand in the Horse, relax the body, regulate the breath, and calm the mind. Bring your hands together in front of the body, palms up and fingers aligned, and slowly raise them up along the front of the body while inhaling slowly and deeply. As your palms rise and your lungs fill, draw in the abdominal wall and slightly contract the anus in order to increase internal pressure on the organs. When the hands reach face level and the lungs are full, turn palms up so that they face the sky, continue to push them up above the head, briefly holding the breath until arms are extended palms up to the sky. Next, relax and release the breath, exhaling slowly as you bring your arms smoothly down the sides in a full circle. When your arms are back at original position and your lungs are empty, turn palms up again in front, and start inhaling as you begin another cycle. Perform at least one dozen cycles, preferably two or three, but do not hurry through them. It's better to do six slowly and correctly than rush through sixty haphazardly.

Benefits: This exercise harmonizes the energies of all the major organ systems by regulating and balancing the Triple Burner. The Upper Burner in the chest governs breathing and circulation, the Middle Burner in the solar plexus controls digestive organs and functions, the Lower Burner in the lower abdomen regulates the excretory and sexual organs. By stimulating and harmonizing their energies, this exercise regulates the vital functions of the organ-energy systems. It enhances the lungs' capacity to assimilate energy from the atmosphere; the heart's circulatory functions; the kidneys' and liver's blood-cleansing powers; the digestive

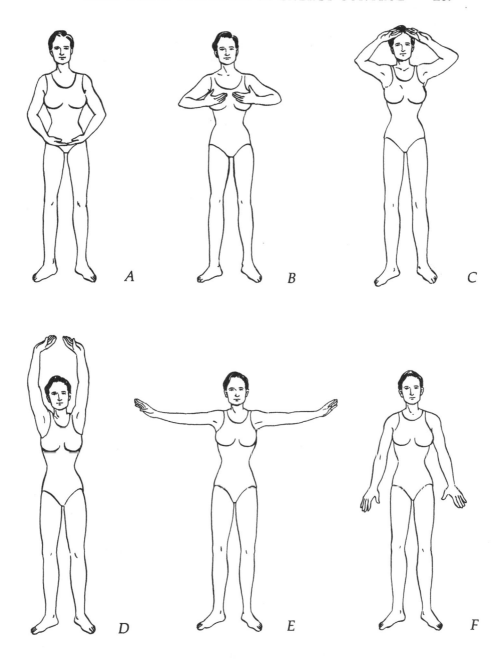

Fig. 18 **Palms raised to heaven to regulate the Triple Burner.**
A. Start raising palms up along torso and inhale.
B. Complete inhalation as palms reach heart.
C. Turn palms up and raise to sky, retaining breath.
D. When arms fully extended, lower to sides and start exhaling.
E. Inscribe full circle with arms, exhaling.
F. Hands return to sides, complete exhalation.

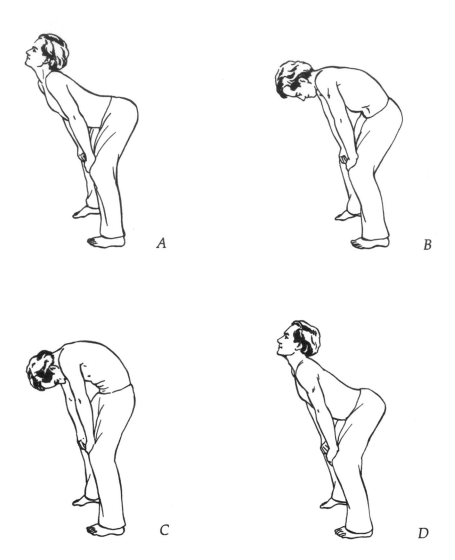

Fig. 19 'Shake the head and wag the tail to extinguish Fire in the heart'

First phase:
A. Extend chin, raise head, bow spine, inhale fully with nose.
B. Tuck chin in, lower head, arch spine, exhale with mouth.
C. Complete spinal arch, head down, complete exhalation.
D. Return to start, inhaling with nose, and repeat.

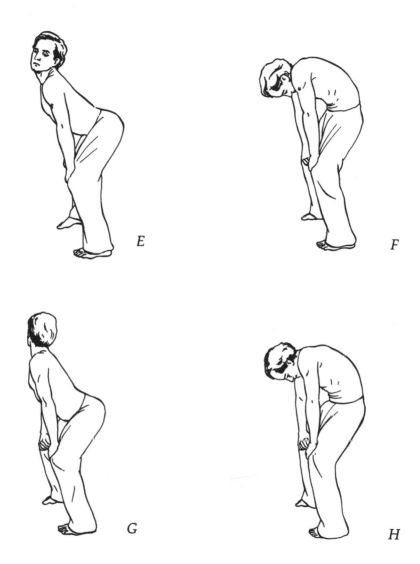

Fig. 19 continued

Second phase:
E. Turn head to left and look over shoulder, bow spine, twist hips to left, inhale fully with nose.
F. Return head to front, tuck chin in, lower head, arch spine up, exhale with mouth.
G. Turn head to right and look over shoulder, bow spine, twist hips to right, inhale fully with nose.
H. Return head to front, tuck chin in, lower head, arch spine up and exhale with mouth.

functions of stomach, pancreas, and spleen; the small intestine's assimilation of nutrients; the excretory efficiency of colon and bladder; and glandular secretions of vital hormones. It also strengthens the shield of guardian energy which envelops the body.

'Shake the head and wag the tail to extinguish Fire in the heart' (Fig. 19)
Technique: This is the fourth exercise in the Eight Pieces of Brocade set. First, adopt the correct posture: feet slightly more than shoulder width apart, toes splayed inwards at about 45 degrees, torso bent forwards, hands placed firmly above the knees for support, with fingers and thumbs on the inside of thighs. In the first phase of the exercise, inhale slowly as you extend the chin out forwards and bow the spine, tilting the butt out and up in back. When your spine is fully extended, tuck the chin down and in against the chest, pull in the butt, and arch the spine up as you exhale through the mouth with an audible 'hah' sound. This phase is somewhat similar to the spinal stretch shown above.

Repeat slowly and smoothly three to six times, then proceed to the second phase: instead of jutting your chin forwards on inhalation, turn your head to the right and look over your right shoulder, while bowing the spine and sticking the butt up and out towards the right side. Try to turn your head and twist your pelvis far enough in the same direction so that your eyes can see your butt; otherwise, just turn as far as possible. Then turn your head forwards again, tuck the chin down and in, and pull in the butt as you arch your spine up and exhale audibly through the mouth. Then do the same towards the left, repeating both sides three to six times.

When finished with the side-to-side phase, perform another three to six stretches in the first phase. When finished, stand erect in the Horse stance, and relax with a few deep abdominal breaths.

Benefits: This is an excellent exercise for stretching and toning the spine and aligning the vertebrae. The alternate bowing and arching of the spine, coupled with the expansion and contraction of the chest, provides direct stimulation to the adrenals, thymus, and spine. By exhaling audibly through the mouth, you expel excess Fire energy from the Upper Burner, which regulates heart and lungs. Excess postnatal Fire energy is regarded as a major cause of disease and degeneration in Chinese medicine, and it's usually caused by excess consumption of food, alcohol, and drugs, by breathing polluted air, and by the aberrant energy of rampant emotions. Audible mouth exhalations combined with the pump action of the upper and lower torsos forces excess Fire energy out through the lungs and mouth. This exercise directly stimulates the kidneys and adrenals, thereby generating cooling, calming Water energy from the original essence stored in the kidney organ-energy system. The immune system functions best when Fire and Water energies are kept in balance; modern lifestyles tend to cause a chronic excess of aberrant Fire energy. This exercise therefore helps the immune system subdue one of its major enemies.

Iron Bridge (Fig. 20)
Technique: Stand in Horse, but with your feet a bit less than shoulder width apart. Slowly bend over forwards, starting with the head and upper spine and working down the vertebrae, letting your arms dangle down loosely. When you are bent over as far as possible without discomfort, let your arms and head hang down completely relaxed and take three slow, deep breaths, drawing the breath down into the abdomen. Since you are bent over forwards, abdominal pressure will shift and cause the breath to push up against the kidneys at the back.

After the third exhalation, slowly start to rise up again on the next inhalation, starting with the lower spine and working upwards, as though pulling up on a zipper.

When your spine is erect and head up, continue without pause to raise your head and arms upwards, then lower your arms down behind and place palms firmly on the lower back below the kidneys as you continue arching backwards, and let your head hang back. Lean back as far as comfortable without straining, and perform three slow, deep, abdominal breaths.

After the third exhalation, straighten up the spine, then raise your arms and extend them straight up over the head on the next inhalation. When your arms are straight over your head, give them an extra stretch upwards, stretching the entire ribcage; swallow hard (even if you have no saliva to swallow), then start exhaling as you point your fingers down towards the ground and bring your hands down in front of the body. Bend the head and neck forwards, and continue bending over towards the ground to commence another cycle.

Repeat three times as a warm-up exercise, or six times as a main exercise.

Benefits: Stretches and tones the spine, aligns the vertebrae, stimulates the flow of cerebrospinal fluid. Deep breathing while bent over forwards provides stimulating diaphragmic massage to the kidneys and adrenals. Arching back in Iron Bridge posture gives a strong boost to kidney and adrenal energy. Expansion and contraction of the front chest cavity stimulates the thymus. Bending back

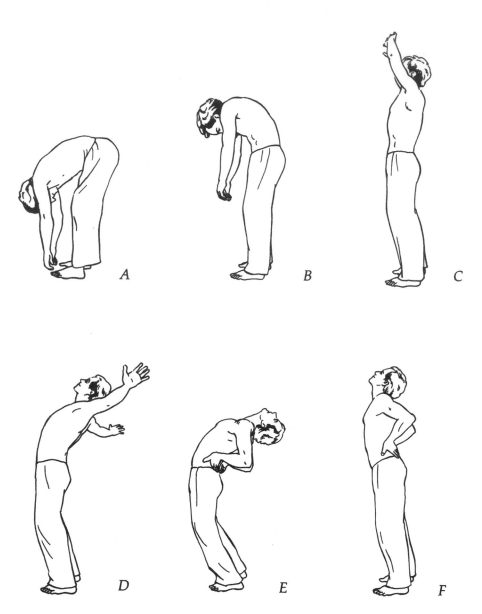

Fig. 20 **Iron Bridge**
A. Bend forwards, knees unlocked, head and arms hanging down; three slow deep breaths.
B. Raise up slowly on inhalation.
C. Continue raising arms up above head, complete inhaling.
D. Bend back slowly, start exhaling, lower arms to back.
E. Iron Bridge stance, palms on kidneys; three slow deep breaths.
F. Straighten up slowly on inhalation.

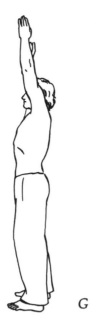

G

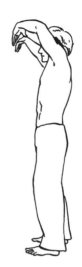

H

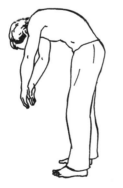

I

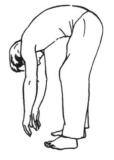

J

Fig. 20 continued
G. Extend arms above head and stretch, complete inhaling and swallow.
H. Turn fingers towards ground, lower arms down along torso, start exhaling.
I. Bend forwards and lower torso towards ground behind arms, continue exhaling.
J. Return to start; repeat three breaths.

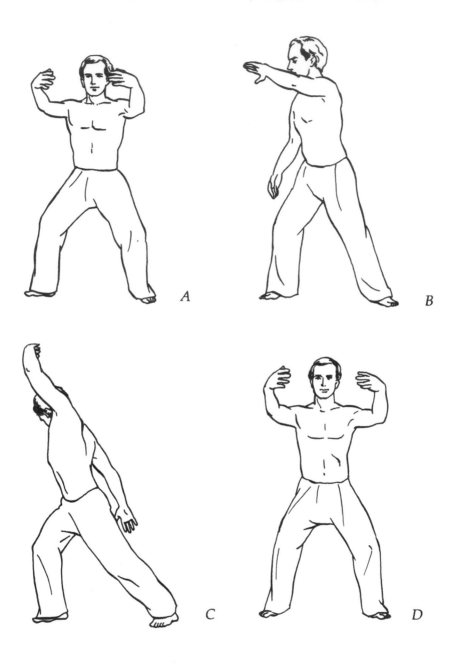

Fig. 21 **Dragon Turns Its Head**
A. Starting posture: Embracing Tree; 3–6 breaths.
B. Slowly turn body to right, inhaling.
C. Extend left palm above head, right palm down along left thigh, turn head to look at right hand; 4 breaths.
D. Return to Embracing Tree on inhalation, then exhale.

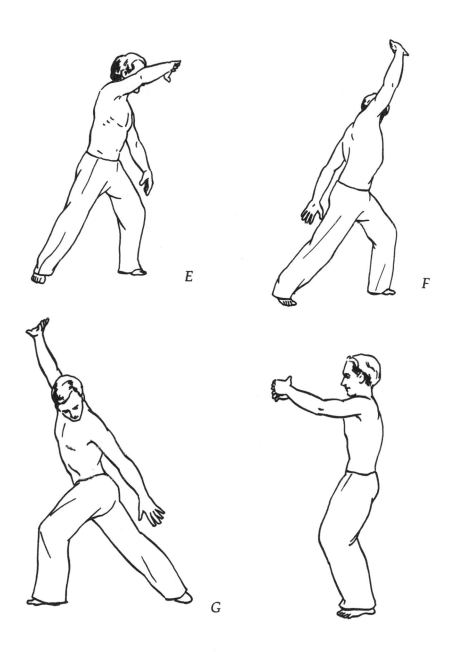

Fig. 21 continued
E. Slowly turn body to left, inhaling.
F. Extend right palm above head, left palm down along right thigh, turn head to look at left hand; 4 breaths.
G. View of extended breathing posture from the other side.
H. Side view of Embracing Tree posture.

and forth while raising and lowering the arms encourages the flow of lymph and aids the circulation of blood to extremities.

Dragon Turns Its Head (Fig. 21)
Technique: This is a basic exercise in the martial-arts form called *ba-gua* ('Eight Trigrams'). It is specifically designed to tone the spine and stimulate the kidney and liver functions. Place your feet in wide stance, toes splayed outwards at 45 degrees. Inhale and slowly raise the arms up to Embracing Tree posture. If you wish, you may practise a few minutes of deep abdominal breathing in this posture, before proceeding.

Next, inhale and slowly turn the body to the right, bringing the left arm above the head with palm facing out and the right arm down to the side with palm facing leg, and turn your head around to look down at the right hand. Note from the illustration that the correct posture calls for a straight line from the upper hand down along the arm and back of head to the lower hand, and onwards down the leg to the foot. This alignment is important.

When this posture is correct, perform four deep abdominal breaths, drawing the breath as deep down into the abdomen as possible, but without straining. This is a very good exercise for practising 'palm breathing': focus your attention to feel and visualize energy streaming in and out of the points in the centre of the palms as you breathe. After the fourth exhalation, inhale and slowly turn back to the Embracing Tree posture, exhale, then turn to the left on the next inhalation, and repeat. Perform at least five or six times on each side, more if you wish.

Benefits: This exercise provides a direct stimulation to the energies of the kidneys, adrenals, and liver. It enhances the blood-cleansing functions of liver and kidneys. Twisting the torso in conjunction with deep diaphragmic breathing provides diaphragmic massage to internal organs, including adrenals, tones the spine, and aligns the vertebrae. Alternate stretching of the rib cage to right and left also stimulates the thymus. Palm breathing in this posture draws fresh energy in directly from the atmosphere through points in the centre of the palms.

The Six-Syllable Secret

The Six Syllable Secret is an ancient form of healing *chee-gung* that uses differently modulated modes of mouth exhalation to cleanse and stimulate the various vital organs. In a book entitled *The Maintenance and Extension of Life*, written by the famous physician

Tao Hung-jing during the fifth century AD, this system is described as follows:

> One should take air in through the nose and let it out slowly through the mouth . . . There is one way of drawing breath in and six ways of expelling breath out. The six ways of expelling breath are represented by the syllables *hsü, her, hoo, sss, chway, shee*. The six ways of exhalation can cure illness: to expel heat, one uses *chway*; to expel cold, one uses *hoo*; to relieve tension, use *shee*; to release anger, use *her*; to dispel malaise, use *hsü*; and to regain equilibrium, use *sss*.

This system works by establishing resonance between the vibratory pitch of exhalation through the throat and mouth and the frequency of a specific internal organ-energy system. When resonance between external breath and internal organ energy is achieved, fresh energy flows freely throughout the particular organ-energy system activated by the syllable used for exhalation. According to the tenets of traditional Chinese medicine and Taoist alchemy, internal organ energies are directly influenced, for better or for worse, by prevailing external energies. Each of the six syllables used to modulate exhalation in this practice establishes the precise energy vibration which the related organ-energy system requires to open up its meridian, expel stagnant energy, receive fresh energy, and restore optimum energy balance.

The version of the Six-Syllable Secret introduced here is provided by courtesy of one of the author's main *chee-gung* teachers, Master Luo Teh-hsiou of Taiwan. It should be practised precisely as presented below.

Important points of practice

Before conmencing practice, it is essential to relax the body completely, calm the mind, and regulate the breath. One should prepare for this practice as follows:

● Stand in the Horse stance, muscles and joints relaxed, arms hanging loosely down by your sides, head held as though suspended from a string, chin drawn slightly in, with a straight line running from the crown of the head down through the perineum and on down to the soles of the feet.

● In addition to calmness, it is very important to remain as loose and relaxed as possible. The entire body should be so relaxed that it

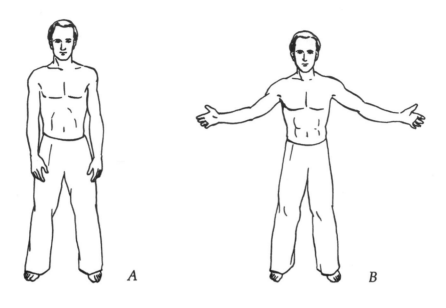

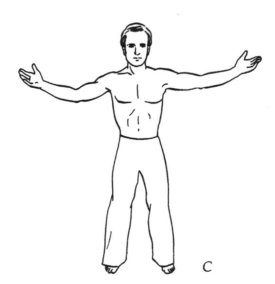

Fig. 22 **Liver/gall bladder syllable:** *hsü*
A. Starting posture: Horse stance.
B. Turn palms up, raise arms to side, grip big toes to ground, inhale.
C. Arms extended to sides, palms up, complete inhalation.

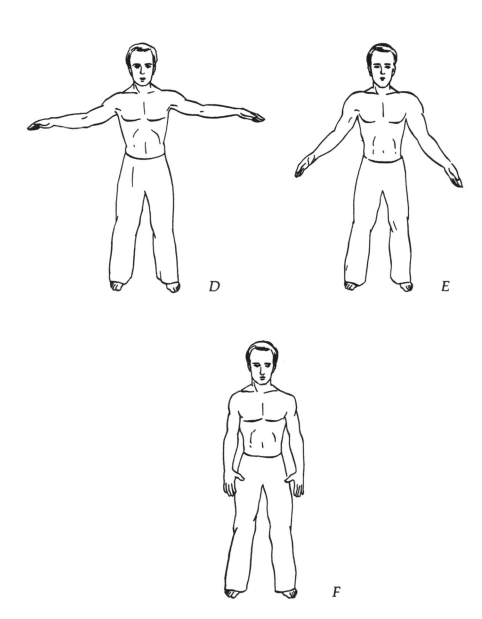

Fig. 22 continued
D. Turns palms down, relax toes, start exhaling with mouth, aspirating 'hsü'.
E. Lower arms down to sides, continue exhalation/aspiration.
F. Return to Horse stance, relax; repeat.

feels as though each and every muscle were being pulled towards the earth by force of gravity.

● Only after attaining a state of total relaxation, calm, and smooth natural breathing, should you begin to practise the Six-Syllable Secret.

● Practise each syllable at least six times, but do *not* sound them out loud. Instead, aspirate each syllable silently in the throat, and use your mind to regulate and guide its vibrational frequency into the related organ. Before commencing aspiration of the syllables, first perform a few deep diaphragmic breaths to expel stale air and stagnant energy, then start by taking a long, slow, deep inhalation through the nose, followed by a long, slow, silent exhalation through the mouth, with lips, tongue, teeth, and throat formed as though to pronounce the syllable.

● It is not necessary to practise all six of the syllables every time you practise. You may select one or two, according to your requirements, and incorporate them into your regular daily *chee-gung* workout. You may also practise the entire set as a complete workout from time to time.

The Six Syllables

Syllable One: hsü (pronounced as 'shoo', with lips pursed, but softened by the umlaut over the vowel)
Element: Wood
Season: spring
Organ: liver/gall bladder
Method: 1) Stand relaxed in Horse. Bring your hands slightly forwards so the palms are facing each other at thigh level. Focus attention on the point between the eyebrows and the point midway between the nipples, in order to open up these vital energy centres, then shift attention to the centres of the palms and the tips of the middle fingers.
2) Grip the ground with the big toes to activate the liver meridian, and start inhaling slowly and deeply into the abdomen, while slowly raising the hands up and out to the sides, turning the palms up towards the sky as you raise them. Focus attention on the middle fingers and palms.
3) When your breath is full and your palms reach shoulder level, turn the palms over to face the ground, relax the grip of the toes on the ground, and slowly lower the arms back down to the sides, while exhaling through the mouth, silently aspirating the syllable *hsü* with pursed lips, and visualizing a stream of energy

flowing up and out from the liver along with the breath.

4) When breath is empty and hands are back down in front, pause and relax for a moment, then grip big toes to ground and commence another cycle on next inhalation.

Benefits: Decongests the liver and clears the liver meridian. Draws fresh energy into the liver and gall bladder. Helps detoxify the liver and stimulate its functions.

Syllable Two: her (pronounced as 'her' but without the final 'r', with mouth open, tip of tongue pressed against lower teeth, and syllable aspirating in the top of the throat on exhalation)
Element: Fire
Season: summer
Organ: heart/small intestine
Method: 1) Stand in Horse and hold the palms facing each other in front in same starting posture as the previous syllable. Commence inhalation and, as you begin to raise your hands up and out to the sides, turn the palms so that they face towards the back, and extend the little fingers outwards as far as possible in order to activate the heart meridan.

2) When your breath is full and the hands reach shoulder level, commence exhalation through the mouth, aspirating the syllable *her* in the top of the throat, while slowly lowering the hands back down the sides with little fingers relaxed. Visualize hot Fire energy streaming up and out of the heart with exhalation.

3) When the breath is empty and your hands are back down in front, pause to relax, then begin the next cycle on the next inhalation.

Benefits: Pacifies and expels excess Fire energy in the heart and clears the heart meridian. Especially effective during hot summer weather or in tropical climates to eliminate symptoms of excess heart Fire, such as insomnia, heart palpitations, profuse sweating, and hypertension. Also benefits the small intestine.

Syllable Three: hoo (pronounced 'who', with the lips rounded and the tongue suspended in mid-mouth, as though blowing out a candle)
Element: Earth
Season: late summer
Organ: spleen and pancreas/stomach
Method: 1) Stand in Horse. Bring your hands out front, just below the navel, with the palms facing up to the sky and the fingers

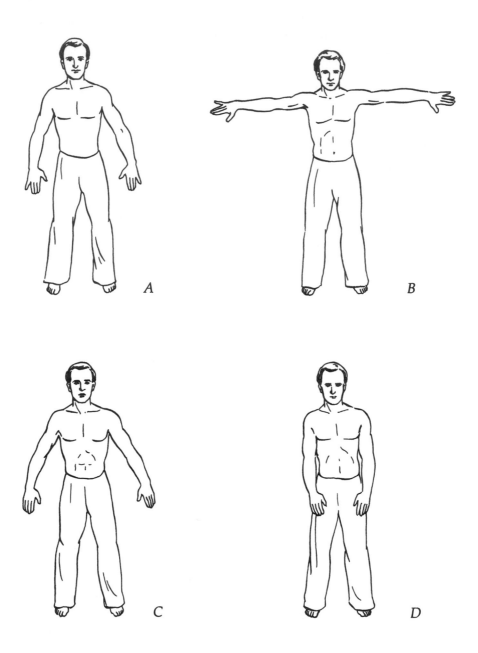

Fig. 23 **Heart/small intestine syllable:** *her*
A. Starting posture: Horse stance, turn palms back, extend little fingers out, raise arms up to sides, inhale.
B. Arms extended to sides, little fingers extended up, complete inhalation.
C. Relax little fingers, lower arms down to sides, exhale with mouth, aspirating '*her*'.
D. Return to Horse stance, relax; repeat.

aligned. Slowly commence inhaling through the nose as you raise both hands up along the centre of the torso.

2) When your hands reach the *tan-jung* point midway between the nipples, and the breath is full, commence exhaling through the mouth and aspirate the syllable, *hoo* as you turn the right palm out and around 360 degrees so that it faces the sky. Continue raising it upwards past the face and above the head, while turning the left palm in and around 180 degrees so that it faces the ground; then push it down the front of the torso back to thigh level.

3) When the breath is empty, right palm is extended up towards the sky above your head, and the left palm is extended down towards the ground below, commence the next inhalation. Turn the right palm down, left palm up, and slowly bring the palms together so that they meet again at the *tan-jung* point midway between the nipples just as the inhalation is complete.

4) When the breath is full and your palms meet at mid-chest, commence the next mouth exhalation and syllable aspiration, and continue pushing the right hand down with the palm facing the ground, while turning the left palm out and around 360 degrees to face upwards again; continue raising it up above your head to full extension.

5) When the breath is empty, the left palm is extended above your head to the sky and the right palm extended down to the earth below, turn the palms over and bring them together again at mid-chest level on next inhalation.

Benefits: Improves the digestive functions of spleen, pancreas, and stomach. Benefits any sort of digestive ailment and helps eliminate bad breath caused by indigestion in the stomach.

Syllable Four: sss (pronounced as in 'hiss', without the initial 'hi-', with your tongue behind the lower teeth and the upper and lower teeth slightly parted)
Element: Metal
Season: autumn
Organ: lungs/large intestine
Method: 1) Stand in Horse, bring your hands out to the front just below the navel, palms up (same as in the previous syllable), and slowly raise the palms up along the centre of the torso as you inhale deeply and slowly into the abdomen.

2) When your hands reach the point midway between the nipples and your breath is full, turn the palms down, around, and up again, so that they are facing outwards to either side, with the fingers

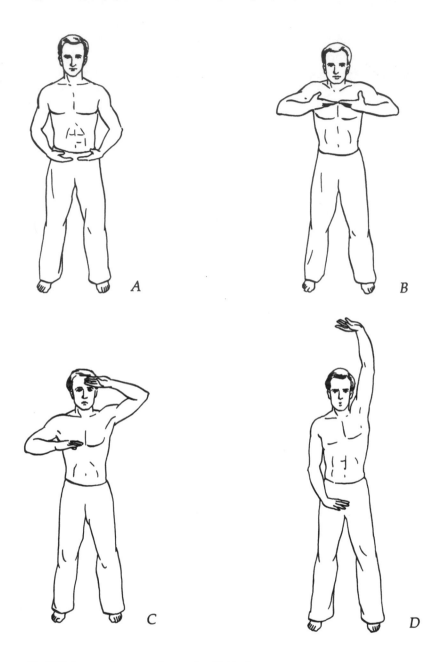

Fig. 24 Spleen and pancreas/stomach syllable: *hoo*
A. Starting posture: Horse stance, turn palms up in front and raise hands along torso, inhaling.
B. Hands reach heart, palms up, complete inhalation.
C. Turn left palm up and raise, turn right palm down and lower; start exaling with mouth, aspirating 'hoo'.
D. Palms fully extended up and down, complete exhalation/aspiration.

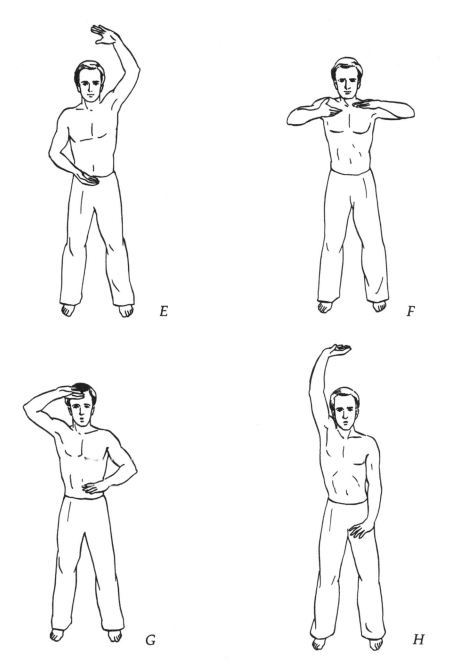

Fig. 24 continued
E. Turn top palm down and bottom palm up, slowly bring together at heart, inhaling.
F. Palms meet at heart, inhalation complete.
G. Descending palm continues down along torso, ascending palm turns out and up and continues rising above head; start exhaling and aspirating 'hoo'.
H. Palms fully extended up and down, complete exhalation/aspiration.

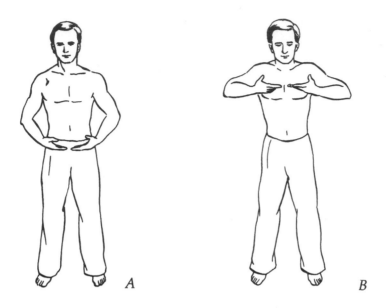

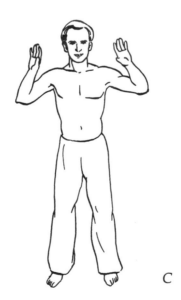

Fig. 25 **Lungs/large intestine syllable:** *sss*
A. Starting posture: Horse stance, turn palms up in front and raise hands along torso, inhaling.
B. Hands reach heart, palms up, complete inhalation.
C. Turn palms out to sides and push outwards, start exhaling and aspirating 'sss'.

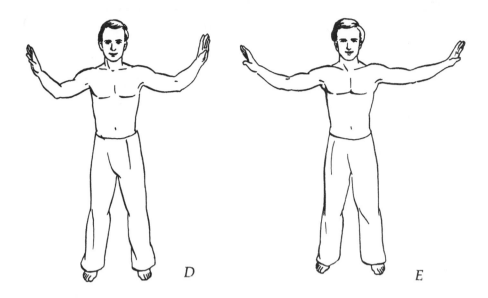

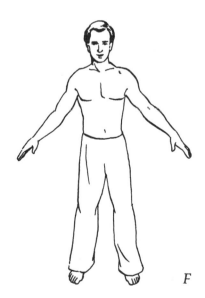

Fig. 25 continued
D. Continue pushing palms out to sides and aspirating until arms extended.
E. Turn palms to ground and slowly lower to sides, continuing exhalation/aspiration.
F. Return to starting posture; repeat.

pointing up towards the sky. Commence exhaling and aspirating the *sss* syllable through the mouth as you push your hands outwards towards the sides, as though pushing open a lift door, with the palms facing outwards. When your arms are extended out to the sides but with the elbows still slightly bent (not locked in full extension), turn the palms down towards the ground and slowly lower the arms back down to the starting position while continuing the mouth exhalation and syllable aspiration.

3) When your breath is empty and your arms are hanging down loose by your sides, pause briefly to relax, then commence another cycle on the next inhalation.

Benefits: Clears congestion from lungs and the lung meridian and stimulates large-intestine energy. Eliminates excess heat from the lungs, enhances lung energy, improves all respiratory functions. Effective remedy for colds, flu, and other bronchial ailments. Also relieves aches in the shoulders and upper back.

Syllable Five: chway (pronounced as in 'way' with a 'ch' in front. Lips slightly pursed on the initial 'ch', then relaxed and open on the final 'way')
Element: Water
Season: winter
Organ: kidney/bladder
Method: 1) Stand with the feet slightly closer together than in standard Horse, arms hanging loosely down by your sides, the palms facing the thighs.

2) Take a deep inhalation, bend your arms and raise the hands slightly up in front so that the palms are facing each other at navel level, then slowly bend your knees and squat down to the ground as you exhale through the mouth and aspirate the syllable *chway*. Try to keep the spine fairly erect as you crouch down, slightly contract the anus, and keep the palms facing each other in front.

3) When your breath is empty and your body is crouched down in a full squat, with your arms wrapped around your legs and the palms facing, commence the next inhalation and slowly rise up to the original posture. Then commence the next exhalation and syllable aspiration as you squat down again in another cycle.

Benefits: Builds up kidney energy, clears the kidney meridian, tonifies the kidneys, and stimulates the adrenal glands. It is a remedy for sexual debility and any kidney or bladder ailment.

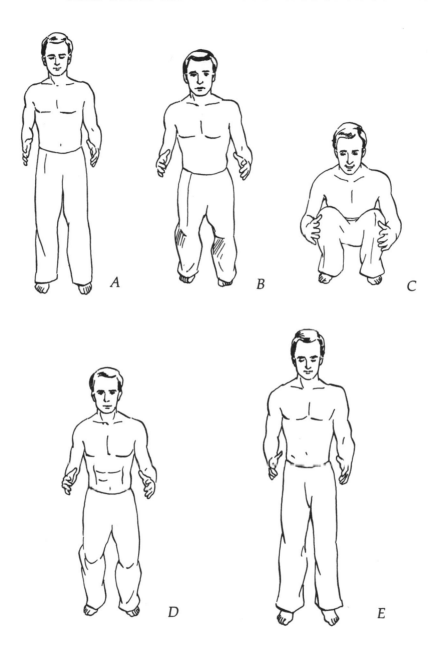

Fig. 26 **Kidney/bladder syllable:** *chway*
A. Starting posture: raise hands up in front, palms facing, take full inhalation with nose.
B. Bend knees and squat down slowly, start exhaling with mouth and aspirate first part of syllable 'choo'.
C. Continue squatting to ground, palms facing in front, and complete aspirating syllable 'way'.
D. Slowly rise up to standing position, inhaling with nose.
E. Return to starting stance, inhalation complete; repeat.

Note: If you have high blood pressure, avoid this exercise until your blood pressure is normalized. If your knees are too weak to perform the squat, wait until you build up your knee and thigh strength with other exercises, before practising this one.

Syllable Six: shee (pronounced 'she', with the teeth slightly parted and the lips formed in a small smile)
Element: Fire
Season: summer
Organ: Triple Burner/pericardium
Method: 1) This syllable exercise is performed in precisely the same format as the exercise 'Palms raised to heaven to regulate the Triple Burner', above. However, when your palms reach full extension above the head, switch the breath over to open-mouth-exhalation mode and aspirate the syllable *shee* as you lower your arms back down the sides.
2) When your arms are back down in front of you, turn the palms up and commence another cycle on the next inhalation.

Benefits: This exercise helps remedy any ailments caused by imbalances or malfunctions in the Triple Burner system, including swollen thyroids, sore throat, hot and cold spells, ringing ears, bloated abdomen, profuse sweating, dizziness, and oppression in the chest. It is a good way to balance the entire Triple Burner system, including respiratory, digestive, and excretory functions. The difference between this and the other exercise performed in the same format is that this one focuses energy specifically on the apertures of the Triple Burner in the chest, solar plexus, and lower gut, whereas the other one circulates energy throughout the entire Triple Burner organ-energy system. Use this one for healing and the other one for overall stimulation of the entire system.

Note: If you have high blood pressure, you should not raise your arms any further than head level on inhalation. Upon reaching head level, turn the palms out and around, then push them out to the sides and lower them back down to the starting position on exhalation.

Two modes of practising the Six Syllables

1) If you are extremely fatigued, weak, or ailing, you may also practise the Six-Syllable Secret using only the aspirated breaths, without the movements of the body. In this case, each syllable you practise

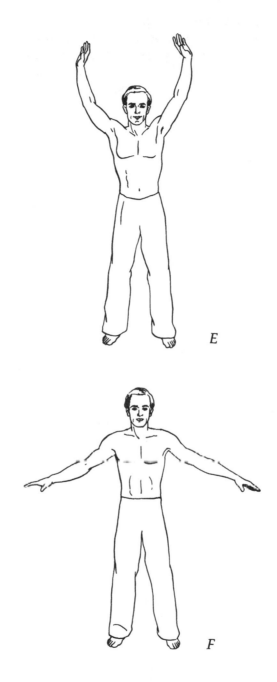

Fig. 27 Triple Burner/pericardium syllable: *shee*
As Fig. 18 (p. 209) until:
D. Start exhaling with mouth and aspirate the syllable '*shee*'.
E. Lower arm down to sides, start exhalation with mouth and aspirate syllable '*sss*'.
F. Continue lowering arms down to starting position and complete exhalation/aspiration.

should be performed at least six times, using only the breath, either standing in Horse, or sitting on edge of a stool with your spine erect. After each exhalation, pause to relax the body, regulate the breath with a few ordinary abdominal breaths, clear the mind, then do another syllable.

2) When practising the syllables in conjunction with the physical movements, be sure not to tense the muscles or tighten the joints. Especially keep the shoulders as loose and relaxed as possible. Use the mind of intent to open up the vital energy points between the eyebrows and midway between the nipples, so that energy may flow freely between head and torso.

Chee-gung hand balls (Fig. 28)

Since ancient times, Chinese calligraphers, painters, *chee-gung* healers, martial artists, and others whose livelihoods depended on strong, well-balanced hand energy and nimble fingers have used this simple but highly effective method for balancing their internal energies, toning the tendons of their hands and arms, and increasing the flow of energy to their palms and fingers. *Chee-gung* hand balls are two balls of equal size and weight, made of steel, marble, agate, or jade. Though expensive, jade is by far the best material, thanks to its capacity to conduct and purify energy.

Held in the palm of one hand, the balls are rolled in a circle by manipulating them with the fingers, counterclockwise in the right

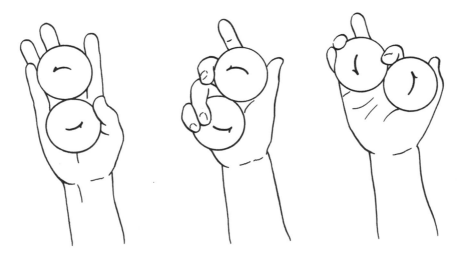

Fig. 28 Chee-gung hand balls.

hand, clockwise in the left. At first you'll feel clumsy doing this, and the balls will clack loudly against each other as you try to spin them round in your palms. But with a week or two of daily practice, you'll be able to rotate them smoothly and swiftly, keeping the balls in contact the entire time, so that they make a smooth humming sound rather than clacking randomly against each other.

Hold the two balls in the palm of one hand with the forearm held away from the body and parallel to the ground. Start the balls rolling by drawing the inside ball towards your body with the little and ring fingers, thereby causing the other one to roll forwards towards the index and middle finger, with the thumb preventing it from rolling off to the outside. Then extend the little and ring fingers forwards again and let the outside ball roll inwards towards them, pulling it towards the body, and continue rolling the balls around in circles. Do this until the tendons in your hand, wrist, and forearm feel a bit sore or numb, then switch hands. You can practise this any time of day or night, while reading or watching a film, on a bus or train or plane.

This exercise is a very effective way to harmonize the Five Elemental Energies and stimulate the organ-energies whose meridians run into the fingers: lungs, large intestine, heart, small intestine, pericardium, and Triple Burner. Balancing internal energies has long been a primary method for preventing disease and degeneration in Taoist alchemy and Chinese medicine. The rhythmic flexing of finger, hand, wrist, and arm tendons increases strength and coordination in the hands, cures and prevents arthritis and rheumatism in all joints from fingers to shoulders, and provides an excellent warm-up prior to practising calligraphy, painting, surgery, massage, or any other skill that requires digital dexterity and a strong flow of energy to the hands.

Cool-down collection and storage set

The set of collection exercises given below should be practised at the conclusion of *chee-gung* workouts. It only takes five to ten minutes and serves to draw the energy you've generated and circulated during the workout back down into the Lower Elixir Field for storage. From there it will gradually flow into the Microcosmic Orbit of the Governing and Conception channels, which serve as *chee* reservoirs, feeding the accumulated energy into the twelve main organ meridians as required. Failure to collect and store energy at the end of a *chee-gung* workout may result in the wasteful loss of energy known as *san-chee*, 'scattered energy', which happens when you leave energy 'floating' in your head, chest, and limbs after a workout. *San-chee* can also cause headaches and dizziness, tingling or numbness in the extremities, congestion in the chest, and other uncomfortable symptoms of scattered and floating energy. Therefore, it's always a good idea to spend a few minutes collecting and storing the energy you've so carefully cultivated during *chee-gung* practice. It's also helpful to pause briefly between each exercise in your workout and perform a few deep diaphragmic breaths standing in the Horse position, with your mind focused on the lower abdomen, in order to collect your energy in the Lower Elixir Field after each exercise. This is an effective way to prevent energy from getting 'stuck' in the wrong place during the course of a workout and enhances the benefits of each exercise, which should begin and end with energy concentrated in the lower abdomen.

While performing these exercises, try to keep your mind focused on the Lower Elixir Field, a point located in the geometric centre of a triangle formed by drawing lines between the navel, perineum, and the point on the lower spine directly opposite the navel (Fig. 29). This point is located at the urinary bladder, which contains electrolytes that can absorb and hold the extra energy cultivated through *chee-gung* practice until it moves into general circulation in the meridian network.

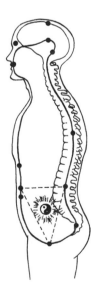

Fig. 29 ***Dan-Tien:*** **Lower Elixir Field, the centre of the human energy system.**

Harmonizing internal and external energies (Fig. 30)
Technique: This is another exercise used in the esoteric martial-arts form called *ba-gua*, or 'Eight Trigrams'. After completing any *chee-gung* set, regardless how long or short, this should be the first collection exercise you perform. Stand in Horse, completely relax your muscles, and perform five or six deep abdominal breaths. Then bring your hands forwards in front of the thighs, palms facing each other, and slowly extend the arms and hands out towards the sides as you commence slow inhalation. Continue moving the hands outwards and upwards, keeping the palms facing the entire time, until the hands are at head level and inhalation is complete. Then, as you commence a long slow exhalation, bring your palms, forearms, and elbows all together towards each other in a single smooth movement, as though you were compressing a big balloon from fingertips to elbows. When the palms and forearms are about six inches apart, start drawing them down in front towards the navel, keeping the palms facing each other as you continue exhalation. When the palms are down below the navel and exhalation is complete, move them out to the sides again as you commence the next inhalation.

There should be no pause between breaths or in the circular motion of arms and hands. It's best to keep your eyes closed during this exercise in order to focus full attention on sensations in the centre of the palms and in the fingertips. Imagine that you are expanding and contracting a big, flexible ball of energy between your palms, or that you have a batch of taffy stuck to the palms, stretching and compressing it with each circular motion.

Perform one or two dozen cycles, more if you wish, at the end of your workout.

Benefits: This exercise harmonizes the internal energies you've generated during a *chee-gung* workout with the external shield of radiant protective energy around the surface of your body. It also draws internal energy down into the Lower Elixir Field for storage until it enters circulation in the Governing and Conception channels. When practised slowly, softly and smoothly, as though your hands were moving through water, this exercise causes a strong interaction between the energy in your hands and the atmospheric energy around them, enabling you rapidly to develop a tangible feel for *chee*.

Ear-lobe and jaw rubdown (Fig. 31)
Technique: Rub the palms together slowly and firmly, holding them up at heart level, until warm. Clasp the ears firmly between the index and middle fingers of each hand, with your palms against the

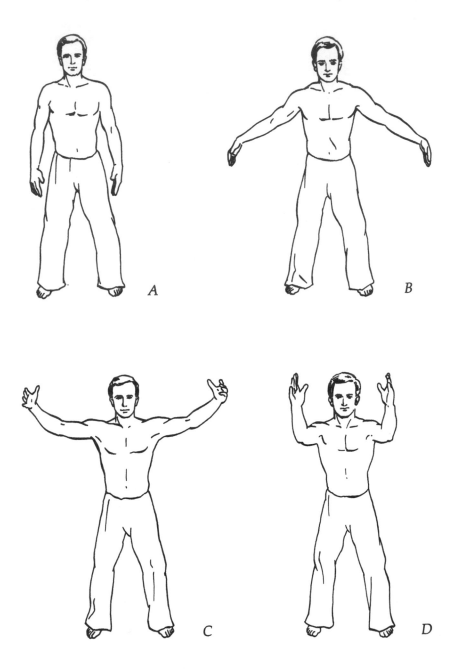

Fig. 30 **Harmonizing internal and external energies**
A. Horse stance, palms facing in front.
B. Extend arms out to sides, palms facing, inhaling.
C. Continue raising arms in wide circle, palms facing, till hands at head level, inhalation complete.
D. Bring palms, forearms, and elbows together in front and start exhaling with nose.

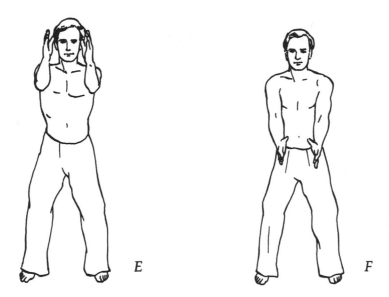

Fig. 30 continued
E. When palms and elbows are about 6 inches apart, bring them down in front, continue exhalation.
F. Palms return to starting position, exhalation complete.

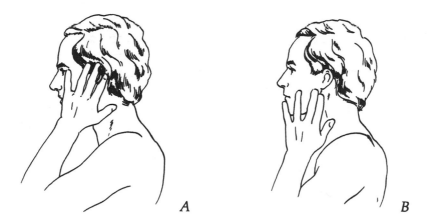

Fig. 31 **Ear-lobe and jaw rubdown**
A. Grasp ear lobes with first and second fingers.
B. Pull down firmly and continue rubbing down jaw line.

jawbone, and rub the fingers down along the ear lobes until the ears are released, then continue rubbing the index and middle fingers about halfway down the jawbone. Repeat at a fairly brisk rate one to two dozen times.

Benefits: This manoeuvre helps draw energy down out of the head and pushes it down the front of the body towards the abdomen. According to Chinese acupuncture therapy, all the vital organs and glands have sensitive energy points located in the shells and lobes of the ears. (It is therefore not a good idea to have one's ears pierced.) This ear massage thus stimulates and balances internal organ energies.

Ear-pressure pop
Technique: Extend the index or middle fingers of each hand and screw them tightly into the hole of each ear, creating an airtight plug. Then yank them abruptly out, causing a 'pop' sound in your ears. Repeat six times.

Benefits: This technique compresses, balances, and releases the air pressure in the Eustachian tubes connecting the ears with the sinus cavities. Eustachian pressure can become unbalanced or obstructed during *chee-gung* practice, and this manoeuvre corrects it. It also drives any excess *chee* floating around in these cavities down and out through the sinus passages.

Back of head and neck rubdown (Fig. 32)
Technique: Rub the palms together till warm, then place one palm on the crown of the head and rub briskly down the back of the head and neck, then down around the side of the neck to the collarbone in front. Follow immediately with the other palm, and continue rubbing down from crown to neck to collarbone alternately with each palm. If you have long hair and wear it tied up in a bun or ponytail, start the rubdown on the back of the neck just below the hair knot. Perform one to three dozen repetitions at a fairly brisk pace.

Benefits: This exercise draws excess energy from the head and neck down towards the front of the body and into the torso, from where it sinks down into the lower abdomen. It also stimulates blood circulation and lymph flow in the neck, energizes the nerves in the neck, and provides a soothing massage to the muscles and tendons connecting head to shoulders.

Tapping the Celestial Drum (Fig. 33)
Technique: Place the palms firmly against the ears, creating an airtight seal over the ears. Cock the index fingers over the middle

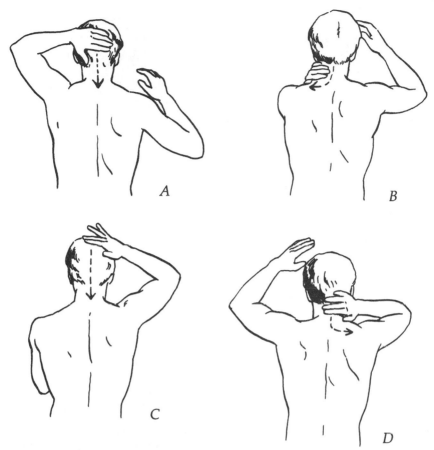

Fig. 32 **Back of head and neck rubdown**
A. Rub down from crown to back of neck.
B. Continue rubbing down side of neck and place other hand on crown.
C. Rub down head and neck with other hand.
D. Continue rubbing down side of neck.

fingers, then sharply snap the index fingers off the middle fingers and onto the back of the skull at the 'Jade Pillow' region, located at the base of the skull where it connects with the top of the neck. This will cause a loud, hollow drumming sound to reverberate throughout your skull and brain. Perform two to three dozen taps per set.

Benefits: This exercise helps drive excess energy accumulated in the head during *chee-gung* practice down into the chest, from where it sinks down into the lower abdomen for storage. This technique may also be employed any time of day or night to clear the mind of random thoughts and balance cerebral energy. Performed immediately before sitting meditation, it not only clears the mind but also

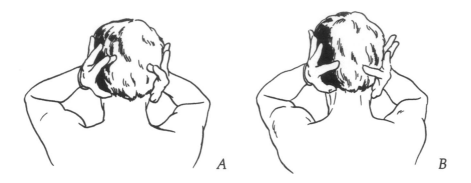

Fig. 33 **Tapping the Celestial Drum**
A. Cross index over middle finger.
B. Snap index finger against Jade Pillow points on back of head.

stimulates the Jade Pillow point to draw energy upwards along the spine from the sacrum into the cranium. Try it whenever you're feeling uptight or bedevilled by obsessive thoughts and conflicting emotions.

Navel rub (Fig. 34)
Technique: Rub the palms together till warm, then place the centre of one palm directly over the navel, with the other palm placed firmly on top of the inside hand. Breathing naturally, rub the palms around slowly in small circles, keeping the centre of the inner palm in contact with the navel and keeping the mind focused there. It helps to keep the eyes closed or half-lidded while doing this. Some teachers specify either right or left palm against the navel and different rubbing directions for men and women, but the author's teachers say that it makes no difference which palm is placed against the navel and which direction one rubs, so do it in whichever manner is most comfortable to you. Perform two to three dozen circular rubbings.

Benefits: This exercise draws energy from the head, chest, and extremities into the navel region, then drives it into the Lower Elixir Field for storage. In the process, energy is balanced and condensed. This technique also stimulates digestion, peristalsis, and other gastrointestinal functions and is therefore a good remedy for indigestion, flatulence, and sluggish bowels.

Standing still
Technique: After performing the collection exercises introduced above, 'don't just do something, stand there!' In other words, adopt

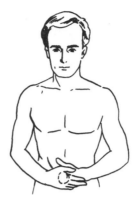

Fig. 34 **Navel rub.**

the Horse stance, totally relax the body, close the eyes, breathe naturally, focus the mind on the Lower Elixir Field, and just stand there quietly for one to three minutes, letting your energy sink and spiral down into the lower abdomen.

Benefits: This is the best way to conclude any sort of *chee-gung* workout, short of sitting down to meditate for twenty to thirty minutes. It serves as a brief but effective standing meditation, during which your internal energies have a chance to calm down and sink into their headquarters in the lower abdomen. It's important to keep your mind clear and calm and your breathing soft and natural during this final coda to your *chee-gung* practice.

Solo 'sexercises' for women and men

The exercises presented below for boosting sexual essence and energy are drawn primarily from Bodhidharma's *Marrow Cleansing Classic* and have three primary purposes:

Stimulate essence Designed to stimulate directly the so-called 'external kidneys' (testicles in men, ovaries in women), these exercises induce the testicles, ovaries, and other sexual glands to secrete elevated levels of sexual essence (i.e. hormones), which are the most potent form of essence in the body. These sexual secretions supply the basic ingredients for refining the 'elixir of life' by means of Taoist internal alchemy.

Convert essence into energy Energy derived from sexual essence is stored primarily in the two reservoirs formed by the leg vessels of the Eight Extraordinary Channels. When this energy is drawn upwards from the legs into the Central and Governing channels by deep breathing, visualization, *chee-gung*, and meditation, the extra sexual essence produced by practice of 'sexercises' is automatically converted into energy and stored in the leg channels to replace the energy that has been drawn up from those channels into the higher energy centres.

Excessive loss of semen essence through frequent ejaculation usually leaves men feeling weak and wobbly in the legs and knees, confirming the ancient Taoist tenet that sexual energy is stored in the leg channels.

Convert energy into spirit This is the final stage of internal alchemy, whereby sexual energy drawn up from the leg channels is further refined and sublimated as it rises upwards through energy centres of the Central and Governing channels into the brain, where it is transformed into pure spiritual vitality. As it rises, it cleanses and energizes the marrow, fluids, and nerves of the spine.

'Sexercises' may be incorporated into regular daily *chee-gung* workouts or practised by themselves any time of day or night. When practising them as part of an overall *chee-gung* set, you should always perform warm-up and cool-down sets before and after the workout. It is not necessary to do complete warm-up and cool-down sets before and after the 'sexercises' on their own, but you should at least prepare your body and energy channels with a few stretches and some deep breathing, and conclude with ten or fifteen minutes of still standing or sitting to harvest your enhanced sexual energy and move it into general circulation through your channels for storage in the lower abdomen. You should never leave hot sexual energy floating in your brain after practising solo 'sexercises'. If you do, you risk what Taoists call 'boiling the brain' with excess *chee*, which can cause headaches, dizziness, and other symptoms.

Bear in mind that anything which enhances sexual essence and energy – be it *chee-gung*, 'sexercises', food, or herbs – simultaneously boosts resistance and immunity, but only if the extra essence and energy are retained, transformed, and circulated internally. This in itself is a good reason to practise 'sexercises' regularly, and for men not to squander their harvest of sexual essence and energy on reckless sexual indulgence.

For women and men

Pelvic thrust (Fig. 35)

Technique: Stand in Horse stance, place hands on hips, and slightly bend the knees. Inhale and slowly thrust the pelvis back as far as possible, arching the lower spine and sticking the butt out. Then exhale and draw the pelvis forwards, straightening the lower spine and tucking the butt in as far as possible. Continue this for two or three minutes. You may also use this as a warm-up exercise.

Benefits: Stimulates and stretches the nerve fibres in the sacral region, thereby stimulating secretions of sexual essence in testicles, ovaries, prostate, and other sacral glands. Limbers and tones the vertebrae and nerves of the lower spine, which regulate sexual functions. Stimulates kidney and bladder organ energies. Draws blood and energy into the sacrum, thereby enhancing sexual energy. Encourages energy to rise up from the leg channels to the perineum, where it enters circulation in the Central and Governing channels. This triggers conversion of sexual essence into sexual energy to replace the energy drawn up from the legs.

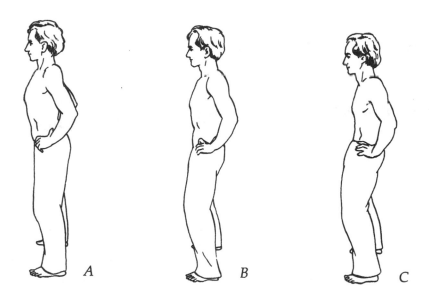

Fig. 35 **Pelvic thrust**
A. **Thrust hips back as far as possible on inhalation.**
B. **Bring hips forwards on exhalation.**
C. **Thrust hips forwards as far as possible on completion of exhalation.**

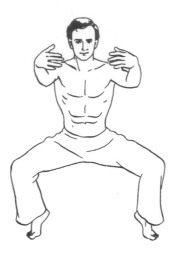

Fig. 36 **Embracing Tree in wide stance on toes.**

Embracing Tree in wide stance on toes (Fig. 36)
Technique: Adopt a wide stance, with feet splayed outwards at 45 degrees. Raise arms into Embracing Tree posture, with fingertips of hands aligned, thumbs up, hands held at throat level. Tuck in the butt, straighten up the back of the neck, and stand up on the toes and the balls of the feet. Breathe slowly and deeply, focusing attention on the fingertips and bones of the hands and keeping the anal sphincter slightly contracted to prevent energy from escaping through that orifice. On inhalation, imagine energy entering in a spiral through the fingertips and spinning up through the bones of the hands into the arms, then down the chest into the lower abdomen, where it accumulates. Then exhale and visualize energy spiralling up the spine from the lower abdomen to the head. This is a good exercise for practising reverse abdominal breathing, which intensifies the effects.

At first you won't be able to hold this posture very long, but as the muscles, tendons, and energy in your legs build up, you'll be able to practise it for increasingly longer periods. Try starting with four to six deep abdominal breaths and work up to a dozen or more.

Benefits: This exercise builds up the muscles and tendons attaching the thighs to the hips and pelvis and draws energy up from the legs and down from the arms and chest into the sacral region, where it stimulates sexual secretions. It strengthens the sexual organs in men and women, builds up the lumbar vertebrae (which regulate sexual functions), and encourages energy to rise up from the leg channels and enter the upper channels via the perineum point, known as 'Confluence of Yin' (*hui-yin*), which serves as an intersection between the upper and lower branches of the Eight Extraordinary Channels.

Jade Hop (Fig. 37)

Technique: This exercise should be performed naked. Place your feet a bit wider than shoulder width apart and parallel to each other. Raise your arms above the head, with elbows bent, shoulders relaxed, and palms facing each other. Straighten up the back of the neck, slightly contract the anus, and start hopping gently up and down at a fairly brisk pace. As you hop, slowly curl the fingers into fists and relax them, repeating rhythmically but at a slower pace than the hopping. For men, the hopping should cause the 'Jade Stalk' (penis) to flap up and down, slapping against the stomach above and the perineum below, while the testicles jounce up and down. For women, the hopping should cause the breasts to bounce

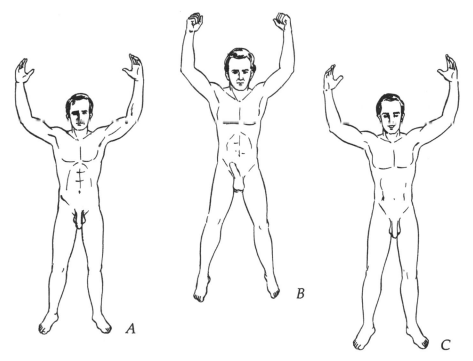

Fig. 37 **Jade Hop**
A. Starting posture
B. Hop up, curl fingers every 2–3 hops.
C. Return to start.

up and down. Continue until you feel winded, which will only take two or three minutes at first; eventually you'll be able to continue for longer periods.

Benefits: For men, this exercise strongly stimulates the testicles and prostate and greatly enhances circulation of blood and energy in the Jade Stalk. For women, it stimulates the ovaries and enhances circulation in the uterus and 'Jade Gate' (vagina). It also stimulates blood circulation and sexual secretions in women's breasts. For both men and women, hopping stimulates the pituitary in the brain and the thymus over the heart. It builds up strength and stamina in the legs, where sexual energy resides, and stimulates the kidneys and adrenals, which play major roles in regulating sexual vitality. It also prevents formation of kidney stones by shaking up the contents of the kidneys, which helps dissolve crystals before they get big enough to cause trouble.

Abdominal and lumbar massage
Technique: Stand in Horse and rub your palms together briskly until they are warm. Firmly massage the entire abdominal region between navel and pubis with circular motions. Then rub the palms to warm them up again and massage the kidneys, lumbar vertebrae, and coccyx with alternate up and down motions. Continue until the entire abdominal and lumbar regions feel warm.

Benefits: Rubbing the palms together fills the hands with energy, which is then transmitted to any part of the body that the hands massage. This exercise energizes and stimulates the entire sacral region, front and back, thereby enhancing sexual secretions and improving sexual functions, and encourages the conversion of sexual essence into energy.

For women only

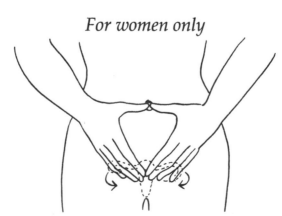

Fig. 38 **Ovary massage: massage ovaries with fourth and little fingers.**

Ovary massage (Fig. 38)
Technique: Stand relaxed in Horse stance and warm up with a few minutes of deep breathing. Rub your palms together till warm, then place thumbs together at the navel, forming a straight line from thumb to thumb parallel to the ground. Then place the tips of the index fingers together to form a triangle. You'll find the ovaries located at the tips of the little and ring fingers. Use those fingers to massage the ovaries in a circular motion thirty-six times in one direction, and thirty-six times in the other. Keeping the hands in this position on the abdomen, follow up with a few minutes of deep abdominal breathing to draw warm sexual energy upwards along the spine into the head, then back down the front into the Lower Elixir Field for storage. Apply the anal lock on inhalation and relax it on exhalation in order to stimulate energy into circulation through the Microcosmic Orbit.

Benefits: Increases sexual secretions from ovaries, stimulates female sexual energy, helps regulate menstrual cycles. If you have ovarian cysts or similar problems, do this exercise two or three times daily, in order to stimulate circulation of blood and healing energy into these tissues.

Thigh-cleft massage (Fig. 39)
Technique: Sit on the ground or floor with your legs extended forwards, feet about 24 inches apart. Rub the palms together till warm, then use the outer edge of the hands (from tip of little finger to wrist) to rub and massage the V-shaped cleft formed where the

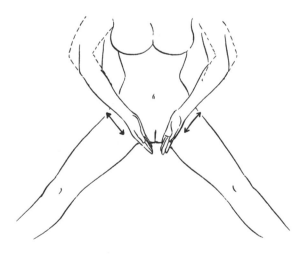

Fig. 39 **Thigh-cleft massage.**

thighs meet the pelvis on both sides of the pubic mound. Massage briskly till it feels warm.

Benefits: Stimulates female sexual energy and vaginal secretions. Good preparation for sexual intercourse or internal-energy meditation. Draws sexual energy up from the leg channels, thereby encouraging conversion of sexual essence into energy.

Foot and ankle twist

Technique: Sit on the ground or floor with legs extended, as in the above exercise. As you inhale, twist the feet and ankles inwards towards each other, then pull them back towards the upper body. Then exhale and let feet relax and return to the original position. Repeat one or two dozen times.

Benefits: This is an old Chinese exercise designed for women after childbirth in order to help tighten up the vagina again. This is meant not only to enhance sexual pleasure, but also to prevent loss of *chee* through flaccid vaginal muscles, a common problem for women after childbirth. Female adepts of Tao must take care to keep their vaginal muscles well toned in order to prevent leakage of energy through this orifice. Practising the anal lock on inhalation enhances the benefits of this exercise.

Nipple massage (Fig. 40)

Technique: Stand in Horse, or sit comfortably on a hard stool or chair, with bare feet planted parallel on the floor. Close your eyes and do a few minutes of deep breathing. Then rub the palms

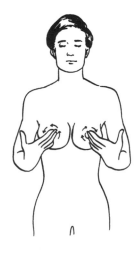

Fig. 40 **Nipple massage.**

together till warm, place the centre of the palms firmly over your nipples, and slowly massage in circles, thirty-six times in one direction, thirty-six times in the other. If you prefer, you may instead use the tips of the index, middle, and ring fingers to massage in circles in one-inch radius around nipples. As you massage, focus attention on the point between the eyebrows, then the throat, then the heart, then the kidneys, and finally the ovaries, drawing warm sexual energy to those centres. Perform one to three sets, as you wish. When finished, stand or sit still for a while with your eyes closed and let energy circulate up the back and down the front.

Benefits: This exercise is often prescribed in cases of frigidity or low libido, because it stimulates female sexual energy. Performed before intercourse, it facilitates female orgasm. It also turns on the entire female endocrine system. By focusing attention on various glandular centres (pituitary in brain, thyroid in throat, thymus at heart, etc.), warm sexual energy is drawn to those points and stimulates those glands. This is also a good way for women to warm up their channels before practising internal energy meditation.

Breast massage
Technique: Adopt the same position as above, rub your palms together till warm, and use the tips of all four fingers to massage the breasts in circles, thirty-six times in one direction, thirty-six times in the other. Massage the entire surface of the breasts, not only around the nipples. Perform one to three sets.

Benefits: Practised daily, this exercise can increase the size of the breasts by stimulating their growth. It also increases sexual energy, heightens sexual sensitivity, and is recommended as a preventive measure against formation of breast tumours. As the breasts get warm and sexual energy builds up, you may use your mind to lead the energy to various vital organs, such as lungs, stomach, liver, or bowels.

For men only

Dragon Pearl testicle massage (Fig. 41)
Technique: Stand in Horse, or sit on the edge of a hard stool or chair, without pants. Rub your palms together till warm, then place the tips of all four fingers underneath the testicles, with thumbs on top, and massage the testicles firmly by rolling them around between fingertips and thumbs. Pressure should be firm but not painful. Roll the testicles thirty-six times in each direction, then relax and

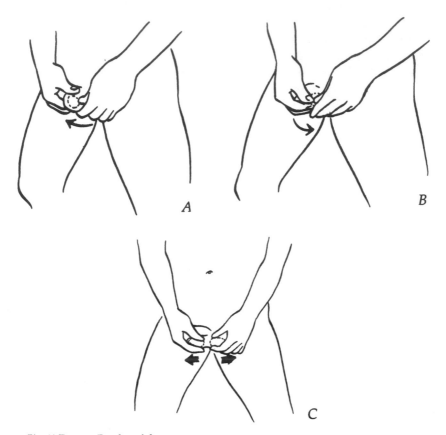

Fig. 41 **Dragon Pearl testicle massage**
A. Using both hands to massage right testicle.
B. Using both hands to massage left testicle.
C. Rolling both testicles around between thumb and index fingers of both hands.

draw energy upwards with abdominal breathing performed in conjunction with anal lock and visualization.

Benefits: Increases production of testosterone, sperm, and seminal fluids and elevates male sexual energy. When energy is drawn upwards from the leg channels, the extra sexual essence produced by testicle massage will be converted to energy and stored in the leg channels.

Dragon Tendon seminal-duct massage (Fig. 42)
Technique: Hold the testicles in the same manner as above, but instead of massaging the testicles, use the tips of the ring fingers and thumbs to locate the seminal ducts above the testicles. When you've found them, roll these tubes around between fingertips and

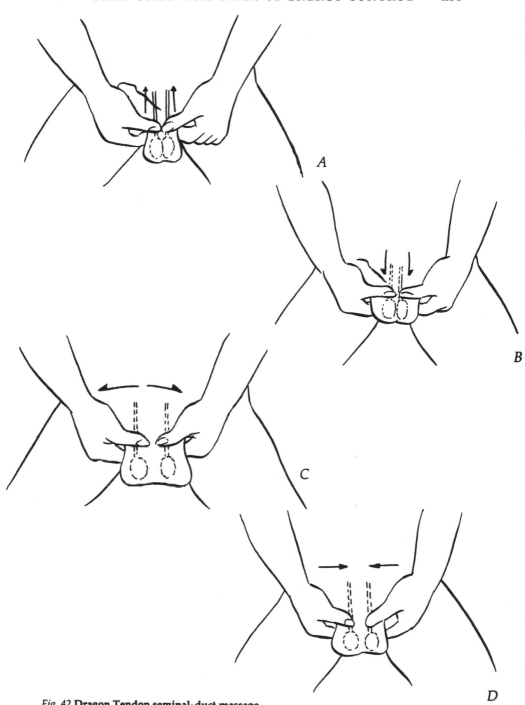

Fig. 42 **Dragon Tendon seminal-duct massage**
A, B. Massaging seminal ducts up and down by stretching and contracting them.
C, D. Massaging seminal ducts side to side by rolling them between thumb and first two fingers.

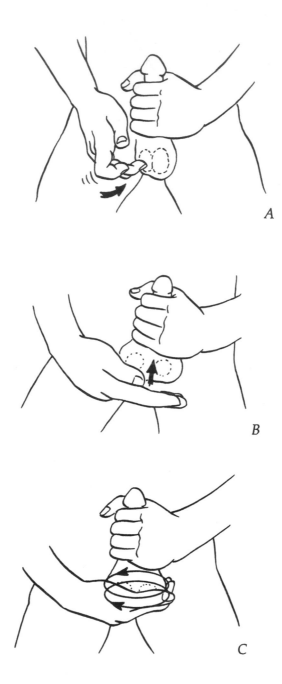

Fig. 43 **Tapping and rolling the Dragon Pearls**
A. Tapping testicles with fingertips.
B. Tapping testicles with palm.
C. Rolling testicles with palm.

thumbs, then pinch and release them, then stretch them downwards like rubber bands. Be careful and be gentle.

Benefits: Clears the seminal ducts of stagnant seminal fluids, tones the tissues of the ducts, and stimulates sperm and semen production.

Tapping and rolling the Dragon Pearls (Fig. 43)
Technique: Stand in Horse, or sit on the edge of a hard stool. Rub your palms together till warm, then use one hand to grasp the penis and pull it upwards and the fingertips of the other hand gently to tap the testicles, so that they bounce up and down. Do one or two sets of thirty-six taps each on each testicle. Then rub the palms till warm again, grasp and lift penis with one hand as above and use palm of the other hand to cup the testicles and roll them around in circles, thirty-six times in each direction. Keep the anus lightly locked during this exercise in order to encourage sexual energy to rise up spinal channels for sublimation in the brain.

Benefits: Stimulates production of semen and sperm, increases secretions of testosterone, tonifies and cleanses the tissues of the testicles, improves circulation in the scrotum. Do not squander these benefits by plowing the extra harvest of sexual essence and energy back into the field of reckless sexual indulgence. Men who practise 'sexercises' should also exercise restraint and regulate ejaculation during intercourse in order to retain the benefits.

Jade Stalk and scrotum stretch (Fig. 44)
Technique: Stand in Horse, or sit on the edge of a stool. Rub your palms together till warm, then encircle the fingers of one hand under and around the entire scrotum, with the thumb over the top of the penis root, until tips of thumb and middle finger meet to form a noose. Inhale deeply, contract the anus and perineum, then pull down firmly on the root of the Jade Stalk and scrotum, stretching the tendons as far as possible without pain. It's important to keep the anus and perineum contracted throughout the duration of the stretching phase. Release pressure, exhale, and relax perineum and abdomen. Repeat a dozen times. Then perform a dozen pulls and stretches to the left and a dozen to the right, remembering to contract the anus and perineum on each stretch. When contracting the anus and stretching the Jade Stalk, mentally visualize energy rising upwards into the internal organs, especially the kidneys, liver, and lungs. Conclude the exercise with a few minutes of quiet standing or sitting, eyes closed, mind focused on

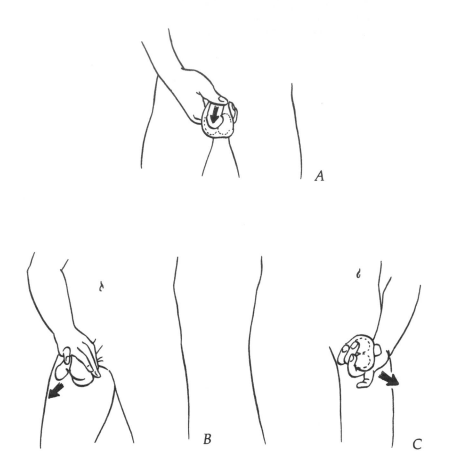

Fig. 44 **Jade Stalk and scrotum stretch**
A. Stretching forwards.
B. Twist and stretch to right.
C. Twist and stretch to left.

raising energy up the spine to the head and back down the front into the Lower Elixir Field.

Benefits: Strengthens the tendons and muscles of the penis and scrotum. Improves circulation in the penis, thereby enhancing sexual potency. Draws warm sexual energy upwards from the leg channels and sacrum into the internal organs and brain. Stimulates conversion of sexual essence to energy.

In addition to the solo 'sexercises' introduced above, the *Marrow Cleansing Classic* also contains a set of exercises for men and women known as 'Genital Weightlifting'. While some teachers have introduced these techniques to beginners in books, others believe that this stage of practice should be commenced only under the personal guidance of a qualified teacher, in order to avoid injury and the arousal of deviant energy. This writer agrees with the latter view, and therefore sexual weightlifting exercises are not included here. However, with a proper foundation in *chee-gung* practice and instruction from a qualified teacher, these exercises are not dangerous and can be very beneficial, but only if practised within the overall context of the Taoist way of life.

By way of brief preview, male genital weightlifting is performed by tying a silk scarf around the root of the penis and scrotum, hanging weights from it, tightly locking the anus and perineum, then raising the weights off the floor and gently swinging them back and forth. Women perform the same exercise by hanging weights from a string attached to a smoothly polished piece of stone, marble, or jade the size and shape of an egg. This is inserted into the vagina, and the weights are lifted and swung to and fro by contracting the vaginal muscles. These exercises build up sexual vitality very quickly, but it is not a good idea to attempt them without guidance from a qualified teacher.

CHAPTER 14

Energy Medicine

> One way of looking at illness is to characterize it as stagnant energy that is not being transformed . . . Holistic medicine may therefore be seen as a system of health maintenance that permits the free, unimpeded flow of energies, the expression of the potential of the whole self.
> Jack Schwartz, *Human Energy Systems* (1980)

The use of energy as medicine to cure and prevent human disease and degeneration has been studied and practised for thousands of years in China and other Oriental cultures. Today, however, it still remains anathema to most practitioners of orthodox Western medicine, in Asia as well as the West, because its efficacy is generally superior to chemical drugs and surgery and threatens their lucrative livelihoods. As the Tao master Shih Chien-wu noted hundreds of years ago: 'Energy is a medicine that prolongs your life. Mind is the aspect of spirit that controls energy. Therefore, if you can learn how to use your mind to control your energy, you may become a wizard.' The last thing allopathic doctors want their patients to learn is how to cure and prevent their own diseases by applying mind over matter through the medium of energy.

The *Internal Medicine Classic* described three forms of energy medicine: magnetic (placing lodestones over ailing organs and energy points); electric (acupuncture); and heat (moxabustion). All three methods work by manipulating the flow and balance of the patient's internal energies. 'Cold' conditions are warmed, 'hot' conditions are cooled, 'full' conditions emptied, 'empty' conditions filled – all by juggling and harmonizing the patient's own energies via the network of meridians and points that channel energy throughout the human system.

The meridians and their vital points have two basic functions.

One is to circulate and distribute energy to organs, glands, brain, limbs, bones, and other tissues of the body. The other is to send warning signals back to the brain whenever an organ is ailing or an area of the body over which a meridian passes is injured. The brain then responds by triggering healing and repair mechanisms via the nervous system. The human healing response is thus regulated by a closed-circuit electrical control system which links the energy system to the nervous, endocrine, and circulatory systems, with the brain serving as the central switchboard.

Sceptical Western doctors continue to deny the existence of the human energy system, simply because they cannot see it, claiming instead that it is nothing more than a manifestation of the nervous system. That's like saying radio waves don't exist because we cannot see them, even though we can easily manipulate them to send and receive audiovisual signals across vast distances. Human energy can similarly be manipulated to send signals throughout the body, which responds to them as precisely as a radio tuned to a particular frequency. For example, needles may be inserted into specific combinations of points to block all sensations of pain to the brain, enabling surgeons to conduct major operations while the patient is wide awake and aware of what's happening, yet feeling no pain. The energy points used for anaesthesia are usually located far from the area of surgical incision. If they were mere extensions of the nervous system, how could they block pain in nerves which are cut at the point of incision? The Taoist view is that the energy system overrides the nervous system because the nervous system operates by virtue of signals carried by neurotransmitters, which are forms of essence, while the energy system functions purely by energy, and, as we've already learned, 'energy commands essence'.

Internal energy

The most basic, primary form of energy medicine is individual practice of *chee-gung*, whereby a person learns how to control energy with mind and use energy to regulate organs, glands, circulation, metabolism, and other vital functions. This is accomplished by switching the autonomous nervous system over from the depleting sympathetic mode to the restorative, calming parasympathetic mode of operation, a switch-over which requires physical relaxation, mental tranquillity, emotional equilibrium, and deep abdominal breathing. This sort of internal harmony lies at the root of all forms of Taoist alchemy, from martial arts to meditation, medicine to metaphysics.

Chee-gung forges a direct link between the conscious mind and the immune system, a link already acknowledged though not well understood in modern Western medicine as 'psychoneuroimmunology'. Master Luo Teh-hsiou cites the 'harmony of the nervous and endocrine systems' as the very essence of *chee-gung* practice, and modern medical science has clearly established a close biofeedback connection between neurochemicals and hormones. Stress and excitement activate the sympathetic circuit of the autonomous nervous system, which triggers release of adrenalin, cortisol, and other action hormones. These hormones then further reinforce sympathetic nervous response by biofeedback, setting up a continuous cycle of depletion and exhaustion. *Chee-gung* in all its forms, from moving exercises to still sitting, counteracts the exhausting stress and excitement of daily life by turning on the calming parasympathetic circuit of the autonomous nervous system, which releases neurochemicals that stimulate secretions of hormones with healing, relaxing, and restorative properties. These hormones in turn sustain secretions of parasympathetic neurochemicals by biofeedback, establishing a cycle of repair and rejuvenation.

Conscious belief, or faith, in the efficacy of the method is a prerequisite for successful self-healing through *chee-gung*, as it is in any form of medical therapy. Only when the mind understands and has faith in the medicine will the medicine work. This principle applies to drugs as well as energy and explains the placebo effect, another phenomenon recognized but not understood by orthodox Western medicine. Give an ailing patient a simple sugar pill and convince him or her that it is a new miracle drug, and more often than not the pill will produce the desired effect. That's because the mind is convinced and therefore mobilizes to take command of energy in order to activate the healing process, which operates entirely by virtue of the patient's own energy. By the same principle, even the most potent, scientifically proven drugs often fail to produce any therapeutic effect whatsoever in patients who have their minds set against those drugs.

Another manifestation of energy in the healing process is the well-known immunosuppressive effect of negative emotions such as grief, depression, and anger. Recall that according to the Chinese medical view, emotions are nothing more than energy in motion. Therefore, when emotional energies are unbalanced and run rampant through the system, they have extremely disruptive effects on the balance and harmony of internal energies, upon which health and vitality depend. When internal energies lose their

natural balance and harmony, the first casualties are immunity
and resistance, which is why restoration of natural balance and
harmony among human energies has always been a primary goal
of therapeutic *chee-gung*.

External energy

When a patient's condition has become too severe and his energy
too weak to effect a cure through individual practice of *chee-gung*,
the next step in energy medicine is to apply an external source of
energy in order to boost and balance the patient's own depleted
and radically unbalanced energies. In China, this was traditionally
accomplished in three ways: medicinal herbs; applying lodestones
(magnetic energy), moxabustion (heat energy), or acupuncture
needles (electric energy) to vital points along the meridians; and
direct transfer of healing energy from healer to patient.

Chinese medicinal herbs work in a different way from Western
chemical drugs, which function solely on a biochemical basis.
Chinese herbs are categorized according to the type of energy they
release when assimilated into the human system and the way that
energy influences the patient's own internal energies. As we have
seen, the Eight Indicators used in Chinese diagnosis and treatment
are indications of various states of energy imbalance, which in
herbal medicine are corrected by prescribing a combination of
herbs. Through their correlations with the Five Elemental Energies,
all herbs have natural affinities for specific organs, glands, and
tissues, and by virtue of their associations with yin and yang, they
either 'warm' or 'cool', 'fill' or 'empty', 'raise' or 'lower', and otherwise adjust human energies. As the great Sung-dynasty master
Wang Che wrote: 'Medicinal herbs contain the finest energies of
mountains and rivers and the purest essences of plants and trees.'
Herbs thus carry the pure essences and potent energies of nature
into the human system, where they do battle with aberrant energies
and restore natural balance and harmony.

Acupuncture, lodestones, and moxabustion all work by manipulating human energy via sensitive terminals along the meridians
called 'vital points'. Depending on which points are used and
how the external energy sources are manipulated, pain may be
blocked, energy stimulated, organs toned up or sedated, emotions
pacified, injuries repaired, and so forth, according to the patient's
requirements.

The phenomenon of healing by hand, which has been taken for
granted in the East, is currently gaining recognition in the West.

China is conducting research on the transfer of energy from healer to patient, a technique known as 'therapeutic *chee-gung*'. Researchers at Jiao Tong University in Shanghai have shown that human energy displays electromagnetic properties when flowing within its own meridians, but takes on characteristics of light energy, somewhat similar to lasers, when emitted out from the body through the hands. Using renowned therapeutic *chee-gung* masters as test subjects, these investigators found that the laserlike beam of energy projected from the healer's hands travelled over distances of 26–165 yards without a drop in power. This human energy beam penetrated 4 inches of leather, 2 inches of wood, 2 inches of brick, and two sheets of iron. This means that human energy beamed from the hands of *chee-gung* masters has greater penetrating power than alpha or beta rays.

The same research revealed that during treatment the frequency of the patient's electromagnetic field becomes identical to that of the healer, indicating that the healer somehow plugs the patient into his or her own enhanced energy field. The healer's own energy is then able to dissolve obstructions in the patient's energy channels, scatter stagnant energy, boost weak energy, sedate excess energy, and otherwise rebalance the patient's energies in order to effect a cure. They also found that *chee-gung* therapy invariably enhanced the patient's immune system by stimulating the production of antibodies, increasing white-cell activity, and raising haemoglobin levels in blood serum. This phenomenon confirms the first tenet of Taoist alchemy, that 'energy commands essence'. It was further discovered that the *chee* emitted from a healer's hands could kill staphylococcus bacteria and hepatitis virus and inhibit the growth of cancer cells in the lungs and liver, but *only when the therapist consciously tried to emit 'killer* chee'. This evidence indicates that the conscious will of the healer determines the type of energy emitted from his hands, which verifies the second precept of Taoist alchemy, that 'spirit commands energy'. In other words, the energy emitted from a healer's hands is a synthesis of energy and information, a precise signal which triggers specific responses in the receiving patient.

The Chinese scientists studying therapeutic *chee-gung* also discovered that the application of healing energy depleted the energy reserves of the healer, indicating that an actual transfer of energy from healer to patient takes place. *Chee-gung* healers must therefore recharge their batteries by practising restorative *chee-gung* exercises and internal energy meditation, otherwise they would fall ill themselves.

Based on their observations, Chinese scientists have developed a *'chee-gung* machine' that simulates both the energy and the information transmitted by energy healers, and this device has proven quite effective in treating hepatitis, apoplexy, paralysis, and other diseases. It also significantly enhances functions of the immune, nervous, and endocrine systems and improves the flow of blood and energy throughout the system. Unfortunately, because of the continued hostility of the Western medical establishment to any form of alternative medicine, the results of this research into energy medicine in China have not become available to Western physicians or patients.

Another ancient Oriental form of energy medicine is *reiki* ('spirit energy'), originally developed in China and Tibet over a thousand years ago, then rediscovered in Japan during the 1800s by Dr Mikao Usui. *Reiki* may be practised on oneself or on others, simply by placing the hands on specific energy points on the body and beaming healing energy into them. In recent years, the Western chiropractor and acupuncturist Dr John Veltheim has begun to conduct training classes and therapeutic workshops in this ancient form of energy medicine. Dr Veltheim could easily be quoting an ancient Chinese medical manual when he states: 'Man is energy. Health is energy in harmony. Disease, be it physical, spiritual, or emotional, is energy out of harmony. By far the best healing systems of the future will be systems that will work by balancing that disharmony at an energy level.'

Electrotherapy

Since human energy shares many fundamental properties with the universal energies of electricity and magnetism, it stands to reason that electromagnetic devices may be rigged to manipulate human energy for therapeutic purposes. Electricity, which always produces a magnetic field, is an effective medium for triggering healing responses in the human energy system. Western scientists have recently made significant contributions to this new field of medical therapy.

The British surgeon Dr Margaret Patterson, for example, has developed a highly effective electrotherapeutic cure for drug addiction by attaching electrodes to both ears of the patient and running a low-level pulsed electric current through their heads. Her therapy has consistently recorded a higher cure rate than the methadone and other chemical treatments currently used in the USA, but when Dr Patterson discussed her technique with the Food and Drug Administration, they flatly rejected it, despite the abundant scientific evidence she presented, once again protecting orthodox American medical ideology as well as the lucrative pharmaceutical industry from competition.

Dr Robert Becker has pioneered electrotherapeutic methods for healing bone fractures by attaching electrical energy sources to the body in order to create pulsed magnetic fields around the sites of fractures. These pulsed fields in turn stimulate the body's own electrically controlled healing mechanisms to reknit the fractured bones. This therapy has shown an impressive 80 per cent rate of efficacy in cases when the bone has failed to reknit naturally.

Electrotherapy has been applied to cancer patients ever since the late nineteenth century. During the 1880s, a French surgeon, Dr Apostoli, reported significant shrinkage in cancer tumours when positive electrodes carrying current of 100–250 milliamperes were inserted directly into the tumours. Dr Björn Nordenström of the Karolinska Institute in Stockholm, Sweden, has been applying similar techniques to cancer patients, using a form of electrically amplified acupuncture. Rapidly growing tissues always display a higher negative polarity than other tissues, with malignant tumours recording the highest negativity of all. Consequently, when positive currents are applied to such tumours, their growth is retarded and they begin to shrink. Dr Becker speculates that this effect is caused by 'a massive shift in the local acid-base [yin-yang] balance with the production of a highly acidic [yang] area within which cells are destroyed'. In Taoist parlance, Dr Becker is saying that the electric current (energy) alters the pH balance (yin-yang) of the tumorous tissues (essence), resulting in the desired therapeutic effect. This boils back down to the old Taoist precept that 'energy commands essence'.

In the June 1986 issue of *East West Journal*, Richard Leviton reported that researchers at California's Loma Linda University School of Medicine found that low-frequency, low-intensity magnetic fields were successful in alleviating chronic pain and healing ulcers in over 1,000 patients tested in sixteen different countries. In 90 per cent of those patients, a significant improvement in blood circulation was also reported. These researchers concluded that every cell in the body is 'a small electric battery' whose energy may be manipulated by exposure to different magnetic fields. Since *chee-gung* practice establishes a low-frequency, low-intensity magnetic field similar to that of the earth, it has a rejuvenating therapeutic effect on each individual cell, as well as on the whole organism.

There are now dozens of different electrotherapeutic devices on

the market: energy synergizers, microwave harmonizers, biocir-
cuit enhancers, alpha-wave stimulators, biofeedback monitors,
negative-ion generators, energy balancers, biomagnetic devices,
field polarizers, electromagnetic-pollution detectors, computer-
radiation protectors, brain-wave synchronizers, light and sound
integrators, and more. These devices are designed for home use
and are well worth exploring, especially if you live in an area with
heavy electromagnetic pollution, such as a big city. Like *chee-gung*,
they tend to balance and harmonize human energies and ward off
the ill effects of abnormal electromagentic fields. However, they
should not be regarded as convenient substitutes for *chee-gung*
exercise and meditation; instead, they should be used as adjuncts to
the alchemy of internal energy cultivation, just as vitamins and
minerals supplement rather than replace healthy diets. No electronic device can ever duplicate human consciousness, and only
human consciousness can control and cultivate human energy.
Gaining conscious control over energy can only be accomplished
through self-discipline, patience, and diligent practice. There are no
short cuts.

'Wind and water'

Another interesting aspect of recent research into the earth's
electromagnetic field and its influences on human health is the new
light it sheds on the ancient Chinese science of *feng-shui* ('wind and
water'), known in Western terminology as 'geomancy'. Long
ridiculed by Western sceptics as hocus-pocus, geomancy remains a
well-respected and frequently utilized science throughout the Far
East. No contractor in his right mind in Hong Kong or Taiwan
would erect a building without first consulting a *feng-shui* master
for precise advice on where to locate windows and doors and how
to arrange rooms and hallways for optimum harmony with the
surrounding energies of the earth and sky. Geomancy sometimes
plays a role in energy medicine by moving a patient from a room
where adverse environmental energies prevail into a room where
the confluence of environmental energies is more conducive to
healing.

Feng-shui masters speak of 'dragon veins' which conduct the
various energies of earth and sky, wind and water, along the
surface of the earth. These might well be lines of electromagnetic
energy interacting with other natural forces, such as wind and
water, sun and moon. It would be well worth while to conduct
scientific research in this field, in order to determine whether

geomancy might play diagnostic and therapeutic roles in medicine, and to develop electromagnetic devices to counteract adverse environmental energies.

Wave of the future

Energy medicine holds the potential to revolutionize health care throughout the world, and it's high time that it did. Despite all the fancy gadgets and high-tech machinery, the expensive new drugs and increasingly complex surgical procedures upon which modern Western medicine depends, this form of medicine is rapidly losing the battle against cancer and AIDS, Altzheimer's and heart disease, and scores of other ailments prevalent in the industrially developed world. Meanwhile, the cost of the complex chemical-mechanistic methods favoured by orthodox Western medicine continues to multiply at a rate that affects the national economies of many countries.

Energy medicine requires little or no equipment, no drugs, no hospitalization, and entails little or no cost to the patient other than time and effort. Based on the proven premise that all healing ultimately takes place within the patient's own energy system, and that all the therapist can do is stimulate the patient's own energies to rally to his or her defence, energy medicine is good news for patients but very bad news for the bloated multi-billion-dollar hospital and pharmaceutical industries, which thrive on public health crises without solving them.

Another good thing about energy medicine is that it enriches consciousness while promoting health and prolonging life. Owing to the inseparable and mutually transformative relationships among the Three Treasures of essence, energy, and spirit – in which energy functions as a bridge between body and mind – energy medicine not only heals the body, it also enhances the mind and stimulates spiritual growth. Antibiotics and surgery certainly don't do that!

Fortunately, when it comes down to the life-and-death issues of health and disease, people are interested only in what works, not in academic arguments and political debates. Since energy medicine, when properly practised, usually works better than chemical or surgical medicine, without extravagant expense or debilitating side effects, it's only a matter of time before the public demands its inclusion into the mainstream of modern medical care.

CHAPTER 15

Spirit

Spirit is master of the body, just as a lord is master of his kingdom. A restless spirit cannot take care of the body, which, when not guided by spirit, wanders down the path to death. However, a tranquil spirit which calmly guides the body is the guardian of health and longevity.
Chin Kang, *On Cultivating Life* (fourth century AD)

In traditional Chinese medicine as well as Taoist internal alchemy, spiritual tranquillity has always been a key factor in human health and longevity. In modern Western medicine, however, mental factors are consistently overlooked, and the somatic links between body and mind are not clearly recognized. Instead, so-called 'mental cases' are sent to the 'shrink' for psychoanalysis, even if their problems are caused by physiological disorders, and physiological disorders caused by spiritual malaise are treated by chemical and mechanical methods.

Even a cursory glance at modern urban life reveals two pervasive factors that always go hand in hand: chronic stress and chronic disease. In a chapter of the *Internal Medicine Classic* entitled 'The Oldest Truth', it is written: 'When one empties the mind and frees it of all desires, the genuine energy arises. If one maintains an undisturbed spirit within, no disease will occur.' What this means is that stress (i.e. 'disturbed spirit') impairs immunity and renders the body vulnerable to disease, a fact often observed but not well understood by modern medicine. The Western medical approach to stress-related disease is to give the patient tranquillizers, which suppress the overt nervous symptoms of stress without in any way alleviating its causes or its physiological side effects.

Tranquillity is in fact the solution to the problem, but not the sort of tranquillity induced by drugs. What is required here is the harmonization and rejuvenation of the Three Treasures by activating the internal alchemy of essence, energy, and spirit. In the first stage of the process, essence is conserved and nourished, then transformed into energy, which in turn is refined and raised to nurture spirit. When spirit is strong and stable, one applies the second stage of internal alchemy, whereby 'spirit commands energy' and 'energy commands essence'. With a strong and tranquil spirit, the adept may consciously harness energy to stimulate essence and heal the body. It is accomplished simply by 'sitting still, doing nothing' and letting nature take its course.

The nature of spirit

Like essence and energy, spirit has its pristine primordial and its conditioned temporal aspects. Primordial spirit, also known as the 'mind of Tao', is the original source of all consciousness, the flame of primal awareness that lights up the mind. It is eternal, indestructible, and immortal, but soon after birth it becomes dormant through social conditioning and the constant distractions of temporal life. As primordial spirit becomes shrouded with layer upon layer of self-woven egohood, it disappears from conscious awareness, and the primal unity of the Three Treasures is torn asunder. Spirit loses its rightful command over energy, which the body instead commandeers for its own sensual gratification and sensory entertainment. Unfettered by spirit, emotions run rampant and random thoughts clutter the mind, further obscuring awareness. Like a leaf in the wind, the temporal mind is blown to and fro by the vagaries of external events, while the body's energies are plundered and dissipated by the Five Thieves of the senses. Small wonder that the body, 'when not guided by spirit, wanders down the path to death'.

The original mind of Tao is like an immaculately clean mirror, clearly reflecting everything towards which it turns its attention. The human mind, by contrast, is like a dirty mirror, bespecked with the dust of greed and lust, smudged with the grime of conflicting emotions, streaked with the haze of conditioned thoughts. The process whereby one recovers the original mind of Tao and restores primordial awareness is called 'polishing the mirror'. This is an introspective process by which one gradually clears away the emotional obstructions, mental obscurations, and physical defilements accumulated since birth, so that the original mind of Tao may once again shine forth and reflect the world as it really is.

This introspective process of clarifying the mind goes beyond words, arguments, and theories. It can be achieved only by practice, not by study; only by 'letting go' rather than 'holding on' to thoughts and ideas; only by integration of conflicting views, not by sectarian differences; only by realization, never by rationalization. As Lao-tzu disclaimed in the opening line of the *Tso Teh Ching*: 'The way which can be spoken is not the real Way.' The sage Lu Tung-pin agrees: 'Words are not true explanations of the Tao. When you have realized the Tao personally, you can dispense with words.' That is why true adepts of the Tao shun sectarian debates and doctrinaire arguments. The 'real way' is not divided by sects and doctrines, for a path that's divided leads nowhere. It is most important to guard against charlatans and imposters in the Tao. In *Vitality, Energy, Spirit*, Thomas Cleary translates Lu Tung-pin's remarks on this issue as follows:

> The mind that understands the Way is entirely impartial and truthful. But because Taoist tradition has gone on so long, personalistic degenerations have cropped up. People attack one another and establish factions of supporters; they call themselves guardians of the Way, but they are really in it for their own sakes. When you look into their motivations, you find they are all outsiders. People like this are rot in Confucianism, bandits in Taoism, troublemakers in Buddhism. They are confused and obsessed.

Fire mind and Water mind

Postnatal spirit, i.e. the 'human mind', has two distinctive aspects, known in Chinese as the 'mind of emotion' (*hsin*) and the 'mind of intent' (*yi*). The mind of emotion is said to reside in the heart and is associated with Fire energy. It is volatile, unpredictable, and easily swayed by external stimuli. The mind of intent resides in the brain and is associated with Water energy. It is cool, calm, and introspective, and when properly cultivated, it provides an infinite source of wisdom by virtue of its link with primordial awareness.

Using intent to subdue and control emotions, or Water to subjugate Fire, is an important aspect of Taoist internal alchemy and an absolute prerequisite for health and longevity as well as for restoring conscious access to the original mind of Tao. Six hundred years ago, the great alchemist and martial-arts master Chang San-feng wrote: 'When wisdom controls desire, you live long; when desire overcomes wisdom, you die early.' In the Taoist paradigm, mental as well as physical health are achieved by maintaining balance between emotions and intent, passion and wisdom, heart and brain, Fire and Water. When the scales tip neither towards one nor the other but strike a homeostatic balance, perfect equilibrium is achieved, yin and yang energies merge, and the Three Treasures are harmonized.

Mind of emotion		Mind of intent
Fire		Water
yang		yin
heart		brain
feelings		thoughts
passion		wisdom
	Balance	
	equilibrium	
	harmony	
	stability	
	clarity	
	vitality	
	health	

Taoist alchemy puts the head in command of the heart, training the wisdom mind (*yi*) to control the vagaries of the emotional mind (*hsin*). The conflict of interests between the head and the heart is a perennial problem of human life, particularly in this age of intellectual rationalization and emotional self-indulgence. In his movie *Crimes and Misdemeanors*, Woody Allen utters the memorable Taoist lament: 'It's very hard to get your heart and head together in life.'

The fact is, only you can 'get your heart and head together' on the same track, no one else can do it for you, and if you don't, you can be certain that they'll gallop off in opposite directions, tearing your life asunder. The problem usually arises at the moment a decision is being made whether to resist or succumb to emotional temptation. The fiery mind of emotion often gains the upper hand at such crucial moments by sheer bluster and bravado, overruling the finer sensibilities and better judgement of the cool, calm mind of wisdom. Then, when things go wrong, as they inevitably do when you let your heart lead your head, hindsight always rules in favour of the wise advice of the head rejected by the devil-may-care heart, but by that time it's too late to change your mind. However, it's never too late to learn a lesson from such experience in order to prevent history from repeating itself.

In the strictly chemical-mechanistic view of conventional

Western medicine, the brain is synonymous with the mind, but in the Taoist view, the brain is only a physical organ through which the mind exerts control over the body. Primordial spirit is formless, boundless, and immortal, but in order to function in the temporal material world it must manifest a temporal aspect, which is called the 'human mind', including emotions and thoughts. In order for the mind to communicate with and control the physical body, it must operate through the brain, which is connected to every organ, limb, and tissue via the network of nerves and energy channels. The brain is a two-way terminal by which the mind exerts command over the body and the state of the body influences the state of the mind. This is the basis of psychoneuroimmunology, in which neurotransmitters represent the mind and brain, hormones represent the body and immune system, and biofeedback provides the balancing mechanism. One of the primary functions of *chee-gung* exercises and meditation is to feed the brain with essence (oxygen- and nutrient-laden blood) and energy (raised up the spine from the sacrum) in order to enhance the power of the spirit's only vehicle of communication and activity on the physical plane, the brain. It's very important, however, to view the brain as part of the body and not confound it with the mind itself, just as a computer, despite its apparent ability to think, is still just a machine that processes information upon command of the human mind.

It is also exceedingly important to distinguish clearly between intellectual understanding and rational knowledge on the one hand, and intuitive insight based on primordial awareness on the other. Intellect and reason are products of the human mind, and can provide us only with practical information regarding the material world of external phenomena perceived by the physical senses. They cannot fathom the mysteries of consciousness itself, nor reveal the true nature of spirit. The problem with existential Western philosophy is that it is based entirely on intellectual speculation and gives no credence to spiritual inspiration. As the 2,000-year-old Taoist classic *Huai-nan-tzu* states: 'While intellect has its uses, it must always remain rooted in spirit.' If we follow only our temporal intellectual minds in conducting our lives, we tend to rationalize our every whim, overwork our bodies, and lead ourselves astray, for the intellect is as ephemeral and finite as the body and has no basis in the eternal and infinite abode of the spirit. 'The temporal mind controls the body,' the *Huai-nan-tzu* continues, 'but the spirit is the precious treasure of the mind. If mind forces body to work without rest, the body will collapse, and if mind strains spirit without respite, spirit will soon become exhausted.

Treasuring these assets, sages do not dare exceed their limits.' Hence moderation, restraint, balance, harmony, and spiritual insight are constant themes in all Taoist texts.

The great flaw of modern Western science is the tacit assumption that whatever one perceives with the senses and interprets with rational intellect provides an 'objective' view of reality. This assumption overlooks two facts. First, all sense perceptions, including those magnified, amplified, and otherwise assisted by high-tech instruments, are subjective views of the world relative to the cultural conditioning and intellectual biases of the observer. Nothing we perceive with our senses makes any sense at all until we interpret it with our own temporally conditioned minds. Second, the only truly objective fact of life is consciousness itself. No two people have exactly the same view of the world. Therefore, the most important science of all is the science of perception and consciousness, which holds the key to all other sciences and which has always been of paramount importance in the traditions of the Orient. Indeed, Buddhism is often referred to as a 'science of mind', and the ultimate goal of Taoist science has always been 'returning to the source' of primordial spiritual awareness.

The difference, then, between Western and Taoist science is that the former takes the rational intellect of temporally conditioned mind as the ultimate arbiter of objective reality, while the latter regards rational intellect as a minor temporal offshoot of a far more omniscient spiritual awareness. And since primordial spiritual awareness is the only enduring, permanent aspect of the human psyche, transcending life and death, time and space, Taoist science regards the intuitive insights it provides to be far more true, objective, and universally valid that the subjective conclusions of rational intellect. Because the conditioning of temporal mind obscures primordial awareness, the first task of Taoist science is to recover the latent powers of primordial spiritual awareness and restore the primordial spirit's rightful command over the Three Treasures of life. The tool for that task is meditation, the materials are your own essence and energy, and the laboratory is your own mind.

In *Essential Points of Alchemy*, composed in the fourteenth century, the Taoist sage Shang Yang-tzu wrote:

> Intellectual understanding and rational knowledge are by nature spiritual obstructions caused by arbitrary confirmation and denial . . . The essence of intellectual understanding and rational knowledge originates in the

six senses, bound day by day with ceaseless sentimental feelings and emotions. The true nature of life lies right at our feet, eternal and immutable existence as it is, endowed with unconditional freedom. An old sage once said, 'The hell realms are pleasant compared to the enormous suffering of having failed to understand the central point of this great matter.'

Taoist (as well as Buddhist) science therefore seeks the eternal, universal light of consciousness that lies hidden like a 'shining pearl' in the heart of all sentient beings. Once the mystery of awareness itself has been fathomed, everything else comes sharply into focus with perfect clarity. As an ancient Taoist maxim says: 'If you can open this one gate, all other gates will open naturally.'

Spirituality and sexuality

In Taoist as well as Tantric Buddhist tradition, spirituality and sexuality are complementary forces, not enemies split into hostile camps as in Judeo-Christian and Islamic traditions. In the Taoist and Tantric view, sex is sacred, and women are revered as the source of all life on earth. Before the rise of Christianity in Europe, sex was held to be as sacred there as in the Orient, as evidenced by the word 'sacrum', the body's sexual centre, which is derived from the same root as 'sacred'.

In terms of practice, sexual essence and energy comprise our most potent tools for progress on the spiritual path. By virtue of the internal alchemy of the Three Treasures, sexual hormones and sexual energy may be refined, transformed, and raised up from the sacrum to the head in order to enhance spiritual awareness. The solo 'sexercises' in the *Marrow Cleansing Classic* are good examples of specific Taoist techniques for converting sexual energy into fuel for spiritual progress.

Sexual passion itself can also provide a springboard for spiritual insight. The experience of sexual bliss is the closest earthly equivalent to the ecstasy of spiritual realization. Both involve the unity of opposites, the dissolution of duality, enormous energy, intense joy, and a sense of completion. It was through sexual union that we came into this world in the first place, and it is through the experience of sexual union that we may gain a fleeting glimpse of that sublime state of primordial unity to which all spiritual seekers aspire. By applying sexual energy to spiritual practice and spiritual insight to sexual activity, both are enhanced, and balanced equilibrium between our spiritual and carnal natures is achieved. Rather than attempting the hopeless task of suppressing sexual desire in their disciples, Taoist and Tantric spiritual masters teach their followers the real facts of life and sex, without sentiment or prurience, and show them how to make spirit and flesh cooperate rather than conflict on the path.

Centuries ago in Tibet, the Sixth Dalai Lama, who preferred the company of women to monks and the taste of wine to butter tea, said something to the effect that 'if one's feelings towards spiritual practice were as intense as one's feelings towards sex, then one would easily become enlightened in this very lifetime'. If one practises sex as well as spiritual life according to the Tao, one will progress rapidly on both paths, without inner conflict, until sexuality and spirituality merge onto the one Great Highway that leads back to the original source of both.

CHAPTER 16

Sitting Still: Meditation

Nourishing the spirit is the highest task.
The Yellow Emperor's Classic of Internal Medicine
(second century BC)

The Taoist sage Chuang-tzu referred to meditation, which the Chinese simply call 'sitting still, doing nothing', as 'mental fasting'. Just as physical fasting purifies the essences of the body by withdrawing all external input of food, so the 'mental fasting' of meditation purifies the mind and restores the spirit's primal powers by withdrawing all distracting thoughts and disturbing emotions from the mind. In both physical and mental fasting, the cleansing and purifying processes are natural and automatic, but the precondition for triggering this process of self-rejuvenation is emptying body and mind of all input for a fixed number of minutes or days.

Meditation is to spirit what diet and nutrition are to essence and *chee-gung* is to energy – an indispensable tool for cultivating and conserving that treasure. Only by 'sitting still, doing nothing' can we muster sufficient mental clarity to focus fully on the difficult task of 'seizing the monkey and catching the horse', which is Taoist parlance for taming and training the two aspects of temporal mind that govern our lives – the mind of emotion and the mind of intent.

Emotions can be especially troublesome: not only are they regarded as major causes of disease in Chinese medicine, but when unbridled by firm intent, they tend to cloud our minds and vandalize our precious reserves of essence and energy. In a passage called 'Governing the Mind', the grand master of the Complete Reality school of Taoism, Lu Tung-pin, addresses this problem as follows, translated here by Thomas Cleary in *Vitality, Energy, Spirit*:

> Since the refinement of the three treasures requires the removal of emotions, it is necessary to govern the mind.

What is governing the mind? The mind is originally pure, the mind is originally calm; openness and freedom are both basic qualities of mind. When we govern the mind, this means we should keep it as it is in its original fundamental state, clear as a mountain stream, pure, fresh, unpolluted, silent as an immense canyon, free from clamor, vast as the universe, immeasurable in extent, open as a great desert, its bounds unknown.

The only way to restore conscious awareness of those pure, primordial qualities of the original mind of Tao is to tame the wild monkey of emotions, train the strong but stubborn horse of intent, and thereby 'govern the mind'. The only way to accomplish this task is by emptying the mind of all thoughts and pacifying all emotions in the solitary silence and still serenity of meditation.

In light of recent discoveries about the human brain and energy system, both the purpose and the methods of traditional Taoist and other Oriental meditation systems make good scientific sense. Practically speaking, what does 'original mind' mean? According to Dr Robert Becker's research, humans have two distinctly different nervous systems. One is the more obvious and recently evolved system of nerves and neurons which controls our physical senses such as eyes and ears as well as our limbs and all motor activities. The other is a more primitive system which controls such basic functions as growth and healing and governs basic biorhythms such as sleep/wake cycles, menstrual cycles, sexual drive, moods, and so forth. The latter system, which is more ancient and 'original' than the former, is highly sensitive to the subtlest fluctuations in the electromagnetic energies of the earth, sun, planets, and stars, but the constant 'mental static' caused by the rational and emotional mind drowns out the subtle, nonverbal input from the original mind and its sensitive network of energy channels.

Almost all mental static – internal dialogue – is generated by the rational, linear thinking of the cerebral cortex, and this is precisely the part of the brain that is stilled and silenced in Taoist and Buddhist meditation. By shutting off sensory stimuli and dissolving all discursive thoughts, the meditator restores access to the subtle input of what Taoists call 'original mind', a relaxed state of mind that is not only calming and rejuvenating, but which also tunes our attention to other, nonrational, non-sensory sources of information and knowledge. The physical senses – the Five Thieves – keep our brains preoccupied processing mundane sensory input, thereby robbing us of conscious access to the more subtle and sensitive faculties of our 'original minds'. Spiritual masters claim that the insights obtained from the 'original mind' in deep meditation cannot be conveyed in terms of rational thought and language, which are products of an entirely different, much narrower mode of consciousness. Only through persistent personal practice may one come to experience the awareness of 'original mind' and tap the vast trove of primordial wisdom and spiritual insight it holds.

A common mistake many beginning meditators make is to leave the tranquillity and equanimity they find in meditation behind on their meditation cushions when their sitting time is up, plunging helter-skelter back into the stress and confusion of daily activities. This sort of meditation practice is fruitless, because the real purpose of cultivating emotional serenity and mental clarity through meditation is to apply those qualities to everyday life, both for one's own benefit and as an inspiring example to others. As the great Sung-dynasty Tao master Wang Che wrote:

Sitting does not mean simply sitting still with eyes shut. This is only superficial sitting. True sitting means that the mind is as still as a mountain at all times, regardless of what you are doing, in activity as well as repose . . . If the mind always gets excited at the sight of external objects and turns somersaults assessing sizes and shapes, then that is an agitated mind and must swiftly be cut short. Do not permit this sort of thing to continue uncontrolled, because it will damage your spiritual power and deplete your life force.

The Japanese Zen master Hakuin agrees: 'Meditation in activity is infinitely superior to meditation in stillness.' The *chee-gung* master Luo Teh-hsiou advises:

It is particularly important for people to practise meditation after the age of forty, in order to draw energy inwards, calm the emotional mind, and cultivate spiritual awareness. Modern life has so many external distractions and so much stress that by the age of forty, most people's energy is scattered and spiritual vitality depleted. A private period of sitting in silent stillness every day replenishes internal energy and restores spiritual vitality.

In China, which has been civilized for so long that its 'modern' period began about 2,000 years ago, the problem of external distractions has long been noted. The *Huai-nan-tzu* states: 'There are myriad sights, sounds, and fragrances, rare products from faraway lands, exotic objects and curios, all of which can distract the mind from its goals, upset the spirit, and disrupt the circulation of blood and energy.'

In the ordinary course of life, people tend to follow their emotional mind and indulge their heart's every whim. Since the emotional mind responds directly to the physical senses, it forces body and mind to react constantly to the ceaseless flow of external sensory stimuli, resulting in a continuous outpouring of energy and attention that depletes the Three Treasures. If by the age of forty one fails to take measures to counteract the outward drain of essence, energy, and spirit, serious problems on all three levels will begin to develop.

Adepts of Tao counteract the external strain and drain of worldly life by practising inner development through the internal alchemy of meditation, which reverses the process of depletion with the alchemy of accretion. The mind of emotions is governed by the Fire energy of the heart, which when undisciplined flares upwards, wastefully burning up energy and clouding the mind. The mind of intent, or willpower, is controlled by the Water energy of the kidneys, which when unattended flows down and out through the sexual organs, depleting essence and energy and weakening the spirit. When you are 'sitting still, doing nothing', the flow of Fire and Water are reversed: Water energy from the kidneys and sacrum is drawn up to the head via the Central and Governing channels, while emotional Fire energy from the heart is drawn down into the Lower Elixir Field in the abdomen, where it is refined and transformed and enters general circulation through the energy channels. On the spiritual/mental level, this internal energy alchemy enables the mind of intent (Water) to exert a calming, cooling, controlling influence over the mind of emotion (Fire).

Although the terms of Taoist internal alchemy may seem exotic, they refer to specific organs, energies, and mental faculties which are activated and manipulated to the adept's advantage during meditation. This aspect of meditation is not a religious practice, but rather an internal method of preventive health care which complements and reinforces external methods such as exercise, diet, nutrition, and herbal supplements.

Practising external techniques without sooner or later practising internal development is pointless, because the emotional heart,

undisciplined by the cerebral mind of intent, will promptly mono-
polize and squander the enhanced essence and energy provided by
external practices in order to indulge its fickle whims. Only
through internal development may adepts master themselves as
well as the external world which constantly impinges upon their
consciousness. As the *Huai-nan-tzu* classic states:

> When one masters the external by means of the internal,
> all matters are settled. Whatever can be achieved inter-
> nally may also be attained externally. When one masters
> the internal, the vital organs are in perfect harmony and
> the mind is calm . . . One gains clarity and insight and
> develops a firmness and strength that do not falter . . .
> When one perceives the world with clarity and thinks
> with a mind free of sensual desires, when energy is stable
> and the will is strong, when one reposes in blissful
> serenity and remains undisturbed by habitual attach-
> ments, then the vital organs will rest in harmony, suf-
> fused with energy that does not leak. Thus the spirit
> protects the body internally without roaming abroad.

Meditation and internal alchemy

The *Book of Classifications*, written by Chang Ching-yueh during the
second century BC, states: 'Spirit is sustained by energy, and energy
is derived from the transformation of essence. Essence transforms
into energy, and energy transforms into spirit.'

Meditation is the third stage of Taoist internal alchemy, whereby
the essence nurtured and conserved through diet, supplements,
and sexual discipline, then converted into energy with *chee-gung*, is
refined, raised, and transformed into spiritual vitality. When the
outward drain of essence and energy has been staunched and
the spirit is strong and replete with vitality, it then takes over
command of energy in order to nourish and protect the body, thereby reversing the ordinary cycle of depletion with a self-cultivated
cycle of accretion. Chang San-feng, the great fourteenth-century
master of alchemy and legendary founder of *tai-chi-chuan*, made
this comment on the benefits of internal alchemy: 'The cycle continues over and over, enabling the spirit to guide the energy and the
energy to sustain the body. At this stage, one no longer requires
complicated exercises and other techniques in order to achieve
longevity.'

In other words, once the transformational process of internal alchemy is complete and spirit takes full command over energy, one may maintain health and promote longevity entirely through the 'internal work' (nei-gung) of 'sitting still, doing nothing', inducing intent to 'guide energy' into circulation throughout the system 'to sustain the body'. However, it takes many years of disciplined practice to reach this level.

In the past, the terminology of Taoist internal alchemy confused many Western translators, who never practised these methods themselves and therefore missed the essential meanings of the terms. Taoist texts speak of the 'medicinal elements' of internal alchemy, using metaphors which many translators took literally, such as 'red lead', 'black mercury', 'cinnabar', 'white snow', 'green dragon', 'white tiger', 'sun rays', and 'moon beams'. In fact, these metaphors simply refer to various aspects and elements of the Three Treasures – essence, energy, and spirit – which are the only real elements of internal alchemy.

Further to confuse idly curious laypeople and, no doubt, nosy 'foreign devils', the vital junctions, or 'passes', used in circulating internal energy were also given mysterious names, such as the 'Yellow Chamber', 'Red Cauldron', 'Mysterious Pass', 'Lead Furnace', 'Flower Pond', 'Dragon Lair', and 'Vermilion Palace'. In fact, these colourful names denote the invisible but highly functional points inside and along the surface of the body, where energy collects, transforms, and enters various channels for circulation. Taoist internal alchemy is actually a highly scientific method of harnessing, controlling, conserving, converting, and circulating essence and energy under the guidance of spirit in order to replace depletion with accretion, reverse disintegration with integration, and counteract degeneration with regeneration.

A term of particular importance in Taoist internal alchemy is the 'firing process', which has nothing at all to do with fire. The fourteenth-century Tao master Chen Hsu-pai wrote:

> The essence of the secret oral transmission regarding the firing process should be sought in true breathing. Breathing originates in the mind: when the mind is still, breathing is harmonious ... You must use spirit to control energy, and use energy to regulate breathing. Like the expansion and contraction of a bellows, the rise and fall of yin and yang, so exhalation and inhalation have their own spontaneous cycles.

The firing process thus refers to breathing, which acts as a bellows to gently fan the 'fire' of energy in the 'cauldrons' of the Elixir Fields. While *chee-gung* exercises focus on the alchemy of essence and energy by coordinating body and breath, still meditation focuses on the fusion of energy and spirit by concentrating the mind on the breath. By focusing the mind, which is the temporal aspect of spirit, on the breath, which is the temporal aspect of energy, one gradually induces a fusion of spirit and energy on the primordial level. Here's how Chang San-feng describes this process, in his commentary on the writings of Lu Tung-pin, translated here by Thomas Cleary:

> It is said that when you breathe out you contact the Root of Heaven and experience a sense of openness, and when you breathe in you contact the Root of Earth and experience a sense of solidity . . . As you go on breathing in this frame of mind, with these associations, alternating between movement and stillness, it is important that the focus of your mind does not shift. Let the true breath come and go, a subtle continuum on the brink of existence. Tune the breathing until you get breath without breathing; become one with it, and then the spirit can be solidified and the elixir can be made . . . Keep your mind on this all the time, without a moment's distraction, and after a long time, when the work becomes deep, there naturally appears a tiny pearl that shines like the sun, silently turning into the light of awareness of the original spirit, beyond conceptual measurement.

As the fusion of energy and spirit progresses day by day, 'fired' by the conscious mental control of breathing during meditation, spirit and energy crystallize to form what is referred to as the 'elixir', 'spiritual embryo', or 'shining pearl'. It is this elixir that the most advanced adepts nurture as a vehicle to carry consciousness out of the body during meditation, and for the final 'flight into space' at the moment of death, when it becomes the basis of spiritual immortality.

For advanced adepts, this level of internal alchemy is the ultimate goal of inner development, known as 'immortality' to Taoists and 'enlightenment' to Buddhists, but it requires many years of disciplined preliminary practice on one's own, as well as personal transmission from an enlightened teacher who has already reached the ultimate goal. Enlightenment also requires a lot of time and energy, which is why the preliminary goals of health and longevity are so important as a basis for higher practices. Health and longevity also enable the adept to fulfil his or her social obligations while cultivating the Tao. Unlike many mystical traditions, which require complete severance of all ties to family and society, Taoism merges worldly and spiritual paths into one broad highway with fast as well as slow lanes, enabling each adept to progress at whatever pace best suits his or her individual requirements. As the fully realized sage Chang San-feng remarked:

> Studying the Tao requires a firm foundation in alchemy. After you have forged a firm foundation in alchemy, you may go back home to work and support your family. After you have fulfilled your obligations to your family and society, you may go to the mountains to seek a teacher in order to complete your cultivation of the great Tao. Adepts who abandon their homes and wives lay waste to their lives and are not worth discussing.

In other words, the Tao may be practised at home within the context of family life just as well as alone in a remote mountain cave. In fact, those who prematurely abandon the world and forsake their fellow human beings deprive themselves of some of life's most important lessons, lessons which can only be learned by plunging heart and head into the turbulent fire and water of worldly life. The adept Liu I-ming wrote 250 years ago: 'The real is concealed within the artificial; the artificial is not separate from the real. Without the false, we cannot realize the true; without the true, we cannot transform the false.'

Without the basic contradictions of life, we lose the contrasts through which truth is revealed. Transcendental truth lies concealed within, not suspended above, the temporal falsehood of worldly life. As Tantric Buddhists put it: 'Nirvana [enlightenment] and samsara [corporeal life] are one.' Marriage, work, food, sex, travel, and other aspects of worldly life hold important, potentially enlightening lessons for the spiritual adept. By abandoning family and society, the adept is 'cutting class' and becomes a truant from the school of life. Only after learning his earthly lessons does the adept 'graduate' from worldly life and qualify for the solitary 'postgraduate' work of higher spiritual practices conducted in the seclusion of remote hermitages under the tutelage of an enlightened master, or guru.

In Taoist and most other Oriental traditions, this stage of practice usually commences after the age of sixty, when familial and social duties have been completed. The only exception is Tibetan Tantric tradition, in which adepts undergo intensive training during early youth, in complete isolation from the world, then return to the world later in life to guide others onto the path. This is a swift but far more difficult path, requiring great discipline and self-sacrifice for the ultimate benefit of others. For most of us, the easy-going Taoist path of early involvement in worldly life followed by gradual withdrawal provides a more practical, albeit much slower, way of arriving at the ultimate goal.

Adepts may study and practise the techniques of health and longevity from books such as this, but cultivating the 'internal elixir' (nei-dan) required to traverse the higher paths towards enlightenment and spiritual immortality can be accomplished only under the personal guidance of a master who has already arrived at the goal. So why even mention the 'elixir of immortality' in books? Chang Po-tuan, progenitor of the Complete Reality school of Taoism, answers this question as follows, translated here by Thomas Cleary:

> The purpose of writing about alchemy, embracing the foundation of creative evolution and penetrating the marrow of the complementary energies of the universe, is to enable practitioners of alchemy to follow the stream so as to know the source, to abandon the false and thereby follow the true, and not wind up forgetting the root and pursuing the branches.

The great masters of the past clearly elucidated the basic practices which confer health and longevity upon the practitioner, while also alluding in symbolic terms to the ultimate goal of spiritual enlightenment, or 'immortality', so that adepts would not roam astray with the newfound powers they discover through the basic practices of internal alchemy. They revealed the stream in order to indicate the direction of the source, showed the branches to indicate the existence of the roots. Below, we'll take a quick look at the preliminary goals of health and longevity as well as the ultimate goal of spiritual enlightenment fostered by meditation practice, then run through a few basic meditation methods which anyone can use to lay a firm foundation in the internal alchemy of 'sitting still, doing nothing'.

Meditation for health and longevity

A bearded yogi, body smeared with ashes, sits in meditative trance, then lies down on a bed of sharp nails, feeling no pain. The nails puncture his flesh, but the wounds don't bleed. The American writer Norman Cousins, weary of the debilitating and therapeutically useless chemotherapy his doctors prescribe for his cancer, abruptly terminates all medical treatment and instead goes out and rents all the Laurel and Hardy, Three Stooges, and Marx Brothers films he can find, then proceeds to laugh himself to full recovery. An old Taoist master in Taiwan suggests to a woman who seeks his advice that she sit in meditation for six hours a day, breathing in a prescribed manner, in order to conquer the uterine cancer which her Western-trained doctors have repeatedly operated on in vain and pronounced terminal. In six months, all traces of her cancer have completely disappeared. All these examples have one common denominator: they manifest the innate human power of mind over matter, a power which can be awakened and cultivated by the practice of meditation, even 'laughing meditation'.

Most people, especially in the West, are unaware of the vital importance of spiritual training to health and longevity: they assume that meditation, philosophy, and 'all that stuff' are only for monks and saints. Consequently, they indulge recklessly in conflicting emotions and permit all sorts of trivialities to disturb the tranquillity of their minds. They allow television, stress, worry, anger, and other mental and emotional distractions to clutter their minds and exhaust their spirits, which consequently lose command over energy and essence. With the Three Treasures out of harmony, each going its own way, the body becomes vulnerable to negative influences, both internal and external.

'Sitting still, doing nothing' turns attention inwards; and in so doing, it also draws energy inwards, because energy follows where spirit leads. When the senses, such as the eyes and ears, are withdrawn from the outside world, energy stops leaking out along with attention, and the Five Thieves are arrested. Instead, energy condenses and circulates internally, healing the body, energizing the brain, balancing the vital organ energies, and enhancing the powers of temporal mind as well as primordial spirit. Practised daily, meditation refills our tanks with essence, recharges our batteries with energy, and rejuvenates our minds with spiritual vitality.

Anyone who doubts the therapeutic benefits of turning attention inwards, or the debilitating effects of pouring attention outwards, can verify these points by conducting the following experimental regimen. For one full month, strictly avoid watching television, and instead devote at least thirty minutes of the time you save each day to 'sitting still, doing nothing', cultivating and concentrating your spirit rather than distracting and scattering it. A few days is not enough to gain the insight, but if you try this for a full month, you will be amazed at how much better you feel, how much stronger your energy is, how stable and well balanced your emotions become, and how clear and calm your mind grows.

Absent-mindedness is becoming common not only among the ailing and elderly but also in middle-aged people under chronic stress. When it occurs in the elderly, Western medicine calls absent-mindedness a symptom of 'senility', or 'senile dementia', and attributes it to declining secretions of vital neurochemicals, a condition which Chinese medicine refers to as 'brain essence empty'. Chinese medicine, which refers to absent-mindedness as 'absent-heartedness', agrees with the initial Western diagnosis of 'brain essence empty', but then takes it a step further. The spirit, exhausted and weakened by chronic stress and constant external distractions, loses command over energy, which consequently leaks out externally along with sensory attention rather than circulating internally. Since energy commands essence, leaking energy results in diminishing essence. In the case of senility, insufficient cerebral energy causes a reduction in the production and circulation of brain essence (including hormones, neurotransmitters, and blood), which in turn impairs cerebral functions, such as memory. And since energy forms the bridge between body and mind, when cerebral energy fails, the bridge linking mind and brain collapses, and the mind roams aimlessly off on its own. As Master Chen Hsu-pai wrote: 'When essence is depleted, energy is exhausted. When energy is exhausted, the spirit roams alone.' By shutting off external sensory leaks and concentrating attention and energy internally, meditation stimulates the production and circulation of 'brain essence', enhances cerebral energy, strengthens the spirit, and improves mental functions, thereby preventing the decline in mental powers commonly associated with aging.

Meditation has many medical applications, both curative and preventive. For example, visualization in conjunction with meditation is a powerful healing technique whereby the patient focuses the mind to visualize healing energy flowing into ailing organs, dissolving tumours, repairing tissues, and so forth. This sort of 'mind over matter' healing, which makes perfect sense in the light of Taoist internal alchemy, is still practised in China, India, Tibet, and other Oriental cultures, but it is regarded as 'voodoo medicine' by the orthodox Western medical establishment.

Still, not so long ago, this internal healing mechanism and its mental controls were also known in the West, and today enlightened Western physicians are beginning to rediscover how to teach their patients to heal themselves. Paracelcus, one of the greatest medical scientists in Western history, wrote: 'To think is to act on the plane of thought, and if the thought is intense enough, it may produce an effect on the physical plane.' He also wrote: 'The human body is vapour materialized by sunshine mixed with the life of the stars.' This remarkably insightful view of the human body agrees with the latest findings of modern physics, to wit that 'vapour' (energy) may be materialized under the influence of light ($E = mc^2$) and that the material elements (essence) of which the body is composed all originated in titanic thermonuclear explosions of stars, or supernovas.

Paracelcus' 'vitalist' school of thought was bitterly opposed by the 'mechanists', who viewed the human body as a chemically operated machine that amounts to no more than the net sum of its parts, any one of which may be chemically treated, surgically removed, and replaced with artificial parts, like a car. The mechanists won the day, and vitalist concepts were erased from Western medical textbooks. Today, despite the abysmal failure of the chemical-mechanist approach to deal effectively with cancer, AIDS, chronic fatigue, mental illness, and other increasingly common modern maladies, the Western medical establishment stubbornly clings to its failed mechanistic system of health care. Consequently, patients must take the initiative to inform themselves and to seek alternative avenues of health care on their own.

Fortunately, hundreds of good books on this subject have been published in recent years, and alternative therapists are cropping up all over the Western world. Meditation is proving to be one of the most effective means of activating the innate link between brain and body in healing. In an article entitled 'Mental Muscle' in the June 1992 issue of *Omni* magazine, Kathy Keeton writes:

> You don't have to resort to hypnotism to begin to use your brain as a weapon in the battle against aging. Programmed relaxation techniques like meditation, which are actually similar in many ways to self-hypnotism, may do the trick in and of themselves. When the psychologists Charles Alexander of the Maharishi International University in Fairfield, Iowa, and Ellen

Langer of Harvard University, taught transcendental meditation (TM) to a group of octogenarians in eight Boston-area nursing homes, 100% of those who practiced TM 20 minutes a day were still alive three years later, while 38% of their peers who did not meditate had passed on. This is reminiscent of legends of Himalayan yogis using similar techniques to live more than a hundred years . . . Alexander is one of a growing body of scientists who believe that we can muster the power of our brains to stay healthy, to heal ourselves when we're sick, and, quite possibly, to extend our life expectancy.

The ultimate goal: 'returning to the source'

For most people, especially those with an active family and social life, health and longevity remain the primary goals of meditation, at least until one's practice and personal lifestyle permit a shot at the ultimate goal of spiritual enlightenment. Known as 'returning to the source', enlightenment involves a fourth and final stage of internal alchemy in which 'spirit transforms and returns to emptiness'. To accomplish this, the adept must spend many years cultivating the internal 'elixir of immortality', or 'spiritual embryo', as a vehicle for projecting consciousness out of the body into the unimpeded freedom of open space.

The 'Supreme Ultimate' (tai-jee) is the original, non-dual, undifferentiated, ineffable source from which yin and yang, the Five Elemental Energies, and all the myriad elements and energies of the universe sprang. It is also the primal source of spirit and consciousness. Meditation provides a method whereby the finite temporal consciousness of the human mind can withdraw its attention from the external world of material phenomena and focus instead on the infinite primordial mind of Tao that lies at the core of all awareness. As human beings, we must work within the limits of the temporal assets nature bestows on us at birth – body (temporal essence), breath (temporal energy), and mind (temporal spirit). Meditation enables us to still the body, regulate the breath, and empty the mind so that we may re-establish conscious awareness of the 'shining pearl' of spiritual light that glows like an eternal flame in the innermost sanctum of our being. In this process, the temporal mind focuses full attention on the breath, which causes energy to merge with spirit on the primordial level. Thus energized, the spirit shines brightly and grows strong, illuminating the adept's consciousness with the primordial light of wisdom. Words fail to capture this experience; at best, words can only allude to it and point out the way to realize it.

There is a very interesting link here between the highest stages of Taoist meditation and the widely accepted theory that the universe was created spontaneously in a 'Big Bang'. The great English physicist Stephen Hawking describes the Big Bang as something that suddenly exploded forth in the utter emptiness of space from an infinitesimally small point, creating all the fundamental forces of the universe, such as light, heat, electricity, magnetism, and the nuclear energies, which then fused to form matter.

Viewed from the Taoist paradigm, the utter emptiness of space is a state known as 'extreme yin'. Taoist texts state; 'When yin reaches its extreme, yang spontaneously arises as a point of light within yin.' All Taoist meditation manuals refer to this sublime state of utter stillness, emptiness, and silence, a state attained by virtue of the fusion of primordial energy and spirit in meditation. When that state reaches its zenith of stillness, a point of light suddenly appears within it, causing thoughts to stir, energies to move, and forms to appear again, in a sort of psychic re-enactment of the creation of the universe within the microcosmic inner universe of the mind. Chang Po-tuan refers to this moment as 'the instant of utter silence preceding the resurgence of positive energy'. Positive energy is light, heat, motion, and other active yang energies, which arise spontaneously within the utter silence, stillness, and emptiness of 'extreme yin'.

Master Han Yu-mo, who teaches Taoist meditation, astrology, and geomancy in Taiwan and Canada, describes this experience as follows in his meditation manual entitled *Orthodox Method for Cultivating Energy and Breath Control*:

> By concentrating my spirit I learned to regulate my breath and found that regulating my breath helped to concentrate my spirit. After practising in this manner for a long time, spirit and energy fused together into one entity and spontaneously entered the realm of void. This is what is known as 'emptiness', or 'non-being'. Whenever I reached the most extreme state of emptiness, I would suddenly become alert and move spontaneously. This is what is known as 'being' . . . This is precisely the method by which everything in the universe came into existence.

The purpose of returning awareness to the original source of creation is to stop the ceaseless cycle of birth and death which is driven by clinging to desire for material forms. When spirit is suffused with energy and enters the 'realm of void', it gains conscious awareness of the primordial source of all creation, and as that awareness grows stronger with practice, it loosens the bonds of desire and delusion which continuously propel the spirit to take form in material realms, only to grow old and die again. The tenth-century adept Tan Chiao wrote as follows on this topic, translated here by Thomas Cleary:

> The fading of the Tao is when emptiness turns into spirit, spirit turns into energy, and energy turns into form. When form is born, everything is thereby stultified.
>
> The functioning of the Tao is when form turns into energy, energy turns into spirit, and spirit turns into emptiness. When emptiness is clear, everything thereby flows freely . . .
>
> Emptiness turns into spirit, spirit turns into energy, energy turns into blood, blood turns into form, form turns into infant, infant turns into child, child turns into youth, youth turns into adult, the adult ages, the aged die, the dead revert to emptiness. Emptiness then again turns into spirit, spirit again turns into energy, and energy again turns into myriad beings. Transformation after transformation goes on unceasingly, following an endless cycle.

'Returning to the source' of creation stops this endless cycle of transformation and reincarnation, permitting the spirit to rest for ever and fully conscious in the infinite, eternal abode of the Supreme Ultimate, the non-dual state of open primordial awareness which preceded the Big Bang and gave birth to 'two things, then three, then ten thousand'.

The 'spiritual embryo' to which advanced Taoist texts refer is primordial spirit brought into conscious awareness by virtue of its alchemical fusion with energy. This 'embryo' is said to be 'conceived' in the 'womb' of the adept's Lower Elixir Field below the navel, where yin and yang, Water and Fire, 'mother' and 'father', unite to recreate the original primordial energy upon which primordial spirit feeds. When the 'embryo' has 'gestated' to a sufficient degree, i.e. when sufficient energy has been transferred from the body and emotional mind into the spirit, it is ready to be raised to the Upper Elixir Field between and behind the eyebrows. This is the 'Spirit Terrace' (ling-tai), from which the adept 'gives birth to the spiritual infant' by sending consciousness soaring into space through the energy aperture between the brows. The adept must practise this 'out-of-body experience' regularly for many years in order to train the 'spiritual infant' to function independently beyond the flesh. As the adept Liu I-ming wrote: 'Nurture it for three years, and you will be able to condense it into material form or diffuse it into pure energy. Appearing and disappearing mysteriously, it will develop into an indestructible diamond body.'

Finally, at the moment of death, the spirit, which has been 'rehearsing' for this moment for years, exits like a puff of steam through the brow or crown, never to return to the festering prison of corporeal existence. Fuelled by the adept's energy, to which it has been fused by years of advanced practice, the spirit carries the adept's fully awakened awareness into the wide open space and total freedom of the 'void', an infinite, luminous realm with feeling but no form, energy but no essence, unimpeded awareness without the burden and limitations of a fragile body trapped in a material realm. Needless to say, this is not an easy task and remains beyond the capacity of most human beings to accomplish, at least until they have garnered sufficient merit and insight from previous lifetimes to meet an enlightened teacher who can awaken them in this life and show them the way to open the gate from the temporal human mind into the primordial mind of Tao. Opening that 'gateless gate' enables one to attempt the final breakthrough and escape the ceaseless merry-go-round of birth and death.

'Immortality' is a word that constantly crops up in Taoist texts on internal alchemy, confusing and misleading many an adept over the ages. In ancient China, there were adepts who spent their entire lives trying to concoct an 'elixir of immortality' from various mineral and plant substances, some of them highly toxic, including lead, mercury, cinnabar, aconite, and datura. These misguided adepts misread the ancient texts, taking the alchemical metaphors and esoteric terms literally and assuming that if the proper elixir could be forged by fire and brimstone, immortality in the flesh could be achieved here and now. Many of them, and their imperial patrons, died prematurely of poisoning.

In true Taoist parlance, 'immortality' refers to a spiritual state, not a condition of physical permanence. In his books on the teachings of Don Juan, Carlos Casteneda refers to the primordial source of creation as the *nagual*, the vast ocean of emptiness in which material worlds take form and dissolve like drops of dew. *Nagual* refers to everything that cannot be expressed in words, which brings to mind the second line of the *Tao Teh Ching*: 'The name which can be named is not the real Name.' Don Juan's teachings are remarkably similar to Taoist alchemy, and they both cite our innate awareness as the only bridge between the awesome emptiness and power of the *nagual* and its material manifestation in the temporal world.

During the course of our lives on earth, our essence depletes, our energy scatters, and our temporal minds fade away along with our bodies, but the shining pearl of primordial awareness that we carry deep in our hearts remains immaculate, indestructible, and immortal. It is this precious treasure that is blown willy-nilly from life to life, body to body, driven by the force of our own delusion and desire for carnal existence. In order to escape this endless cycle of birth and death, pain and pleasure, we must become consciously aware of 'the other world' and reawaken our primordial spirits *during our present lives*, an experience which shatters once and for all the illusions that sustain corporeal birth, carnal life, and physical death. In other words, developing conscious awareness of primordial spirit while still alive in the temporal world is a precondition for achieving enlightenment, or 'immortality', after death. As the fourteenth-century Tao master Wang Wei-yi wrote: 'To know the Tao one must first understand birth and death. If one does not understand birth and death, it is pointless to seek immortality.'

One must come to realize intuitively that birth and death are merely cyclic transitions, transmigrations of the spirit caused by ignorance of spiritual realities, not absolute beginnings and endings. We must realize that what is born and dies is not the spirit but only the physical body which the spirit acquires at birth and the personal ego it evolves to guide the body through life. When we become consciously aware that the primal spirit of primordial awareness 'is not born and does not die', and that the physical world is an impermanent realm of illusion which we create ourselves, then we are finally free. When that ineffable realization dawns in the silent solitude of meditation, enlightenment shimmers on the horizon with indescribable brightness and bliss, permitting us to escape the clutches of cyclic existence and return to rest for ever in the original source of all creation, never again to be born or to die. That is immortality.

Meditation methods

Taoist meditation methods have many points in common with Hindu and Buddhist systems, but the Taoist way is less abstract and far more down-to-earth than the contemplative traditions which evolved in India. The primary hallmark of Taoist meditation is the generation, transformation, and circulation of internal energy. Once the adept has 'achieved energy' (*deh-chee*), it can be applied to promoting health and longevity, nurturing the 'spiritual embryo' of immortality, martial arts, healing, painting and poetry, sensual self-indulgence, or whatever else the adept wishes to do with it. The Tao makes no moral judgements: what the adept does with his or her newfound powers invariably determines the adept's own future fate through the universal law of cause and effect, or 'karma', a Buddhist concept absorbed into the mainstream of Taoist thought by the Complete Reality school.

The two primary guidelines in Taoist meditation are *jing* ('quiet, stillness, calm') and *ding* ('concentration, focus'). The purpose of stillness, both mental and physical, is to turn attention inwards and cut off external sensory input, thereby muzzling the Five Thieves. Within that silent stillness, one concentrates the mind and focuses attention, usually on the breath, in order to develop what is called 'one-pointed awareness', a totally undistracted, undisturbed, undifferentiated state of mind which permits intuitive insights to arise spontaneously.

When you first begin to practise meditation, you will find that your mind is very uncooperative. That's your ego, or 'emotional mind', fighting against its own extinction by the higher forces of spiritual awareness. The last thing your ego and emotions want is to be harnessed: they revel in the day-to-day circus of sensory entertainment and emotional turmoil, even though this game depletes your energy, degenerates your body, and exhausts your spirit. When you catch your mind drifting into fantasy or drawing attention away from internal alchemy to external phenomena, here are six ways you can use to 'catch the monkey', impose intent over emotion, clarify the mind, and re-establish the internal focus of one-pointed awareness:

1) Shift attention back to the inflow and outflow of air streaming through the nostrils, or energy streaming in and out of a vital point, such as between the brows.

2) Focus attention on the rising and falling of the navel, the expansion and contraction of the abdomen, as you breathe.

3) With eyes half-lidded, focus vision on a candle flame or a mandala (geometric meditation picture). Focus on the centre of the flame or picture, but also take in the edges with peripheral vision. The concentration required to do this usually clears all other distractions from the mind.

4) Practise a few minutes of mantra, the 'sacred syllables' which harmonize energy and focus the mind. Though mantra are usually associated with Hindu and Tibetan Buddhist practices, Taoists have also employed them for many millennia. The three most effective syllables are 'om', which stabilizes the body, 'ah', which harmonizes energy, and 'hum', which concentrates the spirit. 'Om' vibrates between the brows, 'ah' in the throat, and 'hum' in the heart, and their associated colours are white, red, and blue respectively. Chant the syllables in a deep, low-pitched tone and use long, complete exhalations for each one. Other mantra such as '*om mani padme hum*', are equally effective.

5) Beat the Heavenly Drum, as described in the previous chapter as a cool-down energy-collection technique. The vibrations tend to clear discursive thoughts and sensory distractions from the mind.

6) Visualize a deity or a sacred symbol of personal significance to you shining above the crown of your head or suspended in space before you. When your mind is once again still, stable, and undistracted, let the vision fade away and refocus your mind on whatever meditative technique you were practising.

Like all Taoist practices, Taoist meditation works on all three levels of the Three Treasures: essence (body), energy (breath), and spirit (mind). The first step is to adopt a comfortable posture for the body, balance your weight evenly, straighten the spine, and pay attention to physical sensations such as heat, cold, tingling, trembling, or whatever else arises. When your body is comfortable and balanced, shift attention to the second level, which is breath and energy. You may focus on the breath itself as it flows in and out of the lungs through the nostrils, or on energy streaming in and out of a particular point in tune with the breath. The third level is spirit: when the breath is regulated and energy is flowing smoothly through the channels, focus attention on thoughts and feelings forming and dissolving in your mind, awareness expanding and contracting with each breath, insights and inspirations arising spontaneously, visions and images appearing and disappearing. Eventually you may even be rewarded with intuitive flashes of insight regarding the ultimate nature of the mind: open and empty as space; clear and luminous as a cloudless sky at sunrise; infinite and unimpeded. Chang San-feng, the great master of martial arts, meditation, and other Taoist arts and sciences, wrote as follows on the three levels of Taoist meditation:

> Relaxing the body refines essence . . .
> Calming the mind refines energy . . .
> Focusing attention refines spirit . . .
> When your spirit is refined, the two
> energies fuse, the three primordials
> combine, and primal energy is naturally
> restored. The three primordials are
> primordial essence, energy, and spirit,
> and the two energies are yin and yang.

In his book *Vitality, Energy, Spirit*, Thomas Cleary translated the following passage from another work of Chang San-feng entitled *Words on the Way*, in which he elucidates the various phases of Taoist meditation:

> 'Freezing the spirit, tune the breath; tuning the breath, freeze the spirit.' This is the starting work. This should be done single-mindedly, continuing from step to step. Freezing the spirit means gathering in the clarified mind. As long as the mind is not yet clear, the eyes should not be closed in meditation. It is first necessary to exert one-self to restore clarity, coolness, and serenity; then one may concentrate on the pocket of energy in the body. This is called freezing the spirit . . .
> Tuning the breath is not difficult. Once the spirit of mind is quiet, breathe naturally; I just keep this natural-ness, and also focus attention downward. This is tuning the breath.
> Tuning the breath is tuning the breath centered on the base of the torso, joining with the energy in the mind, breath and energy meeting in the pocket of energy in the abdomen. The mind staying below the navel is called freezing the spirit; the energy returning below the navel is called tuning the breath . . .

Then apply the principle of using space as the place to store the mind, using dark silence as the abode to rest the spirit; clarify them again and again, until suddenly the spirit and breath are both forgotten, spirit and energy merge. Then unexpectedly the celestial energy will arise ecstatically, and you will be as though intoxicated . . .

The Way is entered from the center . . . Keeping to the center calls for turning attention inward to concentrate on a sphere 1.3 inches below the navel, neither clinging fast to it nor departing from it, with neither obsession nor indifference.

Additional points of practice and posture are described in detail in the chapter on 'Sitting Still, Doing Nothing' in *The Tao of HS&L* and need not be repeated here. Just as all the rules of *chee-gung* practice can be boiled down to the three Ss – slow, soft, smooth – so the main points of meditation practice may be summed up in the three Cs: calm, cool, clear. As for proper postures for practice, Fig. 45 depicts the two positions most frequently used in Taoist meditation: sitting cross-legged on the floor in 'half-lotus' position, with the buttocks elevated on a cushion or pad; and sitting erect on a low stool or chair, feet parallel and shoulder width apart, knees bent at a 90-degree angle, spine erect. The advantages of sitting cross-legged are that this position is more stable and encourages energy to flow upwards towards the brain. The advantages of sitting on a stool are that the legs do not cramp, the soles of the feet are in direct contact with the energy of the earth, and internal energy tends to flow more freely throughout the lower as well as the upper torso. Most adepts use both methods, depending on conditions. When sitting cross-legged, Western practitioners, whose legs tend to cramp more easily than Asians', are advised to sit on thick firm cushions, perhaps with a phone book or two underneath, in order to elevate the pelvis and take pressure off the legs and knees. This also helps keep the spine straight without straining the lower back.

The way the hands are placed is also important. The most natural and comfortable position is to rest the palms lightly on the thighs, just above the knees. However, some meditators find it more effective to use one of the traditional 'mudras', or hand gestures, three of which are shown in Fig. 46. Experiment with different combinations of posture and mudra until you find the style that suits you best.

Taoist meditation masters teach three basic ways to control the

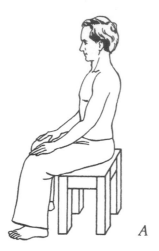
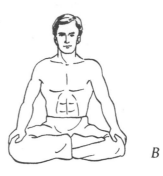

Fig. 45 **Taoist meditation postures**
A. Sitting on stool.
B. Sitting with legs crossed on floor.

Fire mind of emotion with the Water mind of intent, so that the adept's goals in meditation may be realized. The first method is called 'stop and observe'. This involves paying close attention to how thoughts arise and fade in the mind, learning to let them pass like a freight train in the night, without clinging to any particular one. This develops awareness of the basic emptiness of all thought, as well as nonattachment to the rise and fall of emotional impulses. Gradually one learns simply to ignore the intrusion of discursive thoughts, at which point they cease arising for sheer lack of attention.

The second technique is called 'observe and imagine', which refers to visualization. The adept employs intent to visualize an image – such as Buddha, Jesus, a sacred symbol, the moon, a star, or whatever – in order to shift mental focus away from thoughts and emotions and stabilize the mind in one-pointed awareness. You may also visualize a particular energy centre in your body, or listen to the real or imagined sound of a bell, gong, or cymbal ringing in your ears. The point of focus is not important: what counts is *shifting* the focus of your attention away from idle thoughts, conflicting emotions, fantasies, and other distracting antics of the 'monkey mind' and concentrating attention instead on a stable point of focus established by the mind of intent, or 'wisdom mind'.

The third step in cultivating control over your own mind is called

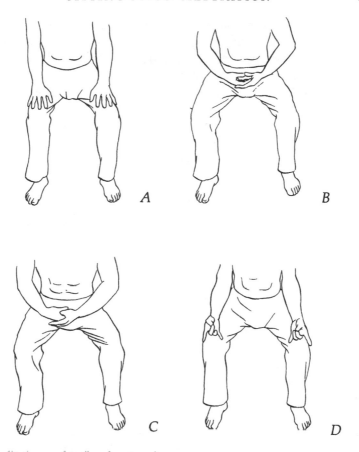

Fig. 46 Meditation mudras (hand gestures)
A. Natural method: hands relaxed on thighs.
B. Traditional Buddhist method: right hand cupped in palm of left, tips of thumbs touching.
C. Traditional Taoist method: left hand (yin) embracing right hand (yang), with left thumb in centre of right palm, or vice versa.
D. Tantric Buddhist method: palms up, resting on thighs, tips of thumbs and middle fingers touching; also called 'Lotus' method.

'using the mind of intent to guide energy'. When the emotional mind is calm and the breath is regulated, the adept focuses attention on internal energy and learns how to guide it through the meridian network in order to energize vital organs, raise energy from the sacrum to the head to nourish the spirit and brain, and exchange stale energy for fresh energy from the external sources of heaven (sky) and earth (ground). Adepts are usually taught to begin by focusing attention on the Lower Elixir Field below the abdomen, then moving energy from there down to the perineum, up through the coccyx, and up along the spinal centres into the head, after which attention shifts to the Upper Elixir Field between the brows. Though this sounds rather vague and esoteric to the uninitiated, a few months of practice, especially in conjunction with *chee-gung* and proper dietary habits, usually suffices to unveil the swirling world of energy and awareness hidden within our bodies and minds. All you have to do is sit still and shut up long enough for your mind to become aware of it.

It's always a good idea to warm up your body and open your energy channels with some *chee-gung* exercises before you sit down to meditate. This facilitates internal energy circulation and enables you to sit for longer periods without getting stiff or numb. After sitting, you should avoid bathing for at least twenty minutes in order to prevent loss of energy through open pores and energy points. If you live in the northern hemisphere, it's best to sit facing south or east, in the general direction of the sun; in the southern hemisphere, sit facing north or east.

Described below are three basic methods which anyone can use to begin meditation practice without personal guidance from a teacher. You could use these techniques to establish a firm foundation in meditation before seeking out a teacher to learn advanced practices. Most meditation masters prefer working with students who have already demonstrated their sincerity by practising meditation and other health regimens on their own for a few years, but only if those preliminary practices are nonsectarian and free of culturally conditioned biases.

Since most readers are concerned primarily with promoting health, enhancing energy, and prolonging life, rather than devoting the rest of their lives to the ultimate goal of spiritual enlightenment, these three methods should suffice to fulfil most of your requirements in meditation. Bear in mind also that the benefits of meditation are cumulative: with continued practice these three methods will produce ever-richer harvests on all three levels of essence, energy, and spirit. As you grow more and more familiar with your own internal terrain, you will find it easier and easier to balance your body, regulate your energy, and clarify your mind while 'sitting still, doing nothing' for about half an hour once or twice a day.

Breath and navel meditation (Fig. 47)
This is the oldest meditation method on record in China as well as India, and it is the method usually taught to beginners. It works directly with the natural flow of breath in the nostrils and the expansion and contraction of the abdomen and is a good way to develop focused attention and one-pointed awareness.

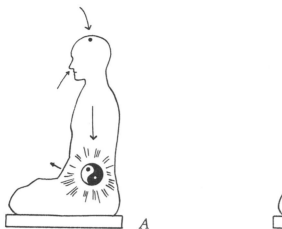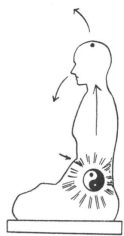

Fig. 47 **Breath and navel meditation**
A. Inhalation: air enters nose, energy enters crown, diaphragm descends, abdomen expands.
B. Exhalation: air exits nose, energy exits crown, diaphragm ascends, abdomen contracts.

Method: Sit cross-legged on a cushion on the floor or upright on a low stool and adjust the body's posture until well balanced and comfortable. Press tongue to palate, close your mouth without clenching the teeth, and lower the eyelids until almost closed.

Breathe naturally through the nose, drawing the inhalation deep down into the abdomen and making the exhalation long and smooth. Focus your attention on two sensations, one above and the other below. Above, focus on the gentle breeze of air flowing in and out of the nostrils like a bellows, and on exhalation try to 'follow' the breath out as far as possible, from 3 to 18 inches. Below, focus on the navel rising and falling and the entire abdomen expanding and contracting like a balloon with each inhalation and exhalation. You may focus attention on the nostrils or the abdomen, or on both, or on one and then the other, whichever suits you best.

From time to time, mentally check your posture and adjust it if necessary. Whenever you catch your mind wandering off or getting cluttered with thoughts, consciously shift your attention back to your breath. Sometimes it helps to count either inhalations or exhalations, until your mind is stably focused. If you manage to achieve stability in this method after ten to twenty minutes of practice, you may wish to switch over to one of the other two methods given below. All three of these methods may be practised in a single sitting in the order that they are presented here, or in separate sittings.

Time: Twenty to thirty minutes, once or twice a day.

Master Han's Central Channel meditation (Fig. 48)

This is an ancient Taoist method modified and taught by Master Han Yu-mo at his Sung Yang Tao Centers in Taiwan and Canada. It is a simple and effective way for beginners rapidly to develop a tangible awareness of internal energy and a familiarity with the major power points through which energy is circulated and exchanged with the surrounding sources of heaven and earth. It relaxes the body, replenishes energy, and invigorates the spirit.

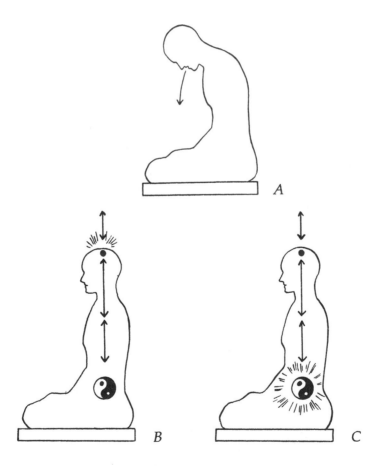

Fig. 48 **Master Han's Central Channel meditation**
A. Start by bending forwards and expelling stale air from lungs through mouth, 3 times.
B. Focus on energy entering crown.
C. Focus on energy filling Lower Elixir Field.

Method: Adopt a comfortable sitting posture. First, take a deep breath and bend forwards slowly, exhaling audibly through the mouth in order to expel stale breath from the lungs; repeat three times. Then sit still and breathe naturally, letting the abdomen expand and contract with each breath. However, instead of focusing attention on the flow of air through the nostrils, focus on the beam of energy entering the crown of the head at a point about two inches above the hairline, called the 'Medicine Palace'. Feel the beam of energy flowing in through this point as you begin each inhalation and follow it down through the Central Channel into the Lower Elixir Field below the navel, then follow it back up the Central Channel and out through the Medicine Palace point on exhalation. The sensation at the crown point is most noticeable at the beginning of inhalation and the end of exhalation and feels somewhat like a flap or valve opening and closing as energy flows through it. There may also be feelings of warmth, tingling, or numbness in the scalp, all of which are signs of energy moving under the scrutiny of awareness.

After practising this method for a few weeks or months and developing a conscious feel for energy as it moves through the Medicine Palace point, you may start to work with other points of exit during exhalation, always drawing energy in through the crown point on inhalation. For example, you may bring energy in through the crown and down to the abdomen on inhalation, then push it back up and out through the 'Celestial Eye' point between the brows. This point usually brings rapid results – a distinct tingling or throbbing sensation between the brows. The Celestial Eye is the point through which adepts with 'psychic vision' perceive aspects of the world that are hidden to ordinary eyesight. The mass of magnetite crystals between the forehead and the pituitary gland is sensitive to subtle fluctuations in surrounding electromagnetic fields. In other words, psychic vision perceives by virtue of its sensitivity to electromagnetic energy rather than the light or sound energy perceived by eyes and ears. So-called 'psychics' are those who have learned how to interpret the electromagnetic signals from the magnetic organ between the eyes in terms of ordinary perception and rational thought.

In addition to the brow point, you may also practise expelling energy on exhalation through the points in the centres of the palms, the centres of the soles, and the perineum point midway between genitals and anus. In each case, look for sensations of warmth or tingling at the point of exit.

After practising this method for a while, your head may start to rock spontaneously back and forth or from side to side after fifteen or twenty minutes of sitting, or else your entire body may start trembling and shaking. This is a good sign, for it means that your channels are opening and that energy is coursing strongly through them. Try neither to suppress nor encourage these spontaneous tremors; instead just let them run their course naturally.

Time: Twenty to forty minutes, once or twice a day, preferably around dawn and midnight.

Microcosmic Orbit meditation (Fig. 49)

This is the classic Taoist meditation method for refining, raising, and circulating internal energy via the 'orbit' formed by the Governing Channel from perineum up to head and the Conception Channel from head back down to perineum. Activating the Microcosmic Orbit is a key stage of practice which paves the way for all the more advanced practices. It fills the reservoirs of the Governing and Conception channels with energy, which is then distributed to all the major organ-energy meridians, thereby energizing the internal organs. It draws abundant energy up from the sacrum into the brain, thereby enhancing cerebral circulation of blood and stimulating secretions of vital neurochemicals. It is also the first stage of practice for cultivating the 'spiritual embryo' or 'golden elixir' of immortality, a process that begins in the lower abdomen and culminates in the midbrain. This is probably the best of all Taoist methods for cultivating health and longevity while also 'opening the three passes' to higher spiritual awareness.

'Opening the Three Passes' is another name for this meditation method and refers to the three critical junctions which pave the way for energy to travel up from the sacrum through the Governing Channel along the spine into the head. A fourth-century Taoist meditation manual states: 'The three passes are vital intersections for the three primordials of essence, energy, and spirit.' Since this is such an important practice, it is worth quoting at length a detailed description of it written in the eleventh century by Chang Po-tuan under the heading 'The Secret of Opening the Passes', translated here by Thomas Cleary in *Vitality, Energy, Spirit:*

> With this settled mind, sit alone in a quiet room, senses shut and eyelids lowered. Turn your attention within, and inwardly visualize a pocket of energy in the umbilical region; within it is a point of golden light, clear and bright, immaculately pure.

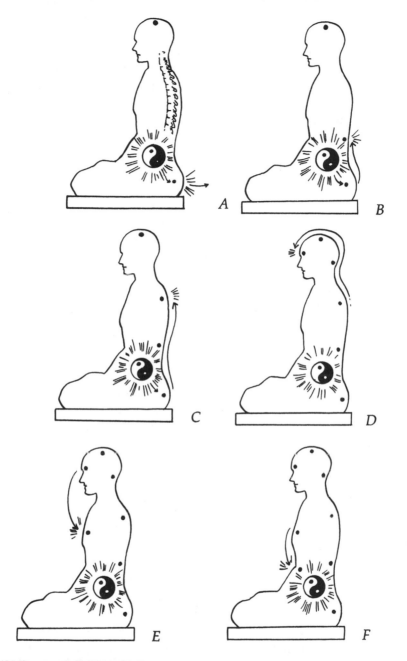

Fig. 49 **Microcosmic Orbit meditation**
A. Focus on energy moving from Lower Elixir Field down through perineum and up to coccyx.
B. Focus on energy moving from coccyx through sacrum to Gate of Life (between kidneys).
C. Focus on energy moving from coccyx through sacrum & Gate of Life to Big Hammer points between shoulders (behind heart).
D. Focus on energy moving from point between shoulders up through Jade Pillow at base of skull to Cavity of Original Spirit in mid-brain and on to Celestial Eye between brows.
E. Focus on energy moving from mid-brow point down to heart.
F. Focus on energy returning down to navel and into Lower Elixir Field.

When you have succeeded in visualizing this light in the pocket of energy, don't let it dim. The breath through your nose will naturally become light and subtle, going out and in evenly and finely, continuously and quietly, gradually becoming slighter and subtler . . . The human body has three posterior passes and three anterior passes. The three posterior passes are in the coccyx, at the base of the spine; in the midspine, where the ribs join the spine; and at the back of the brain.

The pass in the coccyx, at the bottom of the spine, connects with the channels of the genital organs. From this pass ascends the spinal cord, which is called the Zen Valley, or the Yellow River, or the Waterwheel Course, or the Mountain Range up to the Court of Heaven, or the Ladder up to Heaven.

This is the road by which positive energy ascends; it goes right up the point opposite the center of the chest, the pass of the enclosed spine, where the ribs join in back, then it goes straight up to the back of the brain, which is called the pass of the Jade Pillow.

The three anterior passes are called the Nirvana Center, the Earth Pot, and the Ocean of Energy. The Nirvana Center is the so-called upper elixir field. It is a spherical opening 1.3 inches in diameter and is the repository of the spirit. That opening is three inches behind the center of the eyebrows, right in the middle.

The space between the eyebrows is called the Celestial Eye. The space one inch inward is called the Bright Hall. The space one inch farther in is called the Hidden Chamber. One inch farther in from that is the Nirvana Center . . .

The windpipe has twelve sections and is called the Multistoried Tower; it goes to the openings in the lungs, and reaches the heart. Below the heart is an opening called the Crimson Chamber, where the dragon and tiger mate. Another 3.6 inches directly below that is what is called the Earth Pot, which is the Yellow Court, the middle elixir field . . .

The umbilical opening is called the Door of Life. It has seven channels connecting with the genitals. The leaking of sexual energy takes place through these channels. Behind the navel and in front of the kidneys, right in the middle, is the place called the Crescent Moon Jar, or the

Ocean of Energy. And 1.3 inches below that is what is called the Flower Pond, or the lower elixir field. This is where vitality is stored, and it is the place where the medicine is gathered . . .

The secret of conveying energy to open the passes is as follows: Sit as before, closing the eyes and shutting the mouth, turning the attention inward, visualizing the pocket of energy within the body, quieting the mind and tuning the breath. After the breath is settled, only then is it possible to produce the one true energy . . .

Steadily visualize this true energy as being like a small snake gradually passing through the nine apertures of the coccyx. When you feel the energy has gone through this pass, visualize this true energy rising up to where the ribs meet the spine, then going through this pass and right on up to the Jade Pillow, the back of the brain.

Then imagine your true spirit in the Nirvana Chamber in the center of the brain, taking in the energy. When this true energy goes through the Jade Pillow, press the tongue against the palate. The head should move forward and tilt slightly upwards to help it. When you feel this true energy penetrating the Nirvana Chamber, this may feel hot or swollen. This means the pass has been cleared and the energy has reached the Nirvana Center.

After that, move the spirit to the Celestial Eye between the eyebrows, drawing the true energy on to the Hidden Room and Bright Hall, chambers in the brain behind the brows, then finally the Celestial Eye. Then the center of the brows will throb – this means the Celestial Eye is about to open. Then move the spirit into the center of the brows and draw the true energy through the Celestial Eye. If you see the eighteen thousand pores and three hundred and sixty joints of the whole body explode open all at once, each joint parting three-tenths of an inch, this is evidence of the opening of the Celestial Eye.

This is what is meant when it is said that when one pass opens all the passes open, and when one opening is cleared all the openings are cleared.

Once the passes have been opened, then draw the true energy down the pillar of the nose, descending the Golden Bridge. Feeling as though there is cool water going down the Multistoried Tower of the windpipe, do not swallow; let it go down by itself, bathing the bronchial tubes . . .

Then the vital energy will bathe the internal organs and then return to the genitals. This is what is called return to the root.

From the genitals the energy goes into the coccyx, then directly back up to the center of the brain, and from the center of the brain down to the lower elixir field, then going up and around as before. This is what is meant by returning to life.

If you practice this way for a long time, eventually you can complete a whole cycle of ascent and descent in one continuous visualization. If you can quietly practice this inner work continuously, whether walking, standing still, sitting, or lying down, then the vital energy will circulate within, and there will naturally be no problem of leakage. Chronic physical ailments will naturally disappear.

Also, once the inner energy is circulating, the breath will naturally become fine, and the true positive energy of heaven and earth will be inhaled by way of the breath and go down to join your own generative energy. The two energies will mix together, both to be circulated by you together, descending and ascending over and over, circulating up and down to replenish the depleted true energy in your body.

This true energy harmonizes and reforms, so that the vital fluids produced by the energy of daily life again produce true vitality. When true vitality is fully developed, it naturally produces true energy, and when true energy is fully developed it naturally produces our true spirit.

Thus the three treasures of vitality, energy, and spirit experience a daily flourishing of life and fill the whole body, so that the great medicine can be expected to be produced naturally, whereby one can proceed onward to the process of gathering the medicine, thereby to form the golden elixir.

Method: Although the description above is clear and self-explanatory, let's run through it again briefly in less esoteric terms. The first step is to still the body, calm the mind, and regulate the breath. Focus attention on the navel until you feel the 'pocket of energy' glowing in the umbilical region. When the feeling is stable and the energy there is full, use your mind to guide energy down to the perineum and back up through the aperture in the coccyx. Look for feelings of warmth and/or tingling as energy passes through the coccyx. From the coccyx, energy rises up through the sacral bone and emerges into the lowest lumbar vertebra (L5), then travels up to the point along the midspine directly behind the heart, located at the fifth thoracic vertebra (T5). From there, mentally draw the energy up to the Jade Pillow point at the back of the brain and into the 'Cavity of Original Spirit' in the middle of the brain, behind the pituitary. This may cause a throbbing or swelling sensation in your head.

Next, focus attention on the Celestial Eye between the eyebrows and draw energy forwards from the midbrain and out through the point between the brows. This may cause a tingling or throbbing sensation there. You may wish to stay and work with this point for a few minutes, before letting energy sink down through the palate and tongue into the throat to the heart. From the heart, draw it down through the Middle Elixir Field in the solar plexus, past the navel, and down into the Ocean of Energy reservoir in the Lower Elixir Field, where energy gathers, mixes, and is reserved for internal circulation. Then begin another cycle up through the coccyx to the midspine behind the heart and up past the Jade Pillow into the brain.

Breathe naturally with your abdomen, and don't worry whether energy moves up or down on inhalation or exhalation; coordinate the flow of breath and energy in whatever manner suits you best. However, if you reach the stage where you can complete a full Microcosmic Orbit in a single breath, it's best to raise energy up from coccyx to head on exhalation and draw it down from Upper to Lower Elixir Field on inhalation.

If you have any physical problems or discomforts in a particular section of your body, focus your energy at the pass closest to the discomfort and let it throb there for a while. This will help heal and rejuvenate the injured tissues. For example, if you have pelvic problems, focus energy on the coccyx pass; for lower-back pain focus on L5 just above the sacrum; for upper-back and shoulder pain focus on T5, and so forth.

This meditation may also cause the head to rock or the body to tremble, which are signs of progress.

Time: Thirty to forty-five minutes, once or twice a day.

Signs and sensations

As you enter into the regular practice of sitting meditation, you may begin to experience certain signs and sensations that indicate that you are making progress. These sensations occur only when the body is still, the mind is clear, the emotions are calm, the breath is tuned, and energy is flowing smoothly and strongly through your channels. You should not expect these signs to occur, nor try to force them to come or go; just be aware of them when they happen. Furthermore, not everyone will experience the same combination of signs and sensations. They vary according to each individual, your level of practice, the time of day, prevailing astral conditions, and the surrounding environment. Here are the most common sensations experienced by meditators at various stages of practice:

The Eight Sensations
These are physical feelings caused by the enhanced flow of energy through parts of the body normally deprived of sufficient energy, including sensations of warmth, cold, itching, motion, lightness, heaviness, slipperiness, and coarseness. They may be felt in any part of the body, especially the extremities. Make mentally certain that they are not being caused by adverse environmental energies, such as a cold breeze or direct sunlight, or by incorrect posture, such as leaning too far in one direction, or by cramped legs. If this is the case, make the necessary adjustments in your posture and environment, then continue meditating. If the sensations are caused by internal energy circulation, don't worry about them; just let them run their course.

Rocking and trembling
Already mentioned above, this sensation can take several forms – head rocking forwards and back or side to side, torso trembling, limbs shaking, etc. Often it will be experienced as a trembling in the lower abdomen, an indication that the Lower Elixir Field is filling with energy and a sign that energy is ready to enter circulation in the Microcosmic Orbit.

Gurgling abdomen
As energy fills the Lower Elixir Field and circulates in the minor channels of the abdomen, it can cause gas and fluids in the intestines to move, resulting in gurgling sensations in the gut. Often this will be accompanied by sensations of heat in the stomach. As the abdominal channels open up with continued

practice, digestion and bowel functions will improve and the gurgling sensations will gradually disappear.

Lightness
This feeling usually occurs after you have activated the Microcosmic Orbit. Your entire body feels light and airy, almost as though it were nothing more substantial than a cloud. This is caused by the total elimination of all stress and tension in the body, mental tranquillity, energy flowing freely through the channels, and smooth, finely tuned breathing.

Clear light
If you manage to achieve a deep and stable meditative state of mind, you may suddenly feel as though your body has completely dissolved and your energy is merging with the surrounding environmental energy in a mist of clear light or white cloud. Everything solid dissolves into emptiness. This is a very pleasant state and a good sign of progress, but if you try to cling to it by focusing attention on it, it will promptly disappear and ordinary sensations of physical solidity will return. So if it happens, don't get excited, just remain cool, calm, and clear, and let it be.

Abdominal and kidney heat
When your meditation progresses to a more advanced level, you may experience intense sensations of heat in your lower abdomen, as though it were filled with red-hot coals, and/or hot streaking sensations in your kidneys, as though boiling water were pouring through them. The lower abdomen and the kidneys are the primary seats of primordial energy, and extremely hot sensations here are signs of progress in internal alchemy.

Supernatural powers
These signs occur only at the most advanced stages of practice, when the primordial spirit's innate powers are fully awakened and brought under conscious control by the mind. These powers include clairvoyance, whereby the adept can see the future unfold as a natural order of events proceeding from the past through the present into the future, grand visions of the universe, communication with uncorporeal spirits, and the ability to 'read' other people's thoughts by tuning into their brain waves (ESP). These signs are a clear indication that the adept is on the brink of enlightenment and is able to project conscious awareness beyond his or her physical body.

Times to meditate

The best times of day to meditate are during the hours around dawn, noon, sunset, and midnight. Among those times, the best are dawn and midnight, because midnight is when the yin phase of the day (noon till midnight) ends and yang energy begins to rise, and dawn is when yang energy is at its peak. Meditating when yang energy prevails in the atmosphere is far more invigorating and conducive to internal alchemy than during the yin phase of the day, which begins at noon and peaks at sunset. Ideally, one should start meditating about half an hour before dawn and half an hour before midnight, but it's also good to sit any time within an hour or two before or after dawn and midnight. If these hours are inconvenient, then practise any time of day or night that suits your schedule, but try to practise around the same time every day.

There are also certain days of the year when Taoists like to meditate for longer periods than usual, in order to harvest celestial energies raining down from sky to earth during certain favourable configurations of sun, moon, planets, and stars. These times include the nights of the full and new moons, the summer and winter solstices, and other cyclic seasonal dates. On these days it's best to start meditating around 11.30 p.m. and to continue as long as you can. If your legs or spine get cramped, or if you feel restless or stagnant, take a break from sitting and pace around the room slowly in 'walking meditation', then sit down again and continue your still meditation. Meditating on such 'power nights' is a great way to top up your energy reservoirs and revitalize every cell in your body with potent cosmic energies from the sky. Lunar calendars and farmers' almanacs have these days clearly marked for easy reference.

There are also certain times when it is advisable not to meditate, such as during thunder storms, hurricanes, typhoons, extreme heat spells, and other abnormal meteorological conditions, in order to prevent aberrant environmental energies from entering into circulation in the human energy system, where they can cause severe disturbances and imbalances.

'It's all in the mind'

The great alchemist and Taoist sage Lu Tung-pin wrote:

> Although the span of human life is finite, the spirit is infinite. If we view the universe in terms of our human life span, then our lives seem as brief and fleeting as those of

flies. But if we look at the universe in terms of our spirits, then the universe appears as finite as the life of a fly.

It is truly a waste of time and energy to spend our entire lives exclusively focused on the fleeting world of material profit and physical pleasure, for before we know it, our lives are over and death robs us of all our carefully collected worldly gains. At least part of our lives would be better spent cultivating the infinite potential of spiritual awareness, which is the only thing we take with us after death and which is as vast and grand as the universe itself. If we fail to cultivate the conscious spiritual awareness required to qualify ourselves for entry into higher realms, we will die in ignorance and confusion. Our minds, deluded by the accumulated effects of our own misguided activities, will propel our spirits blindly into yet another mortal corporeal existence, over and over again.

Spiritual cultivation is the best – indeed the only – way to 'change the world', for the world is what we perceive it to be. When things are not going well in our individual worlds, we tend to blame the world rather than looking into our own minds for the solutions to our problems, which more often than not are caused by our own wrong habits and misguided activities, mental as well as physical. Cultivating spiritual awareness through the practice of meditation gradually transforms the way we perceive the world, reorders our priorities, broadens and balances our views, clarifies our thoughts, pacifies our emotions, and repaints our mental landscapes. After a while, it appears that the world has changed much for the better, when in fact it is our own consciousness that has changed and thereby improved the view. As an ancient Buddhist adage states: 'When your mind is pure, everything in your world will also be pure.'

Weltschmertz ('worldly pain') is a disease of the mind, not of the world: clear the mind of random thoughts, eliminate paranoid fears, pacify conflicting emotions, harness passions, and the world becomes a beautiful place to live, for suffering and pain are all in the mind of the beholder, not malevolent facts of life. It's easy to blame the world for all our troubles, but in fact we impose our troubles on an innocent world because we are too lazy and ignorant to resolve them ourselves.

Therefore, the solution to worldly problems is not to change the world but to change your mind, and the only way to change your mind is to get to know it, discipline it, and control it, all of which may be readily accomplished through the regular practice of meditation. Indeed, summit meetings between rival world leaders would be far more fruitful and might actually bring lasting peace to the world if, instead of sitting down around a table to talk about 'world problems' from their conflicting points of view, they were to sit down together on cushions and meditate until their minds began to share the same peaceful vision of the world. By changing their own minds, they could change the world for the better on behalf of all of us.

Life is evanescent, the human ego and individual personality dissolve along with the demise of the flesh, and personal memories fade away, but the primordial spirit of consciousness, the shining pearl of pure awareness that lights up our minds, is eternal, immaculate, immortal, and endowed with inconceivable powers which we may awaken and utilize by virtue of spiritual development. It is well worth while to devote some time each day to 'sitting still, doing nothing' in order to get acquainted with the primordial face of your own mind, which is your one and only permanent asset and your only continuous link to the universe. Losing access to that asset and losing sight of that link, as most people do soon after birth, can plunge you into aeons of chaotic rebirths and transmigrations in various unpleasant realms of existence, until you painstakingly garner sufficient merit to qualify once again for human rebirth and another shot at spiritual liberation.

But all that is another story, beyond the earthly concerns of health and longevity which inform this book. Suffice it to say here that every time you sit down to meditate, regardless of the style or purpose of your method, you are coming one step closer to restoring conscious access to your own primordial spirit and one step closer to re-establishing a direct spiritual link to the entire universe and all of its cosmic forces.

'May the Force be with you!'

PART III

The Fruits: Health and Longevity

CHAPTER 17

Immunity

Health is easier to maintain than it is to acquire.
Dr Russ Jaffe (1984)

Most modern maladies are caused by prolonged exposure to a combination of negative lifestyle and toxic environmental factors, including junk food and malnutrition, pesticides, antibiotics, microwaves, chemical pollution of food, water, and air, lack of exercise, and chronic stress. These factors are further aggravated by the failure of modern medicine to recognize them as agents of disease and death, and the consequent failure to take preventive measures against them. By rebuilding immunity, health is naturally restored and disease disappears. If health and immunity are thereafter conscientiously maintained, the individual is no longer vulnerable to disease.

Dr Russ Jaffe, who specializes in the treatment of AIDS, even states: 'I do not believe that healthy people will get AIDS.' This is heresy to the Western medical establishment, but there are significant external factors associated with the groups at high risk of AIDS. Junkies, who do not usually lead healthy lives, have been dying of AIDS-like symptoms caused by blood poisoning ever since the hypodermic needle was invented. Gay men often use immunosuppressive drugs such as amyl nitrite, and antibiotics for venereal disease; anal sex is also a risk factor because when semen is introduced into the anus, it triggers a heavy autoimmune response. In central African countries, where AIDS is thought to have originated, many pesticides and toxic pharmaceuticals, which are now banned in the West and many parts of Asia, are sold cheaply over the counter. In the opinion of traditional healers, therefore, AIDS is caused by a failure to guard the Three Treasures. This does not mean that you need not bother with safe sex, because unsafe sex leads to common VD, which requires heavy antibiotic treatment, which in turn is one of the main destroyers of immune function.

Hospitals do not offer a wholesome environment, either. Despite all the antibiotics, antiseptics, and other chemical weapons used in hospitals to wage war on germs, over 2 million cases of serious infection develop in American hospitals each year, resulting in 60,000–80,000 unnecessary deaths.

The sort of health care required to restore immunity and prevent disease begins at home, not in the clinic, by eliminating factors which impair immunity and cultivating habits which boost it. Though it requires individual effort and self-discipline, preventive health care is always a good investment, in time as well as money, because once you fall ill, it takes a lot more time and costs a lot more money to acquire health again. And every time you lose your health, the road to recovery gets longer and rougher, demanding a growing investment for diminishing returns. By investing in your own immunity now, you ensure your future health and guard your life at minimum cost.

The allopathic approach to treating disease is at least partly responsible for the world's health crisis, because many of the chemical drugs widely prescribed have side effects which are cumulative and impair immunity. The very fact that allopathic doctors dispense antagonistic drugs at the slightest sign of disease or discomfort indicates a basic lack of faith in the innate power of the human body to heal itself. That power is what immunity is all about, so let's take a look at how it works.

Immunity: The body's defence department

Immunity is a manifold defence system which protects the body from external threats such as harmful bacteria, viruses, parasites, and toxins, as well as from internal hazards such as cancerous cells, arteriosclerotic plaque, cholesterol deposits, and free radicals. This defence complex works on all three levels of essence, energy, and spirit.

On the basic physiological level of essence, the body is endowed with numerous glands and tissues that produce immune factors when prompted by proper signals from the brain via the central nervous system. Primary among these defence installations are the following:

Thymus gland

Located behind the sternum near the heart, the thymus produces special immune factors called T-cells, which roam constantly throughout the body in the bloodstream on search-and-destroy missions against foreign invaders.

Bone marrow

The bone marrow is responsible for producing several varieties of white blood cells that attack, kill, and digest foreign invaders as well as malfunctioning pre-cancerous cells. Bone marrow also produces red blood cells, which carry oxygen from the lungs to all tissues of the body. The white blood cells generated by bone marrow also produce specific antibodies to fight specific bacteria and viruses.

Spleen and pancreas

These 'organs' are actually large glands which produce and secrete vital enzymes as required by the body. Diets consisting largely of overcooked and processed foods divert so many enzymes into the stomach and intestines for digestion that immunity is compromised owing to insufficient supplies of enzymes for antioxidant and other immune functions.

Pituitary and pineal

These two tiny glands are located in the midbrain, and their secretions regulate most of the body's basic functions and biorhythms, including immunity. Especially important for immune functions is the growth hormone secreted by the pituitary.

Adrenals

Located on top of the kidneys, the adrenals secrete a wide range of vital hormones involved in sexual functions, immunity, and the fight-or-flight response. The latter response is triggered by stress and severely impairs immune functions. When balanced and undisturbed by stress, adrenals secrete hormones that play important roles in immunity; they also function as 'batteries' for storing the primordial energy which feeds the radiant shield of protective *wei-chee* around the body.

Lymph

Lymphatic fluids absorb toxins and wastes from tissues and blood, transporting them to the colon, lungs, and pores for excretion.

Liver and kidneys
These two organs are responsible for filtering toxins and metabolic wastes from the blood, thereby purifying it so that it can properly perform its nourishing and cleansing functions throughout the system. The liver is also responsible for manufacturing many enzymes that are essential for optimum immunity.

Cerebrospinal fluids
The vital fluids of the spinal cord and brain regulate all communications within the human system and trigger either immunosupportive or immunosuppressive responses by mutual biofeedback with hormones, depending on one's state of mind and emotions. These fluids are the messengers through which mind and body communicate and cooperate to guard health in the cerebro-physical defence system known as psychoneuroimmunology (PNI).

On the level of energy, the body is protected by an aura of radiant energy that envelops the entire body and shields it from invasion by aberrant environmental energies, including such natural elements as wind, heat, and cold, as well as artificial sources such as microwaves, power lines, and electrical appliances. The strength and protective power of this shield depends upon nutrition, breathing, purity of blood, regular exercise, supplements, emotional equilibrium, positive mental attitudes, and other basic factors of health. In addition, each of the 60 trillion cells in the human body generates its own electromagnetic field, which protects the cell from invasion by aberrant energies. When a cluster of cells in a particular tissue lose their electromagnetic shields through extreme toxicity, stress, injuries, heavy-metal deposits, or other adverse factors, they become vulnerable to invasion not only by aberrant energies, but also by pathogens such as viruses and toxins. If the cells are not promptly rebalanced by corrective measures, the cumulative harm eventually reaches their nuclei and causes genetic damage, which in turn can cause cancer and other cellular derangements. While protective energy depends upon nutrition, emotions, mental attitudes, and other factors of essence and spirit, the primary mechanism for enhancing it is deep abdominal breathing and internal energy circulation.

On the level of spirit, immunity is strongly influenced by thoughts, emotions, and attitudes. These mental factors are mediated by biofeedback between the nervous and endocrine systems, which form the powerful immunological mechanisms of PNI. Consistently ignored by orthodox allopathic physicians, who try to impose matter over mind with drugs but feel threatened by the innate powers of mind over matter, the mental factors which trigger the PNI system constitute the human body's most effective and most powerful defence mechanism. By cultivating this innate psychophysiological healing response through meditation, *chee-gung*, and the power of positive thinking, individuals can learn how to cure and prevent disease at home.

In order for the immunological weapons described above to function, they must be properly maintained. Maintaining optimum immunity revolves around the following primary factors:

Clean blood and lymph

Blood plays a front-line defensive role by delivering nutrients and immune factors to diseased and toxic tissues and carrying away metabolic wastes, toxins, and pathogens. Lymph in turn keeps the blood clean and also purifies cellular fluids. The efficiency of their defence functions depends entirely upon their degree of purity, including proper pH balance. Clean blood also depends upon proper maintenance of the liver and kidneys, which filter the blood.

Balanced endocrine function

In order to produce the hormones required for immunity, the entire endocrine system must be maintained in proper balance, for glandular secretions influence one another by biofeedback. Endocrine balance is achieved and maintained by the parasympathetic branch of the autonomous nervous system, and excessive stimulation of the sympathetic branch throws the endocrine system off balance.

Active elimination

In order to keep the body clean, the immune system needs a place to dump all the garbage it dredges from the system. Therefore, all the excretory organs, including colon, lungs, kidneys, and skin, must be maintained in proper working order. Whenever excretory functions are impaired, the body dumps its garbage into joints, body fat, lymph nodes, colonic sacculations, and other nooks and crannies isolated from the bloodstream.

Nutrition

Proper nutrition is absolutely essential for maintaining immunity, for nutrients are the building blocks of human defence installations. Nutrients are also required for antioxidant protection against free-radical damage, rebuilding injured tissues, and metabolic conversion of essence into energy.

Stress relief
Chronic stress is probably the greatest enemy of the human immune system, and effective stress management is therefore crucial to maintenance of immune defences. Stress triggers a chain reaction of immunosuppressive biofeedback between the endocrine and nervous systems, leaving the entire body highly vulnerable to otherwise innocuous pathogens and environmental energies.

Rest
The body requires sufficient periodic rest in order to permit the immune system to 'clean house' and repair damaged tissues. This can be accomplished only when the autonomous nervous system switches over to the parasympathetic branch, as happens during periods of rest and relaxation. 'Rest' does not necessarily mean sleep, though sufficient sleep is also important. Rest is achieved by slowing down the body, deepening the breath, balancing the organ energies, and emptying the mind; all these factors prompt parasympathetic responses and endocrine balance.

Energy
Immunity requires plenty of energy, including nourishing metabolic *ying-chee* to produce hormones, neurochemicals, enzymes, white blood cells, and other highly refined forms of immune essence, and protective radiant *wei-chee* to ward off abnormal environmental energies. This energy must be available at a moment's notice, which means that adequate supplies of it must be stored in the reservoirs of the Eight Extraordinary Channels.

Attitude
The decisive role played by mental factors such as thoughts, moods, feelings, and attitudes in maintaining immunity cannot be overemphasized, but this is precisely the factor most commonly overlooked by allopathic medicine. The so-called 'power of positive thinking' functions by virtue of the biochemical responses it stimulates throughout the immune system through biofeedback. Negative attitudes have an equally powerful suppressive impact on immune functions.

Physiologically, the traditional Chinese view of the human immune system is remarkably similar to the modern Western model. In the Chinese system, the first line of defence is provided by the thymus, adrenals, and spine, followed in order of priority by the bone marrow, blood, brain (pituitary, pineal, and hypothalamus), liver and kidneys, spleen and pancreas. The Chinese, however, also attach great importance to the immunological powers of energy and spirit, which are factors consistently ignored and misunderstood by modern Western medicine, much to the peril of patients. Traditional Chinese doctors and Taoist healers frequently prescribe *chee-gung* to boost immunological response and meditation to mobilize the immunological powers of the mind, usually in conjunction with herbal and dietary prescriptions that work synergistically with energy and spirit. Without sufficient energy, neither drugs, herbs, nor nutrients can be properly utilized in defence of health, and negative mental attitudes such as cynicism, doubt, fear, confusion, and self-loathing can negate the therapeutic benefits of even the most potent medications. While modern Western medicine has a firm grasp of the 'essence' of immunity, it has much to learn from traditional Chinese medicine about the 'energy' and 'spirit' of the human immune system, and the sooner it does so, the better the health of Western societies will become.

Traditional Chinese immunology attaches particular importance to the role of the adrenal glands in guarding health, and recent Western research on the immunosuppressive effects of stress scientifically validates the Chinese view. The Chinese refer to the adrenals as the 'Root of Life' and cite them as the primary source of pure primordial energy, sexual vitality, and immunological resilience. Since they are attached to the kidneys, the technical Chinese name for the adrenals is 'kidney glands', and their functions are directly influenced by kidney organ energy. Fear, for example, is an aberrant emotional energy associated with the kidneys in the Chinese system, and chronic fear is thus regarded as a major suppressant of immune function. This view is confirmed by Western medical science, which cites fear as a form of stress that triggers adrenal secretions of adrenaline and cortisone, two hormones known to suppress immunity severely. When fear or any other source of stress becomes chronic, adrenal burnout soon follows, and the victim acquires a chronic immune deficiency that renders the body easy prey to formerly harmless microbes in the environment. Adrenal burnout and elevated levels of cortisone in the blood are major contributing factors in chronic fatigue syndrome, AIDS, cancer, sexual impotence and infertility, allergies, migraine, and other debilitating conditions. According to the Chinese system, weak adrenals not only impair immunity on the level of essence, they also weaken resistance by cutting the main source of energy which maintains the radiant shell of protective *wei-chee* round the body. And since kidney organ energy governs bone marrow and brain tissue, deficient kidney/adrenal function also impairs production of white blood cells, hormones, and other immune factors in these vital tissues. Therefore, the traditional Chinese view of the kidney/adrenal complex as a primary regulator of immunity that functions on all three levels of essence, energy, and spirit has been confirmed by modern medical science and provides adepts of Taoist alchemy with a powerful protective mechanism that can be cultivated with physical, energetic, and spiritual practices.

As we discussed in Chapter 4 ('The Four Foundations'), traditional Chinese medicine cites four major forms of immune deficiency, or 'immune emptiness': blood, energy, yin, and yang. The term 'empty' refers to a condition of energy deficiency that impairs the vital functions of the organ, gland, or tissue which that particular energy governs. In Western medicine, which does not recognize the roles of bioenergies, various forms of immune deficiency are described directly in terms of the organ, gland, or tissue affected, such as thymus atrophy, adrenal burn out, bone-marrow impairment, cerebral insufficiency, and so forth.

In order to gain a proper perspective on the rapidly growing problem of immune deficiency, we will now discuss some of the primary causes and most effective remedies in terms of essence, energy, and spirit.

Immunity and essence

Until about 1960, the biggest killer of children under the age of fifteen in America was accidents, but now it is cancer. Most cases of immune deficiency begin during childhood with the first glass of pasteurized cow's milk and the first bowl of processed cereal sprinkled with white sugar. The overall physical and mental health of American children has been declining at an alarming rate, and the primary reason for this is their diet. In adulthood, the debilitating effects are compounded by alcohol, drugs (medicinal as well as recreational), contaminated beef, artificial fats, and other factors. Let's take a quick look at some of the most immunosuppressive elements that people routinely allow to enter the inner sanctum of their bodies.

Immunosuppressive elements

Sugar
Refined white sugar triggers the release of insulin from the pancreas. With daily consumption of sugar, the bloodstream is always laced with insulin, which suppresses secretion of growth hormone from the pituitary. Growth hormone is a prime regulator of the immune system.

Hydrogenated vegetable oils
An ingredient in virtually all processed foods, baby formulas, non-dairy creamers, salad dressings, etc., these artificial fats rapidly oxidize in the human system, releasing a deadly barrage of free radicals which destroy cells and cause genetic damage. They impair the immune activity of white blood cells and have been conclusively linked to increased risks of cancer.

Beef and cow's milk
Steroid hormones, antibiotics, and other drugs routinely fed to cattle are absorbed by the people who consume the meat and milk of such contaminated animals, throwing the endocrine system off balance and impairing immunity.

Malnutrition
Malnutrition is a primary cause of immune deficiency throughout the world, not only where people are starving. The most glaring deficiencies in modern diets are essential amino acids and essential fatty acids, both of which are required in the production of immune factors such as white blood cells and antibodies. The thymus gland and lymph tissues, for example, immediately begin to shrink and atrophy when these nutrients are absent from the diet.

Heavy metals
Toxic heavy metals such as cadmium, lead, mercury, and aluminium suppress all branches of the immune system, inhibiting T-cells, B-cells, and antibodies and depressing bone-marrow function. Cadmium also blocks assimilation of zinc, which is an essential element required by the body to manufacture the potent antioxidant enzyme superoxide dismutase, one of the body's most important immune factors. Heavy metals enter our bodies in tap water, contaminated fish, polluted air, fresh produce grown with synthetic fertilizers, and cigarette smoke.

Antibiotics
These commonly prescribed drugs are powerful immuno-suppressors and also destroy the friendly lactobacteria in our intestinal tracts, thereby permitting candida and other harmful yeasts to proliferate throughout the system, where they further inhibit immune functions.

Recreational drugs
Coffee, alcohol, tobacco, opiates, barbiturates, amphetamines, and other popular drugs, when used to excess, severely inhibit immunity by releasing toxic by-products into the blood-stream and suppressing liver function. Coffee has been specifically linked to increased risk of pancreas cancer; the offending agent is not caffeine, but other elements contained in coffee beans. When coffee is consumed together with refined sugar and non-dairy creamer, the immune system gets battered with a triple blow.

Immune deficiency can be prevented and cured by first eliminating as many immunosuppressant elements as possible from your diet and lifestyle, then taking some or all of the following immunity-boosting foods and supplements daily.

Foods

Many common foods have potent immunity-boosting properties when consumed regularly in sufficient quantities, including the following:

Cruciferous vegetables
The members of this family of vegetables, including broccoli, cauliflower, cabbage, Brussels sprouts, and turnips, are rich in betacarotene and protect mucous membranes, especially in the lungs and intestinal tract, from cancer and free-radical damage.

Garlic
Garlic is probably the foremost immune-enhancing food on Mother Nature's menu. It has a wider spectrum of antibiotic activity than penicillin, inhibits many viruses, and helps prevent cancer. It is also one of the richest natural sources of selenium, which is required to produce the potent antioxidant enzyme glutathione peroxidase. It is most effective when consumed raw.

Raw fish
Deep-water fish such as salmon and tuna are rich sources of omega-3 fish oils, which contain the essential fatty acids required to produce immune factors such as white blood cells in the body. They also prevent heart attacks by keeping the arteries clear of cholesterol deposits. These elements are most abundant and easy to assimilate when the fish is consumed raw, but if you prefer it cooked, then lightly steam or poach it.

Seaweeds
Seaweeds are known to lower blood cholesterol, neutralize radiation toxicity, and enhance overall immunity.

Raw almonds
Raw almonds are one of the best natural sources of essential amino acids and essential fatty acids, both of which are required for optimum immunity. For vegetarians, who often become deficient in these vital nutrients, raw almonds are an excellent substitute for meat and other animal products.

Bee pollen
Another good source of essential fatty acids, bee pollen is also loaded with enzymes and other potent nutritional elements which boost immunity. Pollen also helps eliminate many food allergies.

Supplements

Because of environmental pollution and denatured diets, food alone is no longer sufficient to sustain optimum immunity today. Without supplements, the body simply does not get the full range and quantity of vital nutrients and other elements it requires to maintain health and vitality, regardless how much food you eat. Judicious use of the following supplements will supply the elements the body needs most to fight disease, neutralize toxins and free radicals, and guard against premature degeneration of bodily tissues.

Vitamins
Many vitamins function not only as nutrients but also as potent antioxidants. When the body is diseased or distressed, it utilizes vitamins at a far greater rate than under normal conditions, a fact that shows how important these nutrients are to immune functions. Most important is vitamin C, which helps prevent cancer,

counteracts the immunosuppressive effects of cortisol, protects the heart, and boosts overall immunity. The optimum maintenance dose is 2–6 grams per day, and double that amount when ill. Other immunity-boosting vitamins include, in order of potency, vitamin A (preferably as betacarotene), vitamin E, and vitamins B_1, B_5, B_6, and B_{12}.

Minerals

The minerals selenium and zinc are indispensable to the human immune system, because they are required to manufacture antioxidant enzymes, which protect the body from free-radical damage. Zinc, for example, is used to synthesize eighty different enzymes, including the body's most potent anti-aging enzyme, superoxide dismutase. Other minerals essential for immune function include magnesium, potassium, manganese, sodium, copper, and chromium.

Amino acids

Arginine, when taken with synergistic cofactors such as vitamin B_5, stimulates the pituitary to secrete growth hormone, a vital immune regulator. Arginine also enlarges the thymus gland (which produces T-cells), greatly enhances the body's healing powers, and helps prevent cancer. Other immune-boosting amino acids include ornithine, cysteine, taurine, methionine, and glutathione.

Essential fatty acids

These nutrients, including omega-3 fish oils, oleic acid, and caprylic acid, provide the best protection against arteriosclerosis and other forms of heart disease. Since few Americans get adequate levels of these essential nutrients from their food (as clearly evidenced by the fact that heart disease now accounts for 53 per cent of all deaths in the USA), supplemental sources are required. Fatty acids are also essential elements in white blood cells, antibodies, and brain cells.

Enzymes

Since modern diets consist primarily of cooked and processed foods, the body must divert much of its enzyme power to the stomach and duodenum for digestive duty, thereby sharply reducing the availability of enzymes for antioxidant activity and other immune functions. When taken on an empty stomach, enzyme supplements go to work digesting microbes, pre-cancerous cells, toxins, pus, mucus, and other disease-causing agents.

Lactobacteria

Supplemental sources of lactobacteria such as acidophilus, bifidus, and fermented cabbage juice replenish the colonies of 'friendly' bacteria in the intestinal tract. Lactobacteria are the body's only natural defence against candida and other yeast infections, which have powerful immunosuppressive properties. They also facilitate rapid elimination of toxic digestive wastes and improve assimilation of essential nutrients from food.

Herbs

Many herbs have potent immune-boosting properties. In Chinese medicine, the most widely used herbs for enhancing immunity are ginseng, ginkgo, *Astragalus*, *gotu kola*, *Ligustrum*, and *Codonopsis*. The North American herb *Echinacea* (purple Kansas coneflower) is also a highly effective immune-system tonic and was widely used by the Plains Indians to cure and prevent many ailments. Other North American herbs that boost immunity are chaparral (*Larrea divaricata*), yerba mansa (*Anemopsis californica*), and osha (*Ligusticum porteri*). The South American herb *pau d'arco* (*Tabebuia pentaphylla*) enhances the body's ability to resist pathogens and also directly attacks outside invaders. *Shiitake* mushrooms and a rare Chinese mushroom called *ling-jir* also have strong immunity-enhancing properties and are frequently included in herbal formulas that boost immunity. Many of these herbs are currently being used to treat AIDS patients.

Growth hormone

As the human body ages, secretions of growth hormone naturally decline. A synthetic growth hormone that costs about $20,000 per year has recently been shown dramatically to reverse the symptoms of aging in several studies in America. At less cost, you can take other supplements, such as arginine, which stimulate the pituitary gland to secrete elevated levels of natural growth hormone. Another effective growth-hormone-releasing supplement is the drug bromocryptine (sold as Parlodel), which is conventionally used to treat senility, infertility, and other symptoms of growth-hormone deficiency. By taking this supplement, which has no adverse side effects, for a month or two once or twice a year, you can help prevent growth-hormone deficiency and its related symptoms.

Women who have gone through menopause should note that bromocryptine can reverse menopause and restore menstrual cycles and fertility, even in 60–70-year-old women, so if you use it in this stage of life, you should take appropriate precautions against unwanted pregnancy.

Fasting

One of the most effective of all immune-system boosters turns out to be fasting, which all animals do naturally whenever they are ill. When properly conducted, fasting can cure virtually all diseases, including cancer, and completely rebuild the immune system. Fasting is the most effective of all methods for stimulating elevated secretions of growth hormone, detoxifying the blood and all other bodily fluids and tissues, excreting accumulated wastes from the colon and other organs, dissolving tumours and cysts, repairing tissues, and healing internal and external injuries.

Immunity and energy

Aberrant energies always exert an immunosuppressive influence on the human system by upsetting the delicate balance of internal bioenergies upon which immunity depends. Aberrant energies can invade the human energy system from external sources, such as exposure to microwaves, radiation, fluorescent lights, and other forms of electromagnetic pollution, or they can be generated internally by emotional turmoil, toxins, ailing organs, or obstructed energy channels. Either way, the first casualty of aberrant energy is immunity, and the first aid to repairing immune deficiency caused by energy imbalance is the internal alchemy of Taoist energy exercises.

Energy factors that impair immunity

Abnormal electromagnetic fields
We have already discussed in detail the hazards to human health generated by power lines, electrical appliances, and a growing array of electronic gadgets. By suppressing the pineal and pituitary glands and impeding cerebral functions, abnormal electromagnetic fields impair immunity at its central headquarters in the brain.

Microwaves
Not only do microwaves suppress the same glands and tissues as abnormal electromagnetic fields, they also constitute a primary stimulant of the human stress response today. You don't have to be

uptight, paranoid, or stuck in a stressful job or marriage in order to suffer chronic stress. Passive exposure to microwave radiation triggers stress response in even the calmest, most balanced individuals. In laboratory tests conducted on rats, exposure to microwaves at levels twenty times below the current safety standards set in the USA provoked sufficient stress to exhaust the adrenals and cause a complete breakdown of the immune system.

Air pollution
Air pollutants such as motor-vehicle exhaust, smoke, and industrial emissions fill the air with heavy positive ions that negate the activity of negative ions, the tiny charged particles which hold atmospheric energy and carry it into the human system via breath. Air conditioning and central heating have the same effect, robbing the air in closed buildings of vital negative-ion energy. Atmospheric negative-ion energy, along with the energy extracted from food by digestion, constitutes a primary ingredient in True Human Energy. Unless you compensate for such 'dead' air with internal energy practices such as *chee-gung* and deep breathing, your immune system will gradually wind down like a clock, leaving you chronically fatigued and vulnerable to even the mildest pathogens.

Deficient light
Light is the primary source of energy for the pituitary gland, which receives the energy through the retina and optic nerve. Light also influences the pineal gland. Light is required by the body to produce vitamin D, which is why this nutrient is called the 'sunshine vitamin'. Light also regulates many human biorhythms, particularly sleep. The sort of wholesome light that nourishes the body is called 'full-spectrum light', which means that it contains all the wavelengths of natural sunlight. Ordinary light bulbs are deficient in many vital frequencies; the light from fluorescent tubes and television screens is not only deficient, it also vibrates erratically and thereby irritates the pituitary gland and the central nervous system via the optic nerve. Numerous studies conducted in American schools have shown that many of the abnormal behaviour patterns and learning impediments which increasingly impair classroom discipline and education in the USA are quickly corrected when fluorescent lights are replaced with full-spectrum lighting.

Shallow breathing and physical stagnation
Lack of sufficient exercise and shallow breathing create conditions of chronic fatigue and physical stagnation in the human body,

lowering resistance and impairing immunity. Such habits deprive the body of sufficient oxygen, impede circulation of blood, restrict distribution of nutrients, shrink the protective shield of radiant energy around the body, and inhibit internal alchemy.

Emotional turmoil
Frequent outbursts of extreme emotions are regarded as the primary internal source of disease in traditional Chinese medicine, and the new Western science of psychoneuroimmunology has confirmed this ancient Taoist premise. It is well known that grief, for example, such as that experienced after the death of a spouse, renders a person highly vulnerable to disease and degeneration. Emotional equilibrium is a precondition for maintaining strong immunity, and nothing throws human energy off balance more quickly and extremely than sudden outbursts and prolonged bouts of uncontrolled 'energies in motion'.

Fortunately, there are simple and effective ways to remedy and prevent assaults on the immune system by aberrant energies. When practised in conjunction with methods that boost immunity on the level of essence, these 'energy supplements' become even more effective by virtue of synergy.

Energy boosters for immunity

Chee-gung
Chee-gung counteracts the immunosuppressive effects of stress by switching the body over to the parasympathetic branch of the autonomous nervous system. This gives the adrenals a chance to rest and recuperate and stops their secretion of adrenaline, cortisol, and other immunosuppressive hormones. *Chee-gung* also strengthens the radiant shield of energy which protects the body from invasion by aberrant environmental energies, balances yin and yang, Water and Fire, and other polar energies, harmonizes the Five Elemental Energies of the vital organs, and recharges every cell in the body with fresh energy. It greatly enhances circulation, thereby enabling blood to deliver immune factors to all tissues and carry away accumulated metabolic wastes. *Chee-gung* also establishes immune-enhancing biofeedback between the nervous and endocrine systems.

Deep breathing
Deep breathing is an essential part of *chee-gung*, but it also has therapeutic benefits of its own and should be practised at all times.

By practising *chee-gung* daily, one gradually learns how to breathe correctly at all times. Deep breathing causes the diaphragm to massage and stimulate the adrenals with each breath, providing rejuvenating physical therapy to these much-abused glands. It enhances cerebral circulation of oxygen and nutrients, thereby boosting cerebral functions, which in turn maintain immunity. It maximizes assimilation of negative ion energy from the atmosphere and keeps the autonomous nervous system from constantly driving the body into the high gears of the sympathetic branch, which enervates immunity. The great Tang-dynasty physician and Taoist adept Sun Ssu-mo extolled the benefits of deep breathing as follows in his medical masterpiece entitled *Precious Recipes*: 'When correct breathing is practised, the myriad ailments will not occur. When breathing is depressed or strained, all sorts of diseases will arise. Those who wish to nurture their lives must first learn the correct methods of controlling breath and balancing energy. These breathing methods can cure all ailments great and small.'

Energy supplements
Just as there are ways to supplement essence with vitamins, herbs, enzymes, and so forth, so there are ways to supplement energy. Traditionally, quartz crystals and various precious gems have been used to attract positive cosmic energies from the planets and stars and channel them into the human energy system. This is the mechanism by which talismans work. Gold also helps the body to collect and store beneficial environmental energies. In addition to these traditional methods, modern electronic technology has devised a wide range of effective energy supplements, including negative-ion generators, biocircuits, electromagnetic-field harmonizers, pulsed audiovisual aids, and many others. You can find out more about these interesting tools by requesting a catalogue from the supplier listed in the Appendix.

Geomancy
The ancient Taoist science of geomancy (*feng-shui*) calculates the flow of celestial and terrestial energies in a designated area in order to determine the best locations for homes, temples, offices, and other buildings, so that these natural environmental energies harmonize favourably with human energies in order to promote the health and longevity of the occupants and users. Though little understood and often debunked in the West, geomancy definitely works, as anyone who has lived in the Far East for a while can readily attest. Even such common problems as insomnia can often

be completely remedied simply by relocating a bed or sleeping in a different room, and thousands of business firms in the Far East have gone from the brink of bankruptcy to the pinnacle of profit 'overnight' by calling in a qualified geomancer to rearrange their offices, seal off doors that leak energy out, turn the boss's desk to a more favourable angle, and make other adjustments in the flow of the invisible but highly influential energies of sky and earth. If you've tried everything else to no avail, you might give geomancy a chance to improve your fortunes and boost your energies. Wherever you find a sizable overseas Chinese community, you are bound to find a practising geomancer.

Immunity and spirit

Chronic stress is probably the primary cause of immune deficiency in the modern world, especially in the crowded urban centres of industrially developed societies. The human body is equipped to deal with the sort of stress people faced in the preindustrial world, such as crossing paths with a sabre-toothed tiger, tribal warfare, avalanches, floods, and other situations that provoke the fight-or-flight response. In such situations, the adrenal glands spurt adrenaline into the bloodstream and switch the nervous system over to the action mode of the sympathetic branch. The body then responds by fighting, running, or some other high-energy physical reaction, burning off the stimulative hormones and extra glucose pumped into the bloodstream for that purpose, then returning to normal. Such situations occurred occasionally, not chronically, and when they passed, the body naturally recovered its energy and endocrine balance.

Today, the same biochemical responses are triggered hundreds of times throughout the day and night by frustrations in the office, marital strife, repressed rage, bad news on television, exposure to microwaves and abnormal electromagnetic fields, fear, alienation, peer pressures, and other hazards of modern life. However, instead of making high-energy physical responses, people repress their rage, fear, and other negative emotions provoked by stress, thereby failing to utilize the powerful hormones and neurochemicals released into the blood. These potent biochemicals quickly break down into various toxic by-products that poison the system, suppress immunity, and impede other vital functions. Under chronic stress, the body never has a chance to excrete these toxins thoroughly and restore proper balance in essence, energy, and spirit.

Stress is basically a sudden demand on the body to adapt

quickly to a new situation, and therefore it depends largely upon perception and sensory input, which belong to the realm of spirit. However, the effects of stress instantly reverberate down through the realms of energy and essence via biofeedback and the nervous system. Stress thus preoccupies the entire human system whenever it strikes, engaging body, mind, and energy in a vicious circle of tension and turmoil that has no outlet.

In recent years, stress has finally become recognized as a major immunosuppressant and a primary cause of disease. Unfortunately, the tendency of modern Western medicine is to treat stress with tranquillizers, which temporarily relieve the overt symptoms but compound the physiological damage. Stress causes the adrenals to secrete adrenaline and cortisone, the latter being a particularly powerful immunosuppressant, especially in the thymus, lymph nodes, and spleen. Cortisone also impairs production of interferon, one of the body's most potent immune agents. Diseases associated with high cortisone levels include cancer, hypertension, arthritis, stroke, chronic infections, skin diseases, Parkinson's disease, and ulcers. Elevated cortisone is also associated with an increased tendency towards suicide. In *Maximum Immunity*, Dr Michael Weiner states: 'Psychological stress releases powerful hormones that suppress our immune defenses.' In *Eat Right or Die Young*, Dr Cass Igram states the case against stress even more bluntly:

> The role played by stress in the causation of cancer is so great that it would not be an exaggeration to say that 80% or more cancer cases have their immediate origin in some form of mental pressure or strain. Grief, distress, fear, worry, and anger are emotions which have horrible effects on the body's functions. Researchers have discovered that these emotions cause the release of chemicals from the brain called neuropeptides. These potent compounds have a profound immune-suppressive action. Scientists have traced a pathway from the brain to the immune cells proving that negative emotions can stop the immune cells dead in their tracks. This results in part from the release of chemicals from nerve endings. Once this happens, harmful microbes or cancer cells can invade any tissue in the body.

Dr Igram's analysis is virtually identical to the traditional Chinese medical view of negative emotions as potent causes of disease. Since the central nervous system has branches with nerve endings that terminate in the glands which regulate the immune system, there is constant biofeedback between hormones and neurochemicals. The immune system functions much like a sensory organ, responding to external stimuli based on sensory input mediated by the nervous system. A fight-or-flight response from the brain immediately triggers a similar response in the adrenals and other glands, and those glandular secretions in turn sustain continued activity of the neurochemicals that triggered the original stress response. Similarly, calming, soothing neurochemicals stimulate secretion of calming, soothing hormones, which in turn sustain the activity of those neurochemicals through biofeedback. Recall the statement of Master Luo Teh-hsiou of Taiwan that the primary mechanism by which *chee-gung* generates vital energy and rejuvenates the body is by establishing soothing biofeedback between the nervous and endocrine systems. Dr Weiner states in *Maximum Immunity*: 'By learning how to control our mind, subtle hormonal changes emerge that then control our biochemical reality.' Yale University's cancer surgeon Dr Bernie Siegel agrees: 'Psychological and spiritual development are capable of reversing the disease process.' This is virtually a paraphrase of a statement in the chapter entitled 'The Oldest Truth' in the 2,000-year-old *Internal Medicine Classic*: 'If one maintains an undisturbed spirit within, no disease will occur.'

The PNI system can be stimulated into a mode of positive biofeedback which heals the body and restores immunity simply by adopting the right mental attitude. PNI explains, for example, the placebo effect. If the mind can be made to believe that a sugar pill or a capsule of vitamin C is actually a miraculous new drug, it promptly mobilizes the immune system, triggers the healing response, and orchestrates a cure. The 'power of positive thinking' is thus rooted in the physiological and biochemical effects it triggers in the body via the nervous system. As Norman Cousins writes: 'The will to live is not a theoretical abstraction, but a physiologic reality with therapeutic characteristics'.

There are many aspects to positive thinking, foremost among which is will, which the Chinese call *yi* and equate with primordial spirit. But mental factors, such as enthusiasm, are also important in maintaining health. If you are bored or frustrated by your job, hobby, marriage, or other activities, your mind lacks enthusiasm for life, which in turn saps the will to live. Simply by changing your habits or creatively solving the problems that frustrate you, you recover enthusiasm, which in turn stimulates vitality and boosts immunity. A good example of this is the investment banker who late in life contracted 'incurable' leukaemia. As it turned out, he had always wanted to be a concert violinist rather than a banker, but he repressed his dream in order to please his father and went reluctantly to Wall Street. Condemned to death by his doctor's diagnosis, he decided to shuck his pinstriped suit, retired, and learned to play the violin with such enthusiasm that he actually performed on stage before an audience, realizing the dream of a lifetime. Before long, his leukaemia went into what his perplexed doctor called 'spontaneous remission': his renewed enthusiasm for life triggered his psychoneuroimmunological defence system to attack the mutant cells causing his leukaemia.

Visualization is another effective way to restore immunity and heal the body. Carl and Stephanie Simonton of the Cancer Counseling and Research Center in Dallas, Texas, reported a case of a young boy with cancer to whom they taught a therapeutic method of visualization. Day after day, the boy vividly imagined jet fighters zooming into his body to strafe and bomb his tumours, and sure enough, the tumours soon began to shrink and finally disappeared altogether, without chemotherapy, radiation, or surgery. Using this technique, the Simontons have managed to double the survival times of terminal cancer patients under their care. Despite this impressive achievement, however, conventional medicine continues to rely on radical chemical-mechanistic therapies which destroy the human immune system and make the remaining days of terminal-cancer patients utterly miserable.

Visualization is also a key technique in triggering the healing response during the practice of the Six-Syllable Secret healing *chee-gung* exercise introduced in an earlier chapter. The breath mobilizes energy; the lips, tongue, and throat establish the required frequency; and the movements of limbs stimulate the associated energy channels; at the same time visualization directs the stream of energy into and out of the target organ. Similarly, in order to activate 'palm breathing' during *chee-gung* or meditation, all you need to do is visualize energy streaming in and out of the points in the centre of your palms while performing deep abdominal breathing, and soon you can feel it happening. If you can't, it means that you're not concentrating fully on the visualization, that you have serious doubts it will work, or that you're simply not paying sufficient attention to the resulting sensations, any of which factors will negate the effects of the visualization. Mind over matter works both ways: while faith in the method delivers the desired results to the body, doubt obstructs it.

Meditation is a very effective method for boosting immunity and cultivating the power of positive thinking, visualization, and mind over matter. Simply by 'sitting still, doing nothing' for a while each day, you give your mind a chance to retire from the stresses of daily life and explore its own innate powers. Even in the beginning stages of practice, when the 'monkey mind' hops from one trivial thought to another, meditation still boosts immunity on the physiological level by switching the nervous system over to the restful, restorative, immune-enhancing parasympathetic mode. Later, when you've developed a feel for internal energy and learned how to transport it wherever you wish within your system, you can apply that power to heal injuries, balance energies, stimulate glandular secretions, enhance cerebral energy, exchange energy with your sexual partner, dissolve tumours, and other useful purposes.

Though it may sound like a cliché, as so many truths do, love also has great healing powers. Dr Siegel says: 'If I told patients to raise their blood levels of immune globulins or killer T-cells, no one would know how. But if I can teach them to love themselves and others fully, the same changes happen automatically. The truth is: "love heals".'

Love energizes the entire immune system and specifically stimulates the production of antibodies. Lack of love for oneself and others gives rise to negative thoughts and emotions, which, as we've already seen, releases immunosuppressive hormones and neurochemicals into the system via the PNI mechanism. Many people, especially in crowded cities, find themselves stuck in situations they hate but cannot do anything to change, and so they end up hating themselves and others. This results in a state of chronic immune deficiency.

Many of the Chinese medicals texts dating from 2,000 years ago lament the ills of 'modern times' and allude to the traditional 'good old days' another 3,000 years before that. A common theme in these texts is the decline in human health due to careless lifestyles and the deterioration in human relations due to lack of love: degenerative conditions that Taoist alchemy as well as psychoneuroimmunology would link as symptoms of the same syndrome.

In his essay entitled 'Loving People' Chang San-feng, the thirteenth-century master, summed it up by saying: 'Therefore to those who want to know the way to deal with the world, I suggest, Love People.' This is a potent prescription for health and longevity that generates positive healing energy throughout the human system by stimulating the internal alchemy of psychoneuroimmunology.

CHAPTER 18

Vitality

> When the mind is calm and stable, the vitality of life
> circulates harmoniously throughout the body. If the body
> is nourished and protected by this circulation of vitality,
> how can it possibly become ill?
>> *The Yellow Emperor's Classic of Internal Medicine*
>> (second century BC)

In Chinese, the term 'vitality' is expressed by combining the
ideograms for 'essence' (*jing*) and 'energy' (*chee*) to form the word
jing-chee. The combination of 'essence' and 'spirit' in the word
jing-chen also denotes 'vitality'. Vitality is therefore the psychophysiological manifestation of energy and spirit fused with the
vital essence of corporeal life.

Vitality is associated with the potency of vital bodily fluids
such as enzymes, hormones, and neurochemicals, which form a
functional bridge between organic matter and pure energy. Enzyme
activity, for example, releases waves of radiant energy which can
be measured by scientific instruments, and the activity of neurochemicals in the brain is closely associated with the cerebral energy
recorded as 'brain waves' by electroencephalographs. Blood carries
potential energy in the form of negative ions, which are also stored
in the electrolytes of intercellular fluids. Vitality is thus a functional
fusion of biochemicals and bioenergies balanced by biofeedback.

One way in which Taoist internal alchemy enhances human
vitality is by establishing positive biofeedback between the calming
neurochemicals of the parasympathetic nervous system and the
rejuvenating, immune-boosting hormones of the endocrine system.
The neuro-endocrine balance achieved thereby generates the active
vitality associated with organic life.

Vitality is the basis of health and longevity and the foundation of
immunity and resistance. However, after the bloom of youth has

blown, vitality must be carefully cultivated and conserved in order to continue providing the sort of protection it confers naturally during the reproductive prime of life. As James Ramholz writes in *Shaolin and Taoist Herbal Training Formulas*, 'the ideal level of well-being necessitates something beyond what ordinary diet and lifestyle can offer. Only a significantly strong vitality will prevent health problems. Toward this end, many people employ exercise, martial arts, meditation, yoga, *chi-gung*, Tai Chi Chuan, etc., to enhance their health, enrich their lives, and to help foster their spiritual development.'

Cultivating vitality

Since vitality depends on the vigour of all Three Treasures, it may be cultivated by internal as well as external methods, including diet and nutrition, herbs and antioxidants, breathing and exercise, meditation and martial arts. Indeed, vitality is the primary outgrowth of all branches of Taoist internal alchemy and the main indicator of health and immunity in Chinese medicine.

On the fundamental level of essence, diet, nutrition, and tonic herbs have the most direct influence on vitality. The most important nutritional factors are essential amino acids and essential fatty acids, both of which are required to produce the hormones, enzymes, and neurochemicals upon which vitality depends. These basic building blocks must be taken in conjunction with the synergistic vitamin and mineral cofactors the body needs to convert them into 'vital essence'. For example, zinc and selenium are required to produce antioxidant enzymes, and vitamins B_5 and B_6 are the essential cofactors the brain needs to convert amino acids into neurotransmitters.

Food enzymes are another important dietary element for cultivating vitality. The richer the enzyme content of food (such as raw and fermented foods), the less enzyme power the body must divert for digestive duty, resulting in an overall enhancement of vitality. Eliminating 'enzyme robbers' such as refined sugar and starch, hydrogenated vegetable oils, processed foods, and overcooked meats also boosts vitality.

Tonic herbs have been used for thousands of years by Taoist adepts in China for health, longevity, and spiritual development. These herbs work to boost vitality in two ways: first, 'the pure essences of plants and trees' stimulate secretions of vital essence throughout the endocrine system by virtue of their 'natural affinity' (*gui-jing*) for various glands, especially the powerful sexual glands;

second, they release their own vital energies into the human system, thereby balancing human energies and enhancing vitality with 'the most excellent energies of mountains and rivers'.

Vitality may also be cultivated directly on the level of energy. Of all the traditional Taoist disciplines, *chee-gung* is by far the most direct and efficient method of generating the *jing-chee* of human vitality. By establishing positive biofeedback between the nervous and endocrine systems, *chee-gung* enhances the body's innate healing and immune responses and brings them under voluntary control. And *chee-gung* promotes vitality by implementing the first principle of internal alchemy and its corollary: 'essence transforms into energy' and 'energy commands essence'. The former improves the metabolic conversion of nutritional essence into vital energy, and the latter enhances the circulation and distribution of blood, nutrients, hormones, enzymes, and other vital essences by virtue of breath and energy control.

The importance of deep diaphragmic breathing in cultivating and conserving vitality cannot be overemphasized. When properly utilized to regulate breath, the diaphragm acts as a 'second heart' to circulate blood and distribute nutrients and immune factors throughout the system. This extra pump operates entirely by virtue of abdominal and thoracic pressure and takes a big workload off the heart, thereby conserving cardiac energy. Deep breathing also drives nourishing energy (*ying-chee*) throughout the meridian system and strengthens the radiant shield of protective energy (*wei-chee*) around the surface of the body. Since breath is the autonomous vital function over which we can most easily exercise direct voluntary control, it serves as a vehicle for regulating essence and energy with spirit and achieving command of mind over matter. Just as the diaphragm may be viewed as a second heart, so the breath may be regarded as the second pulse of life. Physiologically, the rhythmic synchrony of blood (essence) and breath (energy) depends upon the functional harmony of lungs and heart and constitutes the body's primary source of vitality. Nothing establishes that harmonic synchrony more swiftly and efficiently than *chee-gung*.

Vitality manifests itself on the level of spirit as *jing-shen* ('essence-spirit'), which may be cultivated by the practice of meditation. In Taoist meditation, sexual energy from the sacrum is raised up along the spinal channels into the head, where it is refined into cerebral energy and transformed into spiritual vitality. The enhanced cerebral energy derived from meditation stimulates production of vital neurochemicals and improves all mental functions, including memory and learning, intelligence and awareness, perception and thought. Like physical vitality, spiritual vitality is fuelled by the pure, potent energies associated with secretions of vital essence in the body. While the *jing-chee* of physical vitality comes mainly from the energy associated with hormones and enzymes, the *jing-shen* of spiritual vitality is generated mainly by the cerebral energy associated with neurotransmitters and secretions of the pineal and pituitary glands in the brain.

Facets of vitality

One of the most important facets of vitality is the protective role it plays in health. As a functional fusion of essence and energy, vitality is the foundation of immunity and resistance. As we have discussed in previous chapters, immunity relies largely on secretions of various forms of vital essence, such as hormones, enzymes, white and red blood cells, T-cells, and cerebrospinal fluids. Resistance to aberrant environmental energies is provided by the radiant shield of guardian energy that emanates from and envelops the surface of the body. Thus immunity and resistance represent the total protective power provided by the combination of essence and energy, which are the two pillars of vitality.

The fusion of essence and energy is also the basis of sexual drive and potency. One of the great benefits bestowed by the regular practice of Taoist health regimens is sexual vitality, which has always been regarded as a primary indicator of health and immunity in traditional Chinese medicine. Nature has designed the human body to maintain its reproductive sexual potency at all costs, in order to ensure the propagation of the species. Therefore, whenever sexual essence and energy are depleted, especially in the male immediately after ejaculation, the body promptly tries to restore sexual potency by producing more sperm, semen, and sexual hormones. If any of the vital nutrients required for this task are missing or deficient, which is often the case, the body 'borrows' them from other organs, glands, and tissues, particularly from the cerebrospinal fluid and sexual glands. Sexual excess therefore causes a constant drain of vital nutrients and hormones from the brain, spine, and adrenals as the body struggles to maintain sexual potency and fertility. This is primarily a male problem, because only the male of the species loses his potent semen-essence during intercourse. Nature has designed the female in such a way that sexual activity does not deplete her vital resources, thereby ensuring her ability to nourish and protect her offspring.

Since nature gives top priority to sexual vitality, other facets of vitality such as immunity, resistance, and cerebral functions are the first to suffer whenever sexual excess depletes the body's limited resources of essence and energy. Therefore, when sexual potency itself finally fails, it means that the situation is already extremely grave because the body has totally depleted its resources and can no longer replenish its own sexual essence and energy. Sexual impotence in males is almost always associated with immune deficiency, low resistance, lassitude, fatigue, cerebral insufficiency, and other symptoms of depleted vitality.

Like so many other aspects of the Tao, vitality also has its own functional trinity, manifested as immunity and resistance, sexual potency, and mental vigour. Like the Three Treasures, all three aspects are closely linked and mutually interdependent, each reflecting the condition of the others. By cultivating vitality through diet and nutrition, *chee-gung* and meditation, and other Taoist disciplines, you enhance all three facets of the trinity − immunological, sexual, and cerebral − and by virtue of internal alchemy, including the mechanisms of psychoneuroimmunology, the essence and energy from any one of these branches of vitality may be transformed and transferred to sustain another. This can work for you or against you, depending on whether you cultivate and conserve your essential resources or scatter them to the wind.

CHAPTER 19

Clarity

When the spirit is clear, knowledge is enlightened . . .
When the spirit is clear, truth is apparent . . .
When the spirit is clear, habitual desires cannot deceive
it . . .

Wen Tzu Classic (first century BC)

Taoist philosophy views the human mind as a mirror that reflects the world around it – a dewdrop on the lawn of life. The clarity of the images that it reflects, and of the thoughts those images provoke, depends primarily on the clarity of the mirror, not on intelligence. 'People use still water rather than moving streams as mirrors,' states the *Wen Tzu Classic*, 'because still water is clear and calm.' When the mind is clear and calm, the images it reflects are real and the knowledge it gathers is true. When the mind is agitated and confused, it's like throwing a stone into a still pond, or holding a camera with a shaky hand: the images it reflects are distorted and do not accord with reality.

When the mirror of mind is streaked with the dust of trivial thoughts and shaken by conflicting emotions, it distorts everything it reflects, leading the spirit astray. Under such conditions, intellectual knowledge is not only useless, but often dangerous, for intellect rationalizes everything the mind reflects. If the mind's reflections of the world are gross distortions of reality, the intellect nevertheless treats them as though they were true and uses them as a basis for rationalizing behaviour. Religious warfare is a good example of how intellect manipulates different reflections of the world in order to rationalize such contradictory behaviour as the slaughter of fellow humans 'in the name of god'. Western societies, with their blind faith in rational intellect and scientific method, are particularly vulnerable to the hubris of the temporal human mind, which utilizes reason to justify behaviour based on emotional responses to distorted perceptions.

Since all sensory perceptions are filtered through the mind, mental clarity is as important to human knowledge as a clear lens is to the photographs recorded by a camera. When the mind is cluttered with trivia and programmed with fantasy, it cannot deal realistically with the complexities of life.

Mental clarity is not simply a matter of being alert and perceptive. It is a matter of sweeping clear the veils of conditioned biases and egocentric preferences and perceiving the world through the immaculate mirror of primordial awareness, or 'the mind of Tao'. This is not an easy task, for human beings view the world through the culturally conditioned lens of the human mind, formed by parents and society. In order to deal with this problem and develop methods for 'polishing the mirror' of the mind, the sages and yogis of China and India applied the scientific method to the subject of perception itself. According to this 'science of mind', whatever enters our conscious awareness via sensory channels is a subjective impression of the world relative to the point of view and cultural conditioning of the viewer. The only objective fact recognized by the science of mind is the fact of consciousness itself. By scientifically analysing the nature of awareness and how it functions through sensory perception, the mental sciences of Hindu, Buddhist, and Taoist tradition have devised highly sophisticated techniques whereby an individual may erase his or her arbitrary egotistical biases, discard acquired cultural conditioning, and perceive the world through the crystal-clear lens of primordial awareness, rather than the culturally tinted filters of the temporal human mind. Even a single momentary glimpse of ultimate reality reflected from the immaculate mirror of primordial awareness suffices to banish for ever all acquired illusions and permanently alter the adept's consciousness, and it is to this spontaneous flash of fully illumined awareness that all adepts of higher spiritual paths aspire.

One of the most fundamental principles in the 'science of mind' is that the perceiver, the perception, and the perceived are all inseparable aspects of one and the same process. Since the psychophysiology of perception is much the same in everyone and the perceived world is an external factor which everyone shares and no one can change, the only aspect of the process that you can control and focus in order to obtain clear reflections of reality is the perceiver, i.e. your own mind. By keeping your mirror well polished, you prevent distortions in the images it reflects and gain crystal-clear views of the scenery and scenarios of life.

A detailed discussion of the Buddhist and Taoist 'science of mind' is beyond the scope of this book. However, the basic principle of this science, which is clarity, has abundant applications in worldly life and may be cultivated to anyone's advantage without abandoning the world and retiring to a frosty cave in the Himalayas. Clarity can eliminate family strife, improve job performance, prevent aberrant behaviour, and distil magic from the mundane, all by simply taking a little time each day to 'polish the mirror' of your own mind and see things clearly.

Cultivating clarity

The two most important factors in cultivating clarity are calmness and equanimity. Hypertension and emotional imbalance cloud the mind with a form of aberrant energy which traditional Chinese medicine refers to as 'muddy energy' (juo-chee). Like mud stirred up from the bottom of a clear pool of water, muddy energy rises up from the internal organs and obscures the clarity of cerebral energy in the head whenever stress, tension, or uncontrolled emotional reactions are permitted to disturb the human energy system. Anger, for example, causes 'rebellious' hot energy to rise up from the liver, fear arouses cold Water energy from the kidneys, excess worry stirs up muddy Earth energy from the spleen and stomach, and so forth. Whenever this happens, it's like fogging a clear mirror with steam, or streaking it with water, or smearing it with mud: whatever images it reflects are distorted.

Mental clarity can be achieved and maintained only when internal energies are balanced and calm. Recall the second principle of internal alchemy – 'energy transforms into spirit'. This means that the mind depends on energy for sustenance, and the quality of energy therefore determines the quality of mental functions. Agitated, imbalanced energy gives rise to an agitated, imbalanced mind. Calm, balanced energy sustains a calm, balanced mind, and this is the basis of mental clarity. Returning to the metaphors of camera and mirror: when the hand that holds them is calm and steady, the images they reflect will be clear and accurate. The same applies to the mirror of mind: when the energy which sustains it is calm and stable, the images it reflects are clear and lifelike.

On the fundamental level of essence, clarity may be cultivated by taking various nutrients, herbs, and other supplements with specific affinity for the brain. The most important nutrients for enhancing cerebral functions are essential amino acids and essential fatty acids. Amino acids are required to produce the vital neurotransmitters which relay messages between the cells of the brain and the central nervous system, while fatty acids are important elements in the cellular structure of neurons and in cerebrospinal fluid.

Herbs that enhance circulation to the brain and stimulate the pineal and pituitary glands boost mental clarity with extra cerebral essence and energy and help promote the command of brain over body, mind over matter. The most effective herbs for this purpose include ginseng, ginkgo, *gotu kola*, *Epimedium*, *Astragalus*, and cayenne. All these may be taken together in one formula, and their effects may be further boosted by using them in conjunction with synergistic nutrients such as choline, phenylalanine, vitamins B_5 and B_6, vitamin C, and zinc.

Nootropic drugs, which were specifically developed to enhance cerebral functions, are a modern adjunct to the traditional herbs and nutrients used for this purpose and may be taken in conjunction with them. To enhance cerebral circulation and stimulate synthesis of brain proteins, hydergine is the best nootropic agent. To improve memory and learning capacity, piracetum is the top choice, and, for a quick clarifying cerebral boost, vasopressin nasal spray usually does the trick.

None of these supplements will do you much good, however, unless you take measures to keep your bloodstream clean and its pH well balanced. Polluted blood is one of the major and most often overlooked causes of disease, degeneration, chronic fatigue, failure of nutritional and herbal therapy, emotional depression, and mental confusion. Whenever the blood is toxic, the toxins it carries circulate through the brain as well as every other tissue in the body, and the blood's capacity to deliver oxygen and nutrients to the cells and carry away metabolic wastes for excretion is severely impaired. It is difficult to maintain mental clarity when the brain is riddled with heavy metals, acids, carbon monoxide, food additives, free radicals, and other toxins carried by the blood. By far the most effective method of purifying the bloodstream is to undertake an occasional fast, preferably a seven-day fast once or twice each year. Another good way is to consume nothing but freshly extracted vegetable or fruit juices for a few days each month. This balances blood pH and accelerates the excretion of toxic wastes from all bodily fluids and tissues.

Moving up to the invisible but highly functional realm of energy, *chee-gung* cultivates clarity in three ways. First, by virtue of energy's command over essence, *chee-gung* gives a tremendous boost to cerebral circulation of oxygen and nutrients via the bloodstream. By flooding the brain with essence and energy, *chee-gung* also stimulates secretions of vital neurotransmitters and brain hormones. Second, *chee-gung* acts as the bellows in the internal alchemy of energy transformation and transportation. It draws potent sexual energy up from the sacrum into the spine, where it is condensed and refined, then upwards into the brain, where it boosts cerebral energy and is transformed into spiritual vitality. Third, *chee-gung* immediately switches the autonomous nervous system over from the depleting action circuit of the sympathetic branch to the restorative, calming circuit of the parasympathetic branch. This soothes the entire central nervous system, balances the endocrine system, harmonizes emotional energies, and calms the chronically overactive cerebral cortex, thereby establishing the calmness and equilibrium required for mental clarity.

Since clarity belongs to the realm of spirit, meditation is the most direct method for cultivating clarity. The entire alchemy of meditation may be summed up in three words which appear over and over again in Taoist lore and literature: 'Empty the mind.' To empty the mind means to establish the cerebral silence and emotional equilibrium required for mental clarity by stopping the internal monologue of discursive thought, arresting the Five Thieves of sensory distractions, and eliminating the turmoil of uncontrolled emotional reactions. In short, to empty the mind means to 'polish the mirror', thereby permitting clear reflections of external phenomena and spontaneous insights into the true nature of reality.

In terms of brain anatomy, it is the cerebral cortex that must be stilled and silenced in order to achieve mental clarity and spontaneous insight, for this is where the rambling train of nonstop thought hoots and toots noisily through the mind, drowning out the more subtle sensitivities of intuitive insight. Meditation effectively muzzles the cerebral cortex, allowing other, more sensitive parts of the brain to engage consciousness.

When disciplined adepts cultivate clarity to its highest levels through meditation and other practices, they sometimes develop perceptive powers which transcend the ordinary senses. Known as 'extrasensory perception' (ESP) in English and *shen-tung* ('spiritual breakthroughs') in Chinese, these extraordinary powers include clairvoyance, clairaudience, the ability to 'read' the thoughts of others, spontaneous visions, universal insights, and the capacity to communicate with spirits. Such powers arise only in the highest stages of spiritual practice and are sure signs of progress on the path, but they also pose a potential threat to the final breakthrough of spiritual enlightenment by tempting the adept to misuse them for personal profit and pleasure.

The spiritual lore of Asia is laced with warnings against abusing ESP for material gain, and many an adept has fallen from grace this way. This level of practice, which indicates that the adept is on the brink of enlightenment, is also where 'black magic' and sorcery begin. It's an advanced manifestation of clarity and the final cross-roads on the path to enlightenment: one wrong step at this stage can negate a lifetime of practice by propelling the adept onto the egocentric path of earthly power. True adepts of the Tao therefore disregard these powers – except when required to help others in emergencies – and continue instead to carry their practice beyond this stage to the ultimate goal.

CHAPTER 20

Equanimity

Too much Fire dries you up.
Too much Water drains you out.
This imbalance can be controlled only
by cultivating equilibrium.

Chang Po-tuan (eleventh century AD)

Equilibrium refers to the state of homeostatic energy balance in which all of the body's vital organs function harmoniously and the Three Treasures of essence, energy, and spirit are conserved rather than depleted. As we have seen, energy forms a bridge between body and mind and the fulcrum which keeps physiological and psychological functions in balance. When 'too much Fire' or 'too much Water' prevails, when yin and yang fall off balance, and when the Five Elemental Energies of the organs lose their natural harmony, both body and mind manifest 'dis-ease', physical and mental functions falter, and immunity and resistance are impaired.

In cultivating equilibrium, the aspect of energy with which Taoist alchemy works is emotional energy, or 'energy in motion'. In Chinese medicine, the Seven Emotions are regarded as primary internal causes of the energy imbalances which render the body vulnerable to disease and degeneration. Each emotion is associated with a paired set of vital organs and the elemental energy which controls it. Of all the various energies associated with human life, emotional energies are by far the most difficult to control, and when permitted to run rampant, they disturb the mind, impair immunity, and sap vitality, drying up and draining out your essence and energy. Unlike cerebral energy, which is housed in the head, emotional energy resides in the heart and does not listen to reason. Only sheer force of will can control it.

Taoists refer to the emotions as a monkey. Playful, mischievous, restless, and totally unpredictable, the 'monkey mind' of emotion swings from one extreme to another, responding unthinkingly to external stimuli conveyed by the five senses. We've all heard the old jingle 'Monkey see, monkey do'. That's precisely the way human emotions react to the world. All emotional energies are provoked by sensory perceptions. If we hear something that we perceive as an insult, we instinctively react with anger. If we see something we regard as sexy, we respond with lust. If we receive disturbing news, we react with anxiety. In each case, the emotion is triggered by an external event, conveyed into consciousness by sensory channels, and unleashes an internal wave of energy that floods through the system like water from a burst dam, knocking organ energies off balance, upsetting yin and yang, triggering emergency stress responses, and alarming the mind. When in the throes of an uncontrolled emotional reaction, both body and mind are rendered powerless to resist it, for the Chief Hooligan emotion sucks all your energy into its wake as it stampedes through your system.

Besides robbing us of health and vitality, emotions constitute the greatest obstacle to spiritual cultivation by diverting energy and attention from internal development to external distractions, and by provoking behaviour that contradicts our best intentions. Our emotions constitute our own worst enemies, yet not only does Western medicine overlook the severe pathological consequences of emotional imbalance, Western philosophy romanticizes emotions as heroic impulses to be indulged rather than recognizing them as primitive instincts that must be controlled by the higher sentience of human awareness. Herein lies one of the most fundamental differences between Eastern and Western tradition, for Eastern philosophy clearly identifies emotions as obstacles to spiritual development, pollutants to mental clarity, spoilers of human relations, and enemies of intent and reason. When Asians remark that Westerners have 'hot feelings', what they mean is that they overreact emotionally, thereby 'overheating' human relations with unrestrained emotionally energy.

Anyone who doubts the self-destructive power of uncontrolled emotional reactions need only consider 'crimes of passion' in order to get the point. Crimes of passion are the ultimate manifestation of the age-old conflict between the heart and head in human life. A minor squabble ignites a major temper tantrum, and in the fit of anger which follows a man murders his own wife or best friend. A loved one has an accident and dies, unleashing such an overwhelming flood of grief that the bereaved commits suicide. A husband finds his wife in bed with another man and becomes so consumed with jealousy that he grabs a gun and shoots them both. These things happen every day and are classic examples of how uncontrolled emotions, i.e. lack of equilibrium, can cause people to do things which they had no intention whatsoever of doing, destroying their own and other lives in order to indulge momentary emotions. The Chief Hooligan and Five Thieves consort with our basest instincts and consistently provoke behaviour which runs counter to our own better judgement and long-term interests. The only way to arrest these troublemakers and protect ourselves from their criminal conduct is to cultivate equilibrium and exercise equanimity.

Cultivating equilibrium and equanimity

Equanimity is the mental manifestation of emotional equilibrium and a basic prerequisite for spiritual development. Like all elements of internal alchemy, equilibrium and equanimity are mutually dependent. Without emotional equilibrium, it is impossible to maintain mental equanimity, and without mental equanimity, it is impossible to cultivate emotional equilibrium.

Compared with the task of taming and training the wild monkey of emotion, other Taoist practices are a breeze. Cultivating emotional equanimity requires constant vigilance and a strong leash of self-discipline, lest the monkey break loose and steal the carefully cultivated fruits of your practices. Unlike other violations of practice, such as too much food or sex, indulging in emotional outbursts such as anger, lust, fear, or jealousy can unravel a lifetime of disciplined conduct and has been the downfall of many an adept just as he or she approached the brink of the final breakthrough.

Equilibrium is not meant to be achieved by annihilating emotions, any more than celibacy is meant to be maintained by castration. Cultivating equilibrium means applying discipline and awareness to prevent one's emotions from running wild. It means keeping internal energies in balance by regulating one's emotional reactions to external stimuli. In terms of internal alchemy, it means harnessing the heart with the head, rather than letting the heart gallop out of control; it means controlling Fire with Water, rather than letting Fire burn up all your essence and energy; it means guiding emotions with wisdom and subordinating instinct to intent.

As a basic form of human energy, emotions are an important resource, but they must be trained and transformed so that they support rather than obstruct spiritual development. In Tibetan

Buddhism, enlightenment is realized by the fusion of compassion and wisdom. Without the warm emotional energy of compassion, wisdom is cold and calculating. Without the clarity and insight of wisdom, compassion is a noble intention that can never be effectively put into practice.

And what is compassion? Compassion is a selfless form of passion, a self-indulgent emotion transformed by wisdom into empathy for the suffering of others. The emotional energy of compassion is every bit as potent as ordinary passion, but rather than scattering energy and disrupting equanimity with bouts of unrestrained emotion, compassion focuses energy and motivates intent to apply one's wisdom and other resources towards helping people. In Tantric Tibetan tradition, the compassion cultivated by the transformation of ordinary emotional energy is also known as 'skilful means', for it enables adepts skilfully to utilize their mind and energy for the benefit of others as well as for their own spiritual development.

While meditation and *chee-gung* are helpful in cultivating equanimity because of the clarity and self-control they foster, they are not enough to regulate emotional reactions fully. The only effective way to control emotional reactions and firmly establish equilibrium is by exercising equanimity on a daily basis during ordinary situations and activities. This type of practice is known as 'meditation in action'. Your emotional life is the testing ground for your meditation. If anger, fear, lust, envy, and other conflicting emotions continue to disturb your peace of mind, upset your internal energy balance, obscure your mental clarity, and lead your behaviour astray, it means that you have failed to apply the virtues and insights experienced in meditation practice to your ordinary daily activities. This is a common problem, and one way to overcome it is to try to impose a brief pause between perception and response, especially in emotionally sensitive situations, so that the wisdom mind has a chance to regulate your reactions before the emotional mind commits your energy to a rash and irrevocable behavioural response. This pause between perception and reaction is the principal trick employed to tame the monkey and slip the noose of mental discipline around its neck.

One of the best forums for cultivating equilibrium and exercising equanimity is marriage. The close quarters and personal intimacy of marriage provoke the full spectrum of emotions, and the only way to prevent the emotional monkey from tearing a marriage to shreds is to cultivate equanimity and learn how to lead the heart with the head. Like sexual yoga, which should also be a part of every marriage, 'emotional yoga' requires restraint and vigilant regulation of emotional reactions, so by practising one, you also develop the discipline and intent to practise the other.

Emotional equilibrium is probably the most difficult of all the Taoist virtues to cultivate, but it is indispensable to progress on the path, especially in the higher stages of practice. Without it, your emotions will consistently coopt all your energy and counteract all the commands of your wisdom mind. Reason is of little use here, because reason is commanded by the temporal ego, which indulges the emotional mind and rationalizes behaviour in order to satisfy its whims. Only firm intent and alert awareness can muster the will-power required to liberate yourself from the simian clutches of the emotional mind, which clings to the human ego as the proverbial 'monkey' of drug addiction clings to addicts.

In order to cultivate equilibrium and achieve equanimity, the first step is to recognize emotion as a robber of health and vitality and a poison to spiritual development, rather than to indulge it as a romantic impulse. Not only does this mean avoiding negative emotional responses such as anger, fear, and envy, it also means forgoing the emotional exaltation and self-aggrandizement of worldly success. The tenth-century adept Tan Chiao wrote as follows on this point in *Transformational Writings*, translated here by Thomas Cleary:

> Emotion in the heart is like poison in a substance, like fire latent in reeds – one ought to be aware of this. Therefore, as superior people do their work, they do not feel exalted when given status, do not feel aggrandized when honored, do not pay attention when treated familiarly, do not become suspicious when treated with aloofness, and cannot be abased. Thus they cannot be moved by emotions.

CHAPTER 21

Longevity

When the Three Treasures of essence, energy, and spirit remain calm, they nourish you day by day and make you strong. When they are hyperactive, they deplete you day by day and make you old.

Wen Tzu Classic (first century AD)

Longevity is the sweetest fruit on the Taoist tree of health. Not only does it enable you to enjoy the other fruits of your practice, such as health, vitality, clarity, and equanimity, it also supplies you with the extra time and experience required to traverse the higher paths of spiritual development and take a shot at the ultimate goal of enlightenment, or 'spiritual immortality'.

'The reason people die so young these days,' states the *Classic of the Plain Girl*, 'is that they no longer know the secrets of the Tao.' That was written over 2,000 years ago, as China entered its 'modern age' and people began to 'lose the Way'. Straying far from the Great Highway of health, longevity, and spiritual awareness, people prefer to wander down the dead-end byways of worldly desires, where they're snared by the emotional machinations of the Chief Hooligan and deceived by the sensory tricks of the Five Thieves. Ever since civilization divorced man and woman from nature, human life has lost its natural harmony.

According to the Taoist view, nature designed the human body to live an average life span of about 100 years, and if we take measures to prolong our lives, we should be able to extend our life spans to 150 years or more. There are many examples in Chinese history of Methuselahs who lived even longer than that, the most recent case being a Taoist adept and master herbalist from southwest China named Lee Ching-yuen, who lived to be over 250 years old.

Lee Ching-yuen was born in 1678, during the seventeenth year of the Manchu emperor Kang Shi's reign. He left home at an early age and travelled around southern China with a group of itinerant herb traders, from whom he learned the basics of herbalism. Subsequently, Lee had the good fortune to meet several highly accomplished Taoist masters, who taught him internal alchemy and *chee-gung* and showed him how to utilize diet and herbal supplements for health and longevity.

Though not a strict vegetarian, Lee consumed very little meat and also limited his intake of grains and root vegetables. His daily diet consisted primarily of lightly steamed vegetables, fresh fruit, and tonic herbs. The herbs he recommended most highly for promoting health and prolonging life were ginseng, *gotu kola, Polygonum multiflorum*, and garlic. Nor was Lee Ching-yuen celibate: over the course of his long life he married fourteen times, and by the time of his death in 1930, he counted almost 200 living descendants within his extended family. After his death, modern scholars confirmed his identity, traced his life all the way back to the year of his birth, and conclusively verified his lifespan.

Lee Ching-yuen's life demonstrates how well Taoist longevity techniques work when properly practised. The point here is not only to add years to your life, but also to 'add life to your years', i.e., to maintain your health and vitality until the very end of your days. Lee Ching-yuen continued to take long hikes in the mountains until the final years of his life, remained sexually active for over two centuries, never became senile, and died with all his own teeth and most of his hair. These days, few people even reach the age of sixty in that condition.

Modern Western medicine likes to claim that it has extended the human lifespan by over twenty years since 1900, but this claim is based entirely on a dramatic decline in infant mortality, not on better health or longer life for adults. Several studies have shown that the average beggar in India and peasant in Mexico are healthier than the average American college student, and few people in Western societies today reach old age with their bodies and minds intact. While it is true that thanks to life-saving medical technology a baby born in America today stands a better chance of survival than in Africa or the Middle East, the USA now ranks thirty-seventh in the world for the life expectancy of a twenty-year-old person. In an article published in the *New York State Medical Journal*, Dr Norman Joliffe points out that 'although in America the life expectancy at birth is near the best of any civilized country in the world – at the age of 40 life expectancy in America is near the bottom'. The overall health of the entire population of America –

from children to the elderly – is appallingly poor and continues to deteriorate. Consider, for example, the following facts:

● 98 per cent of Americans have some form of dental disease, and over 20 million adults have lost all their teeth.
● Over 250 million cases of acute respiratory illness are reported each year in the USA, and almost as many cases of gastroenteritis (acute inflammaton of the stomach and intestines).
● Over one million cases of pelvic inflammatory diseases plague American women each year.
● In 1900, cancer was the cause of 5 per cent of American deaths; today it accounts for over 20 per cent.
● 25 per cent of the American population suffers from chronic high blood pressure, and cardiovascular diseases now cause 53 per cent of all deaths in the USA, compared with only 18 per cent in 1900.
● 25 per cent of the population of the USA suffers some form of chronic depression, anxiety, or other emotional disorder, and the homicide rate in the USA is over ten times higher than in Britain or Japan. Rape, child abuse, and other forms of violent assault are also on the rise in America.

These are only a few examples of the current health catastrophe in the USA, but they certainly suffice to confirm what the Taoist master Chang San-feng said 600 years ago, that 'medical science can make a nation sick', for it is by the negligence of conventional American medical care that this crisis has arisen. That negligence includes the failure to recognize the true causes of most human ailments, the failure to institute preventive health care, and the failure to permit American physicians as well as patients to benefit from alternative medical theories and therapies.

Even American presidents are beginning to succumb to the health crisis sweeping through the USA: Ronald Reagan had to have a section of his colon removed with its precancerous growths caused by the standard American diet; former president Bush, as well as his wife and dog, suffers from some sort of autoimmune ailment; and President Clinton is a junk-food enthusiast with allergy problems. Compare their health to that of Chinese leaders such as Deng Hsiao-ping, who still manages to stay healthy enough to wield power in China at the age of eighty-eight, despite a life-long tobacco habit. In Asia, all influential 'movers and shakers' such as presidents and prime ministers, military leaders and corporate tycoons, combine Eastern and Western medicine, traditional therapies and modern technology in their personal health care, with obviously beneficial results.

In Taoist tradition, the primary purpose of cultivating physical longevity is to provide the adept with more time and experience to complete his or her spiritual practices, not simply to live it up for a few extra years or decades. If your sole purpose in prolonging your life is to enjoy extra years of sensual self-indulgence, then you're wasting your time and energy with these practices, because the self-discipline and restraint they require preclude that style of life. Those who wish may spend their entire lives cavorting with the Five Thieves and Chief Hooligan and die young but fully sated.

Another reason for prolonging corporeal life, in Asian tradition, is to enable accomplished masters to continue their teachings and pass their insights on to their disciples. Indeed, in the Mahayana schools of Buddhism, the purpose of enlightenment itself is to help others find the path and arrive at the same goal, not to 'ascend to heaven' all by oneself. Fully enlightened masters who forgo the freedom and bliss of the 'spiritual immortality' they've painstakingly earned through countless lifetimes of suffering, and choose instead to return again and again to this 'dusty world' in order to liberate others from suffering, are known as 'bodhisattvas', or 'awakened ones,' and without them the rest of humankind would have no one to look to for spiritual guidance. Bodhisattvas appear in many guises in all cultures and societies, not only Buddhist, and they teach according to the traditions and needs of the people among whom they are born. By prolonging their lives as long as possible, these spiritually enlightened teachers are able to continue their good works in this world and share their wisdom with others, but this is only possible when their longevity is founded on health and vitality.

There's no point living to the age of ninety-five, if the last twenty-five years of your life are spent confined in a hospital ward or nursing home. And using modern medical technology to keep 'basket cases' alive, at enormous expense and trauma to their families, is a wretched abuse of medical science, whose limited resources would be much better spent keeping healthy people healthy and curing the curable.

Cultivating Longevity

Longevity is the net result on the physical plane of practising the Taoist disciplines introduced in this book and in The Tao of HS&L. Below, we'll briefly review some of the most important factors in cultivating the sort of longevity that also sustains health and vitality.

Environment

The most important environmental factors are the quality of the air and the nature of the prevailing ambient electromagnetic field. Heavily polluted air impairs longevity and vitality by depriving people who breathe it of the vital atmospheric energy carried by negative ions. Steel-reinforced concrete buildings, air conditioning, and central heating also negate the vital atmospheric energy of air. Proximity to electric power lines, transformers, microwave transmitters, and other sources of artificial electromagnetic fields inhibit the functions of the pineal, pituitary, and other parts of the brain and impair immunity by knocking human energy systems off balance.

Diet and nutrition

Standard modern diets of processed and overcooked foods impair health and longevity by depriving the body of the vital nutrients and enzymes it requires to repair and protect itself. This problem is further aggravated by the digestive distress and toxic by-products caused by improper food combining, such as mixing starch and protein or eating fruit after a big meal. Taoist diets should observe the rules of trophology (food combining), eliminate all processed foods, and include at least 30–50 per cent fresh raw food. Proper diet must also include pure water that is not contaminated with heavy metals and toxic chemicals.

Emotional equilibrium

Emotional equilibrium and mental equanimity are mutually dependent factors without which it is impossible to maintain the healthy balance of internal energies upon which longevity is based. Uncontrolled emotional reactions severely impair vitality and immunity, damage the internal organs by disrupting their energies, distract the mind, and exhaust the spirit. The older one gets, the more important emotional equilibrium becomes in sustaining life. In the modern world, chronic stress is the greatest robber of the equilibrium required to cultivate longevity.

Sexual discipline

Of particular importance to males, sexual discipline conserves and cultivates internal energy and permits the transformation of sexual essence into energy and sexual energy into spiritual vitality. Taoist sexual yoga is an effective method for exchanging and balancing vital energy with a partner and cultivating the sexual vitality that prolongs life. By continuing to practice sexual intercourse into advanced age in such a way that it promotes rather than undermines sexual vitality, one prevents the body from triggering the genetic 'planned obsolescence' which nature uses to eliminate weak, physically deficient specimens from the gene pool.

Supplements

Diet and exercise alone are no longer sufficient to combat environmental pollution, sustain health and immunity, and cultivate longevity. Antioxidant supplements, especially vitamins and minerals, are essential in protecting the body from critical cumulative damage by free radicals. Enzyme supplements are required to deal effectively with enzyme-dead diets, and tonic herbal supplements stimulate the endocrine system to secrete the vital hormones required for longevity.

Exercise and breathing

Regular daily exercise of the slow, soft, rhythmic variety keeps the joints limber, tones tendons and muscles, and promotes circulation of essence and energy throughout the system. Deep breathing acts as a 'second heart' to circulate blood, switches the nervous system over to the rejuvenating, immunity-boosting parasympathetic circuit, enhances nourishment and cleansing of tissues by blood, and stimulates positive biofeedback between the endocrine and nervous systems. Together, soft exercise and deep breathing form the basis of chee-gung, which remains one of the most important of all Taoist disciplines for promoting health and prolonging life.

Fasting

Fasting is by far the most effective method for purifying the blood, organs, and all bodily tissues, and in this age of pervasive pollution it is more important than ever in warding off premature degeneration of the body due to toxicity. In laboratory tests on rats and other animals, periodic fasting has proven to extend average life spans by up to 50 per cent.

Clarity

Mental clarity is essential for cultivating longevity, for without it the adept cannot muster the discipline and understanding required to sustain Tao practices. Clarity improves sensory perception as well as mental conception based upon perception. Clarity prevents the adept from being fooled by the Five Thieves and promotes the mental equanimity required to cultivate emotional equilibrium. Clarity also permits the adept to distinguish the true from the false, keep the head in command of the heart, regulate the Fire of emotion with the Water of wisdom, and stick to the Great Highway of Tao rather than getting distracted by life's byways.

Longevity and immortality

Ever since the dawn of Taoist alchemy, adepts have been confounding longevity and immortality, on both the physical and the spiritual planes. Physically, corporeal immortality is impossible, for all forms of composite matter sooner or later disintegrate and return to an amorphous state of pure energy or inert elements. The human body can be cultivated to live a lot longer than the average human life span, but it cannot live for ever.

On the spiritual level, in which fully conscious immortality can be achieved, some adepts still make the common mistake of believing that they can indefinitely extend the existence of their own personal egos after the death of their physical bodies. This is merely wishful thinking provoked by the ego's deluded desire for incarnate immortality. In fact, in order to achieve the sort of spiritual immortality associated with full enlightenment, one must first annihilate the ego in this very life, prior to death, for the ego is the source of the desires and delusions that obscure enlightened awareness and draw the spirit back to corporeal existence time and time again. If at the moment of death one is still deceived by the delusions and desires the ego weaves in the mind, those delusions and desires are carried over to the 'other side' and become the driving force which determines the circumstances of one's next incarnation.

After death, the physical body decomposes into its constituent elements and returns to the earth, 'dust to dust', while the spirit goes to 'heaven', 'hell', 'purgatory', or whichever formless realm its own proclivities and past actions ('karma') dictate. Unless the spirit has shed the delusions and desires of ego and become fully enlightened before death, it sooner or later gravitates towards another material world and takes rebirth in corporeal form. And what happens to the ego, or 'self', during this merry-go-round of cyclic existences? As a mental phantom created by the human mind to go along with its physical body, the ego dissolves along with the body at death, and no power in heaven or earth can make it last beyond the demise of its host. As the ancient Taoist *Huai-nan-tzu* classic puts it: 'Spirit belongs to heaven, and the body belongs to earth. When the spirit returns to its home in heaven, and the body returns to its roots in earth, then where is the individual self?'

The basic lessons which form the basis of enlightened awareness can be learned only in the 'school of hard knocks' of corporeal life, but the ultimate goal of spiritual immortality can be realized only beyond the limitations of the body. As an old Taoist adage says: 'Without the body, the Tao cannot be attained; with the body, truth cannot be realized.' According to Taoist and Buddhist views, the sole purpose of cyclic corporeal life is spiritual evolution, and the driving force behind reincarnation is karmic tendencies accumulated from life to life through activities prompted by ignorance, lust, greed, envy, anger, and other desires and delusions. As long as we fail to correct these spiritual defects and evolve to higher awareness, we must continue taking the same 'classes' over and over again. Longevity therefore accelerates spiritual evolution and paves the way to spiritual immortality by prolonging our attendance in the 'school of life', allowing us to study under the private tutelage of accomplished masters, and enabling us to complete the curriculum required to 'graduate' to the higher realms reserved for the spiritually enlightened.

The body is therefore the vehicle for longevity, while the spirit is the vehicle for immortality. It is extremely important to realize, however, that the spiritual vehicle by which immortality is achieved is not the personal ego, but rather the 'shining pearl' of primordial awareness which the ego suppresses from infancy till death under the guise of 'self'. Rather than identifying you as a unique individual separate from all others, the primoridal spirit identifies you as one and the same as all others, a drop of water in the ocean of universal consciousness. Enlightenment is achieved when we identify our minds with the ocean rather than the drop, at which point we realize the ultimate truth and our awareness expands to embrace the entire universe.

The Way of Tao leads us unerringly to the gate of that realization, but we can only cross the threshold of that gate and abide for ever in the immaculate, infinite, immortal realm of primordial spirit by leaving our desires and delusions behind with our bodies when we die. Spiritual immortality can be achieved only after completely conquering the desires and delusions that propagate cyclic physical existence. This is what is meant by reaching for the infinite from the finite, realizing the truth by recognizing the false, distilling the real from the artificial, and attaining permanence through impermanence.

Earth thus becomes a stairway to heaven, and the impermanence of corporeal life becomes a mode for cultivating the permanence of spiritual awareness. The more time you have to live in this life as a mortal being on earth, the greater are your chances of earning the merits required for a permanent berth as an immortal spirit in 'heaven'. The Taoist view of 'heaven' is not the same as the Judeo-Christian and Islamic concept of a private pleasure club in the clouds reserved exclusively for members of the same faith, who enjoy eternal bliss there as Mr Smith or Miss Jones. For Taoists, 'heaven' is the entire universe itself, and 'ascending to heaven' means clarifying and expanding one's awareness to become *one* with the source of all creation. In order to do this, you must leave your ego behind in the dust along with your body at death, and in order to do that, you must achieve enlightened awareness in the body here and now. As the *Wen-tzu Classic* put it 2,000 years ago: 'Though the body dies, the spirit is immortal. When you use the permanence of spirit to respond to the impermanence of life, you transcend the temporal limits of time and space. The impermanent returns back to the nonexistence from which it arose, while the permanent coexists for ever with the entire universe.'

PART IV

The New Hybrids: Grafting East and West

CHAPTER 22

The New Medicine

Traditional and Western physicians should abandon their prejudices and value the differences between their systems. They should treasure the mutual common sense of both systems, discard what is useless or harmful, and strive for the full growth and development of the best aspects of both systems, so as to incorporate the two in bringing forth a new medical science.

Chen Li-fu, China Medical College, Taiwan (1984)

Throughout the world today, traditional physicians are quietly conducting a revolution by combining modern medical technology with traditional holistic therapies to create an innovative new approach to human health care known as the 'New Medicine'. While orthodox Western medicine continues to rely blindly on increasingly complex and costly technology that treats the human body as though it were a mindless machine and often causes more problems than it solves, practitioners of the New Medicine are culling ancient medical archives in the light of modern science to resurrect traditional tried-and-true therapies deliberately suppressed since the turn of the century by advocates of the allopathic, chemical-mechanistic approach to health care. By boldly blending the best of East and West and discarding 'what is useless or harmful' in both, these medical pioneers are forging a hybrid medical science in which the main criteria for judging the value of treatments new and old is their actual efficacy. It is precisely because of the New Medicine's efficacy in practice that the orthodox Western medical establishment expresses such virulent hostility to it, for, like all revolutions, the new medical revolution threatens to depose reigning authorities and establish a new order of priorities.

In China, Japan, Korea, and other Oriental countries, as well as

Russia and Scandinavia, the New Medicine is progressing by leaps and bounds, thanks to a pragmatic attitude towards science tempered by a healthy respect for tradition, which allows them to absorb the new without tossing the old into the rubbish bin. In China, the New Medicine has enabled medical authorities to keep a population of more than one billion impoverished people in better health than the average affluent American, as numerous studies have revealed, at a per capita cost that amounts to a small fraction of what the average American pays for health care. Known as 'barefoot doctors', teams of health therapists trained in the hybrid methods of the New Medicine roam far and wide across China, creatively combining herbs and drugs, acupuncture and surgery, massage and injections in their treatments and approaching each patient as a unique case rather than simply 'going by the book' as so many Western physicians do. To be sure, modern Western medical technology has played an important role in the health and vitality of East Asian societies, but only because it has been used within the context of traditional concepts and therapies, not as a substitute for them. By contrast, cultural and conceptual biases as well as professional hostility towards traditional Eastern systems of health care continue to deprive many Western societies of safe, effective, and inexpensive therapies.

Clearly recognized in the East but consistently overlooked in the West, the health of each and every individual is a vital factor in the overall health of an entire nation. One reason for the East Asian economic boom has been human energy. The medical science which prevails in a particular nation determines the health of its citizens and thereby also has a decisive influence on the behaviour and performance of the nation as a whole. Chang San-feng, the Taoist master of meditation, medicine, and martial arts, succinctly summarized this point 600 years ago:

> Medical science can energize a nation, but it can also make a nation sick. Medicine can bestow life, but it can also kill. Therefore, one must be very careful about its application . . . I recommend that those who study and teach the social sciences incorporate a comprehensive study of medical science in their programmes . . . One should never underestimate the importance of medical science.

The New Medicine restores the long-neglected human factor in medical care without discarding useful technological innovations.

Instead of waiting until disease has already established a foothold in the body, then treating the superficial symptoms with stop-gap chemical nostrums, the New Medicine shifts attention to the prevention of disease by applying holistic methods which enhance the body's own natural defence mechanisms. When disease invades the body despite preventive measures, the New Medicine uses modern diagnostic technology to 'follow the stream' of symptoms back to the source of the disease, then treats it with traditional therapies that stimulate the body's internal healing mechanisms. The New Medicine bodes ill for hospitals, pharmaceutical firms, and allopathic physicians whose livelihoods depend upon treating rather than preventing disease, but it's the light at the end of the tunnel for people who are sick and tired spending their lives groping through the darkness of one disease after another with drugs and surgery that cost a fortune without providing any lasting relief. It's also good news for health professionals who take seriously the Hippocratic oath to devote their lives to the prevention and alleviation of human suffering. As Master Chang San-feng wrote: 'Physicians should handle medical emergencies without using them to promote their own reputations and should treat suffering without thinking about how much money they'll get paid for it.'

An ounce of prevention

They say that 'an ounce of prevention is worth a pound of cure', but in light of the growing virulence of modern diseases, the exchange rate is more like an ounce to a ton. Timely preventive measures often make the difference between life and death or, worse yet, between life and the long suffering and slow death of chronic disease and debility.

Preventive health care has always been the hallmark of traditional Chinese and other Oriental medical systems. An often quoted passage from the *Internal Medicine Classic* states:

> Wise physicians don't wait until after diseases arise to treat them, but instead they treat them before they arise. They don't wait for conditions to run out of control, but instead they treat them before they run out of control. Administering medicine to diseases that are already established and treating conditions that are already out of control is like starting to dig a well after you're already dying of thirst, or raising an army after you've already

been invaded by the enemy. Would such measures not be too late?

Traditional physicians regard disease as a failure of preventive health care, not as an opportunity to test new drugs on patients. Western patients are as much to blame for their plight as physicians, for they simply do not want to bear responsibility for learning about health, nor are they willing to exercise the discipline required to protect their own health, so they depend on doctors to fix their bodies whenever something goes wrong, much as they depend on mechanics to repair their cars. (And like mechanics, allopathic doctors depend on high-tech hardware and noxious chemicals as the tools of their trade.) Chang San-feng cited this problem 600 years ago in China:

> I suggest that physicians carefully question their patients regarding the onset and development of their diseases, rather than using their patients' diseases to test new drugs. I also suggest that ailing patients try to understand the causes of their own diseases before going to see physicians, rather than blindly risking their lives to test physicians' skills. Patients are to blame for risking their lives to test physicians skills, and physicians are to blame for testing new drugs on patients.

Throughout the entire 5,000 years of recorded history in China, prevention has remained the guiding principle in maintaining human health, and the essence, energy, and spirit upon which health depends were prized and protected as the true 'treasures' of life. Health was regarded as a primary responsibility of the individual, and disease as a mistake in lifestyle. The greatest value traditional Chinese health care holds for modern medicine lies in the many simple but effective methods Chinese physicians developed for cultivating mental and physical health, balancing essence and energy, preventing disease and degeneration, and prolonging life. They recorded their discoveries in the medical archives of ancient China, which remain as valid today as they were then.

Modern medicine has completely lost sight of the vital role played in human health by nonphysical factors such as thoughts, emotions, internal energies, and external environmental aberrations. Many common chronic ills, such as migraine headaches and high blood pressure, are caused and sustained by anger, stress, marital discord, overexcitement, and other uncontrolled emotional responses, which play havoc with the delicate balance of essence and energy. At best, drugs can only provide temporary symptomatic relief for such problems, but they do nothing to eliminate the root causes, and often they further aggravate the underlying biochemical imbalances provoked by stress and emotional turmoil.

The vicarious violence experienced by watching television, for example, provokes physiological responses in the body of the viewer, especially in the brain and endocrine system, and the debilitating biochemical imbalances caused by emotional responses to such sensory onslaughts can be detected by laboratory tests on blood plasma. While sex and violence in television and films provide cheap thrills for the viewer and big profits for the producer, they do so at great cost to human health, though often those costs remain hidden for a long time. In traditional Oriental societies, pregnant women were carefully screened from viewing or hearing any unpleasant sights or sounds, especially those which arouse anger, fear, grief, or any other extreme emotional response, in order to prevent adrenaline, cortisone, and other hazardous biochemicals from being released and transferred to their developing foetuses via the bloodstream. This may have prevented mental, emotional, and physical abnormalities in their offspring.

Food has become a cause of disease rather than a guardian of health in the modern world. Once regarded as the central pillar of life and the most effective of all medicines, food is now a major contributing factor in cancer, heart disease, arthritis, mental illness, and many other pathological conditions. Virtually monopolized by agricultural and industrial cartels, public food supplies are processed and packaged to produce profits and prolong shelf life, not to promote health and prolong human life. It seems incredible that public health authorities permit the unrestricted use of hydrogenated vegetable oils, refined sugar, chemical preservatives, toxic pesticides, and over 5,000 other artificial food additives that have repeatedly been proven to cause cancer, impair immunity, and otherwise erode human health, while restricting the medical use of nutrients, herbs, acupuncture, fasting, and other traditional therapies that have been shown to prevent and cure the very diseases caused by chemical contaminants in food and water.

Misguided medical practice causes more malaise than it cures, as evidenced by the documented fact that many cancer patients who decline conventional treatments such as chemotherapy, surgery, and radiation and opt instead to let nature take its course actually live longer than those who accept chemical-mechanistic therapies.

Conventional cancer therapies damage the blood, liver, and immune system so severely that if they fail, as they usually do, the patient no longer enjoys the option to try alternative holistic therapies, which can work only in conjunction with the body's natural defence mechanisms. Therefore, if you get cancer, consider alternative therapies first, because even if they don't help you, at least they won't harm you, and you can always let conventional doctors try to poison, burn, or cut the cancer out of your system later if you wish.

Modern medicine has been further led astray by the growing tendency to fragment health care into increasingly narrow byways of specialization. It conducts a constant witch-hunt for viruses and other microbes to blame for our ills and uses the human body as a battlefield against them. Rather than preserving health and preventing disease, this approach waits for disease to strike, then wages war on it with ever more lethal weapons. In an editorial that appeared in the April 1987 issue of the *New England Journal of Medicine*, the pressing need for 'more realistic conventions' in modern medical care was stated as follows:

> Science is a hard taskmaster, and in the light of mounting evidence that suggestions of toxicity are for the most part ultimately confirmed by painstaking scientific inquiry, perhaps it is time to reexamine whether scientific standards of proof of causality – and waiting for the bodies to fall – ought not to give way to more preventive health policies that are satisfied by more realistic conventions and that lead to action sooner.

The bodies have already started to fall. Meanwhile, scientific and political expedience continue to obstruct the implementation of preventive health policies which hold the only hope of stemming the rising tide of human disease and degeneration. Below, we'll take a brief look at the most obvious travesties of modern allopathic medicine, then discuss some of the innovative new approaches to health care being forged by the New Medicine by fusing modern technology with traditional therapy, grafting Eastern philosophy with Western science, and applying an ounce of prevention to thwart a ton of pestilence.

Cures that kill

The chemical drugs so freely prescribed by practitioners of allopathic medicine relieve the overt symptoms of disease, particularly pain, but do nothing to eliminate the root causes, which often lie hidden far from the symptoms. People easily grow dependent on these drugs, using them continuously until they develop a tolerance to them, then switching to stronger chemicals. Often the drugs themselves further aggravate the condition, or cause other ailments in related organ-energy systems. The next step is usually surgery.

Antibiotics, which are potent immunosuppressants, are prescribed for dozens of common ailments. In the process of killing the bacteria for which they are prescribed, they also kill off all the 'friendly' lactobacteria in your intestines, severely impairing digestion and assimilation of nutrients at a time when your body needs them most. Lactobacteria are the only elements in the body which keep candida and other harmful yeast infections under control, so whenever you take a course of antibiotics, candida have a field day and spread like wildfire throughout your system. A primary effect of candida infection is suppression of the immune system, which means that the very drug you're taking to combat disease is impairing your only natural defence against it.

Antibiotics rob you of vital nutrients, thereby further aggravating whatever condition you're taking them for. Among the many nutrients which they destroy are vitamin B_{12}, B_6, and B_1, vitamin K, folic acid, iron, calcium, and magnesium. When taken in combination with corticosteroids, which are also frequently prescribed for all sorts of ailments, they knock the immune system out cold. During the 1970s, a combination of antibiotics, especially tetracycline, and corticosteriods was popularly taken by gay males prior to visiting the notorious bath houses in San Francisco, Los Angeles, and New York. They did this in the mistaken belief that it would protect them from contracting skin and venereal diseases. It was among frequent visitors to the gay bath houses of these three cities that AIDS was first identified, the primary symptom and cause of death being *P. carnii* pneumonia. In the December 1984 issue of *Infection and Immunity*, Peter Walzer reported: 'Rats administered corticosteroids, a low-protein diet, and tetracycline spontaneously developed *P. carnii* pneumonia within about eight weeks through a mechanism of reactivation of latent infection.' Low-protein diets are common among drug users, because drugs, including antibiotics, impair the digestive system's capacity to break down and process complex proteins, which are primary dietary sources of the amino acids the body needs to produce enzymes, white blood cells, hormones, and other immune factors.

In light of the evidence against antibiotics, you should think twice before using them, and when you do, you should increase your daily dosage of vitamin and mineral supplements to replenish lost nutrients and also take a supplemental source of lactobacteria, such as Rejuvelac, to restore the friendly intestinal flora destroyed by the antibiotics.

The drugs commonly prescribed for high blood pressure are another example of so-called 'cures' that aggravate the condition they are supposed to eliminate. Normal blood pressure depends in part on adequate supplies of the minerals potassium, magnesium, and sodium in the blood. The drugs prescribed for this condition promote rapid urinary excretion of these very minerals, thereby prolonging the problem and causing continued dependency on the drugs. Several studies have shown that people with moderately high blood pressure who take no drugs at all for the condition live longer than those who take the prescribed drugs.

Arthritis medications are another case in point. Arthritis is often caused by intestinal toxins that are absorbed into the bloodstream by osmosis through weak sections of the intestinal walls. In order to prevent these toxins from poisoning the bloodstream, the blood deposits them in joints, where they accumulate, form crystals, and cause arthritis. Commonly prescribed arthritis medications such as aspirin have long been known to cause intestinal bleeding, thereby further weakening the intestinal walls and permitting even more toxins to seep from the intestines into the bloodstream. This further aggravates the arthritis, driving the patient to take even more of these drugs for symptomatic relief. The primary causes of stomach and intestinal bleeding in hospital emergency-room cases in the USA are the drugs prescribed for arthritis.

Virtually all children in the West these days are inoculated with vaccines which doctors claim will protect them from polio, diphtheria, measles, and other dangerous diseases. However, in his book *Medical Nemesis*, Ivan Illich reported:

> The combined death rate from scarlet fever, diphtheria, whooping cough and measles among children up to fifteen shows that nearly 90% of the total decline in mortality between 1860 and 1965 had occurred before the introduction of antibiotics and widespread immunization. . . By far the most important factor was a higher host-resistance due to better nutrition.

In other words, by the time children began to be inoculated with various vaccines, the mortality rate for the diseases targeted by the vaccines had already dropped by 90%, and the primary factor in the enhanced resistance children have developed to these diseases is nutrition, a therapy which allopathic doctors consistently ignore.

As for polio, Dr Herbert Ratner reported as follows in the journal *Child and Family* (1980, vol. 19, no. 4):

> Suffice to say that most of the large polio epidemics that have occurred in this country since the introduction of the Salk vaccine have followed the wide-scale use of the vaccine and have been characterized by an uncommon early seasonal onset. To name a few, there is the Massachusetts epidemic of 1955; the Chicago epidemic of 1956; and the Des Moines epidemic of 1959.

In fact, vaccines often destroy one's natural immunity to the diseases for which they are administered. In the December 1983 issue of *Let's Live*, Dr Robert Mendelsohn reported: 'Prior to the time doctors began giving rubella measles vaccinations, an estimated 85% of adults were naturally immune to the disease for life. Because of immunization, the vast majority of women never acquire natural immunity or lifetime protection.'

One of the most dangerous drugs ever put on the market is AZT, which is currently being prescribed to anyone who tests positive for HIV. AZT is a failed anti-cancer drug that was developed during the early 1970s. The primary side effects of AZT are severe anaemia, a condition which impairs immunity, and destruction of bone marrow, which is the tissue responsible for producing two types of white blood cells that are essential components of the immune system. This means that AZT causes the very condition of immune deficiency which it is supposed to cure, and that people who take it are likely to develop rather than prevent AIDS. Lippincott's *Drug Facts and Comparisons* (1988) warns: 'Significant anemia may require a dose interruption until evidence of bone marrow recovery is observed.' The 23 July 1987 issue of the *New England Journal of Medicine* reports that out of 140 patients taking AZT in a controlled test, '21% required multiple red-cell transfusions' and that 'serious adverse effects, particularly bone marrow suppression, were observed'. If you happen to test positive for HIV, don't panic, because according to statistics, the likelihood of your contracting AIDS is less than 5%. On 27 April 1992, the UPI wire service reported that Dr Luc Montagnier, the French scientist who first identified HIV in 1983, had come to the conclusion that HIV is not the cause of AIDS: 'HIV infection doesn't necessarily lead to AIDS,' said Dr Montagnier. The report went on to state that 'the HIV virus might not even be involved in some cases of AIDS, while in other cases people with HIV might never contract AIDS.' Rather than causing AIDS, HIV 'might instead be only an agent that stimulates other microbes already existing in humans that cause the symptoms known as AIDS'. Therefore, 'an HIV vaccine is unlikely to work, and popular treatments such as the drug AZT actually could hasten the onset of AIDS'.

The list of medical mayhem caused by allopathic medicine could fill several books. Anyone who's seen a friend or relative die of cancer after submitting to radiation or chemotherapy knows how devastating these can be. Furthermore, statistics clearly reveal that these radical therapies do not significantly prolong the lives of cancer patients, and often shorten them instead. They give patients false hopes for survival and make the last days of their lives utterly miserable. The same goes for spinal surgery, an increasingly popular technique in Western hospitals, despite a recorded failure rate of 80 per cent.

Still, the tide is slowly turning in favour of the alternative therapies practiced by the New Medicine. When your life is at stake and everything your doctor recommends only nudges you closer to the grave, you don't give a hoot what the health authorities think. Your only concern is to find a remedy that works by shopping around for alternative therapies. If anyone tries to deny you that right, vote him or her out of office!

Branches of the new tree.

The New Medicine is a hybrid tree of health grafted together from the strongest branches of medical science and medical philosophy, Western technology and Eastern metaphysics, modern tools and traditional wisdom. Replacing the fragmented view of human health adopted by specialized modern medicine with the holistic approach of traditional healers, the New Medicine treats the human body as a balanced living organism in which all functions are mutually dependent, rather than a machine in which defective parts can be removed and replaced.

Herbalism

Grafting modern science with traditional medicine has always been the key to progress in human health. Of the modern medications currently used in Western allopathic medicine, 85 per cent were originally derived from the natural herbs used since ancient times in traditional medicine, then later synthesized into various chemical analogues. Ephedrine, for example, which is the primary modern medication used for bronchial disorders, is a synthetic analogue of the herb ephedra, which has been used for the same purpose for over 5,000 years in China. However, no chemist can produce an exact replica of a natural substance, and chemical analogues have more dangerous side effects and less healing power than natural substances. Therefore, the current trend in the New Medicine is to use modern chemical technology to produce highly refined, strongly concentrated extracts of natural herbs, rather than synthetic analogues, and these patent remedies are proving to be both highly effective and perfectly safe. Thanks to the extensive clinical experience accumulated in China and recorded in pharmacopoeias and medical texts over the past 5,000 years by traditional herbalists and healers, contemporary physicians and pharmacists have learned how medicinal herbs affect the human body and how they work to fight disease. Based on this precious legacy, contemporary herbalists are using the latest modern technology to develop a whole new arsenal of natural remedies for modern maladies. Some of the most effective of these technologically upgraded Chinese herbal medicines are introduced in the chapter on 'Remarkable Remedies'.

The principle of synergy in human metabolism is one of the most important contributions of traditional medicine to modern health care. Known and practised for thousands of years in Chinese medicine, synergy has only recently been discovered by Western medical science. All Chinese herbal prescriptions contain four functional varieties of herbs, precisely balanced and blended for maximum metabolic synergy. The chief component and most active ingredient is referred to as the 'imperial' herb, and it provides the primary therapeutic punch against disease. The 'ministerial' herb or herbs are added to enhance the effects of the imperial component and facilitate its absorption and circulation in the body. To these are added 'assistant' herbs, whose duty is to counteract any potential negative side effects of the primary ingredients. A team of 'servant' herbs are also included to coordinate and enhance the therapeutic benefits of the entire formula. The correct combinations and proper proportions for blending synergistic herbs into specific formulas for specific diseases are based on thousands of years of trial and error, carefully codified for posterity in Chinese herbal manuals. In fact, many of the oldest written records preserved intact throughout China's long history are medical texts, and these are so complete and comprehensive that they are still required reading for students of traditional Chinese medicine today. Only recently, however, has Western science started to take a serious look at this ancient treasure trove of medical wisdom.

Synergy has manifold applications in the New Medicine. For example, while conventional allopathic physicians rarely dispense dietary advice along with the powerful drugs they so casually prescribe, traditional doctors always do so, for they know that various foods can either synergistically boost or antagonistically hinder the therapeutic benefits of medications. Even aspirin, which Americans consume to the tune of 15 tons per day, must be used with caution and in accordance with sound dietary advice owing to its interaction with various nutrients, which function as 'medicine' once they are absorbed into the system. Aspirin can cause critical deficiencies in vitamin C, vitamin A, calcium, and folic acid when used daily and should therefore be taken in conjunction with extra supplements of these nutrients. Choline, an amino acid often prescribed for poor memory, absent-mindedness, and other cerebral deficiencies associated with senility, is therapeutically impotent unless taken in conjunction with a large dose of vitamin B_5. Choline is the basic building block the brain uses to produce the neurotransmitter acetylcholine, deficiencies of which are associated with symptoms of senility, but without the synergistic presence of vitamin B_5, the brain cannot convert choline into acetylcholine.

Synergy is also the guiding principle in a branch of the New Medicine created by grafting modern nutritional science with traditional herbal medicine to produce remedies whose therapeutic benefits surpass the sum of their parts. For example, the choline and B_5 nutrient combination prescribed for cerebral deficiencies becomes even more effective when blended with ginseng, *Epimedium*, ginkgo, and other cerebroactive herbs, and the effects of traditional Chinese herbal formulas are further enhanced when blended with synergistic nutrient cofactors. Recent research in this branch of the New Medicine has led to the development of many new remedies that blend the best of traditional herbal formulas with the purest, most potent synergistic nutrients, producing cures that surpass the powers of herbs or nutrients alone.

As modern medical science unravels its therapeutic mechanisms, traditional herbal medicine is providing new insights and practical remedies for modern maladies. The Institute of Biotechnology at Hong Kong's Chinese University is screening thousands of medicinal plants from ancient Chinese pharmacopoeias to determine their pharmaceutical properties, and is discovering a lode of potent remedies for problems as diverse as malaria, acne, cancer, and AIDS.

Malaria, for example, which conventional Western medicine

has been treating with chloroquine and quinine, has recently developed new strains that are resistant to these drugs. Consequently, malaria is once again on the rise in the tropical and subtropical regions of the world. Ancient Chinese texts extol the benefits of *ching-hao*, a variety of wormwood related to tarragon, as a remedy for malaria, and recently a potent, highly refined extract of this herb's active ingredient, dubbed 'artemisinin' by Western biochemists, has proven so effective that it can even reawaken comatose patients suffering from advanced cerebral malaria. Intravenous injections of this compound have cut the mortality rate from cerebral malaria in half.

Skin diseases are particularly troublesome for modern allopathic medicine, but an ancient and simple Chinese herbal remedy brewed from peonies, bamboo, and liquorice cleared up hundreds of cases of severe eczema that resisted modern medications in tests conducted by dermatologists at the Royal Free Hospital in London. Conventionally treated with corticosteroids, which have dangerous side effects and can seriously impair immunity, the crusty skin and itchy rash associated with severe eczema vanished in 75 per cent of the patients treated with this safe and inexpensive herbal remedy. Significantly, this remedy was administered in conjunction with strict dietary guidelines which completely eliminated beef, cow's milk, and shellfish from the diets of the patients being tested.

Chinese herbal medicine may even provide an effective remedy against the symptoms of AIDS. A wild cucumber called *tien-hwa-fen* has yielded a potent extract called 'compound Q', which has restored the ability of some AIDS patients to produce the immune cells destroyed by the disease. Other immune-system boosters such as ginseng, ginkgo, *Astragalus*, *gotu kola*, and *Ligusticum* are also being used to rebuild the immune systems of people suffering from various forms of immune deficiency.

Acupuncture

In addition to working with essence, the New Medicine also works directly with energy and spirit, two important aspects of the human organism which are entirely ignored by allopathic medicine. Acupuncture, for example, is being studied and practised throughout the Western world now, both in its classical form and with new techniques enhanced by modern science. At the Karolinska Institute in Sweden, Dr Björn Nordenström is using electronically enhanced acupuncture to shrink malignant tumours in cancer patients by inserting the needles directly into the tumours and running a pulsed current through them. The enhanced electro-magnetic field produced around the tumours by the charged needles kills the rapidly dividing cancer cells without harming normal cells, which are less active than cancer cells and therefore not as sensitive to external electromagnetism. The pulsed currents also enhance blood circulation around the tumours, drawing in white blood cells, enzymes, and other immune factors to dissolve and carry away the dead cells and toxic residues of the tumours.

The New Medicine has also combined traditional acupuncture with modern surgery as an effective substitute for chemical anaes-thesia. There are specific points on the body that block all pain signals to the brain, and others that stimulate the secretion of endorphins within the brain. Endorphins are natural opiates, some of them 200 times more potent than morphine, but without the immunosuppressive and respiration-inhibiting side effects of morphine. The combination of pain-blocking and endorphin-releasing points provides such effective anaesthesia that surgeons can perform open-heart and open-brain surgery without resorting to any sort of chemical painkillers. Not only does this avoid the extremely debilitating immunosuppressive side effects of chemical anaesthesia, it also permits the patient to remain fully conscious and communicate with the surgeon during surgery, an obvious advantage to patient as well as surgeon. Patients who undergo radical surgery with acupuncture anaesthesia heal their wounds and recover their vitality much faster than those who opt to be knocked out by the conventional chemical method. According to Shuji Goto, head of the Tokyo Sanitary Academy, acupuncture awakens our innate self-healing response, which is far more effec-tive than any drug, and it does so without contaminating the body with external toxic agents.

Electromagnetic therapy

Electromagnetic energy is becoming an ever more important thera-peutic tool in the New Medicine. In England, Dr Margaret Patterson's electromagnetic brain therapy for drug addiction has consistently recorded a much higher cure rate than the conven-tional methadone and other chemical treatments still used in the USA, and Dr Robert Becker of upstate New York has developed several therapeutic electronic devices, including a highly effective unit that counteracts stress, balances vital energies, and enhances cerebral functions by delivering pulsed microcurrents to the body through electrodes placed behind the ears. Dr Glen Rein of

Stanford University has found that pulsed scalar fields can significantly enhance immunity by stimulating production of T-cells, which are the main immune factors suppressed by AIDS. He reports: 'The effect we observed was a very, very pronounced stimulation of the growth of these lymphocytes or T-cells to the tune of twentyfold with the scalar field!'

In this age of pervasive electromagnetic pollution, it may become necessary to 'fight fire with fire' by installing therapeutic electromagnetic devices in homes, offices, and schools. Negative ion generators, which recharge the air of polluted cities and climate-controlled buildings with the bioactive energy of negative ions, are already a common feature in offices, factories, hotels, and private houses in Japan, and this may account in part for the high productivity of Japanese business and industry.

Electromagnetic therapy, when properly administered, seems to work primarily by stimulating and enhancing the body's own internal healing mechanisms. Owing to environmental toxicity, electromagnetic pollution, denatured diets, chronic stress, and other debilitating factors of modern life, the natural human healing response is frequently suppressed or impaired, even in apparently healthy people. As Dr Robert Becker's research has proven, this healing response is regulated by a closed-circuit electrical system which links the human energy network with the nervous system. It stands to reason therefore that electrical stimulation is an effective means of rebalancing human energies, restoring immunity, and re-awakening the natural healing response.

Heliotherapy

Heliotherapy, which utilizes the energy of light as a 'nutrient' as well as a 'medicine', is another ancient therapy revived and scientifically enhanced by the New Medicine. Without sufficient doses of full-spectrum light, the pineal and pituitary glands cannot function properly, inhibiting secretions of the vital hormones which regulate the endocrine system and orchestrate human biorhythms. (This branch of the New Medicine is discussed in detail in the chapter on 'Taoist Healing Arts' in *The Tao of HS&L*.)

Astrology

Recent research into the nature of the earth's electromagnetic field and the influence of its fluctuations on human health and behaviour throws new light on the ancient practice of astrology, which

Taoists have always regarded as a legitimate science. It is a scientific fact that shifting positions of the sun, moon, planets, and stars cause subtle but significant fluctuations on the magnitude and pulse of the earths electromagnetic field, and Dr Becker's research has clearly established that even the slightest fluctuations in these fields have a significant impact on the pineal and pituitary glands and other portions of the brain, thereby influencing emotions, immunity, sexual drive, and other vital functions regulated by cerebral essence and energy. While charlatans abound in this field, there are also many astrologers who are renowned for the accuracy of their predictions regarding the effects of various planetary and stellar configurations on human behaviour. In Chinese astrology, emphasis is focused on the practical implications of various astral forces on an individual's emotions, energies, and overall health, as well as on such abstruse factors as 'fate' and 'fortune'. Stripped of its arcane terminology and re-examined in the light of modern electromagnetic science, astrology could become an important diagnostic and preventive tool in the New Medicine, as it always has been in the traditional health-care systems of China, India, and other ancient Oriental cultures. Indeed, since these forces have such significant influences on our health and behaviour, ignoring them only hinders our ability to control the course of our lives and guard our health. As Dr Becker points out in *Cross Currents*: 'The implications of this work are considerable. It would seem that we may not be the free agents we like to think we are. Our thoughts and actions are, at least to some extent, determined by electromagnetic fields in the environment that we cannot sense and that we remain unaware of to our peril.'

Team work

In the hybrid system of human health care practised by the New Medicine, the doctor and patient form a 'team', with the doctor serving as 'coach' and the patient as 'player'. The doctor teaches the patient the rules of the game, but only the patient can play, and whether he wins or loses depends primarily on his own performance, although as in all games the talent of the coach can make a crucial difference in the outcome. This system of health care poses an obvious threat to orthodox allopathic doctors and pharmaceutical firms, who thrive on treating disease, not preventing it. But it is also a big challenge to patients, who have grown accustomed to relying on allopathic doctors for a quick fix whenever something goes wrong, and who prefer to blame 'foreign agents' for all their ills, rather than accepting personal responsibility for having failed to prevent them by letting their guard down. In order for the New Medicine to take root in the world, patients as well as doctors are going to have to change their attitudes towards health and start digging their wells *before* they're dying of thirst. As the *Tao Teh Ching* notes: 'Before an omen arises, it is easy to take preventive measures . . . Deal with things in their formative state; put things in order before they grow confused.'

The great American football coach Vince Lombardi, whose teams rarely lost a game, taught his players the same simple principle and utilized the same winning strategy that guides the New Medicine. He said: 'The best offence is a good defence!'

CHAPTER 23

The New Alchemy

> Instead of preventing diseases only by protecting the individual against their agents, we must, by artificially increasing the efficiency of his adaptive functions, render each man capable of protecting himself.
>
> Alexis Carrel, *Man the Unknown* (1935)

Webster's dictionary defines 'alchemy' as a 'chemical science and speculative philosophy whose aims were the discovery of a universal cure for diseases and the discovery of a means of indefinitely prolonging life'. The search for health and longevity has been in progress in the East as well as the West ever since the dawn of human history, and today it continues unabated as scientists gradually unravel the mysteries of disease and degeneration and forge weapons for 'artificially increasing the efficiency' of each individual's capacity to protect him- or herself.

The difference between alchemy and ordinary chemical science is the 'speculative philosophy' which informs alchemy and links it to fields of knowledge beyond the purely chemical-mechanistic paradigms of conventional modern sciences. Albert Einstein, the quintessential image of the modern scientist, said: 'The gift of fantasy has meant more to me than my talent for absorbing positive knowledge.' Flights of fantasy often provide the crucial sparks of creative insight that inspire scientific discovery, and such syncretic fusion of science and philosophy yields knowledge that is far more complete than either one alone. 'In times to come,' wrote the Nobel laureate Werner Heisenberg, 'it will often be difficult, perhaps, to decide whether an advance in knowledge represents a step forward in physics, information theory, or philosophy.'

Health and longevity are primary concerns of men and women everywhere, and alchemy addresses those concerns by applying scientific methods to questions raised by philosophical speculation.

'Aging and death do seem to be what Nature has planned for us,' says the gerontologist Bernard Strehler. 'But what if we have other plans?' Artificially increasing resistance to disease, aging, and death reflects the mind's capacity to transcend nature and transform its forces to human advantage. The time has come for the scientist and the philosopher once again to put their heads together to harness the ever more awesome powers unleashed by science and technology to principles and purposes that serve rather than sabotage human interests. Since health and longevity rank so high among human interests, science and technology should promote those goals, not hinder them. That's what the 'New Alchemy' is all about.

Free radicals: public enemy no. 1

In 1956, Dr Denham Harman of the University of Nebraska first proposed what is now known as 'the free-radical theory of aging'. This quantum leap in medical knowledge was, predictably, ignored by the medical community for two decades, until the evidence supporting his view became so overwhelming that it was impossible to deny.

Free radicals are highly reactive molecules with an unpaired, or 'free', electron in their outer orbits, a condition of imbalance which turns these fragmented molecules into extremely unstable and biochemically dangerous agents. Chemical compounds, like people, achieve stability by virtue of energy balance; in the case of chemicals, balance depends on the pairing of electrons. When a molecule loses an electron, it becomes electrochemically unbalanced, biochemically unstable, and extremely 'radical' as it seeks to regain stability by violently 'stealing' an electron from another molecule. Every time a free radical attacks a normal molecule in order to steal an electron, it unleashes a cascade of new free radicals, each of which then attacks other molecules, generating an uncontrolled chain reaction of biochemical damage to cells and tissues.

Dr Harman describes free-radical activity as a sort of ongoing 'internal radiation' which relentlessly attacks and destroys cells and tissues, causing the various symptoms commonly attributed to aging: wrinkled skin, 'age spots', cataracts, arthritis, hardened arteries, senility, cancer, and other degenerative conditions. Diseases and degenerative conditions associated with aging and attributed to free-radical damage include arteriosclerosis, hypertension, arthritis, cancer, heart disease, glaucoma, cataracts, Altzheimer's disease, loss of memory and strokes. Aging is therefore not a chronological process determined by the passage of time, but rather a biological process determined by the rate at which free radicals destroy cells, damage tissues, and impair vital functions.

Human beings have always been subject to free-radical damage, because free radicals are natural by-products of normal metabolism. In fact, free radicals play an important role in cellular defence systems by destroying bacteria and viruses, breaking down chemical pollutants, and neutralizing toxins. The damaging side effects of normal free-radical production within the body are kept under control by scavenger enzymes specifically designed for this purpose.

The problem today is that there are so many artificial new sources of free radicals that the body's natural defence mechanisms can no longer prevail. Common external sources of free radicals include nuclear radiation, X-rays and microwaves, toxic metals such as aluminium and cadmium in public water supplies, smog, chemical food additives, cigarette smoke, motor-vehicle exhaust, and, perhaps most prevalent of all, the oxidation of artificial fat-substitutes such as hydrogenated vegetable oils in bodily tissues.

All fats and oils produce free radicals when they oxidize (combine with oxygen) and break down. The free radicals produced by oxidation of fat molecules are called 'lipid peroxides'. Natural fats such as butter, meat, and cold-pressed nut oils oxidize much more slowly and produce far fewer free radicals than polyunsaturated fats made with hydrogenated vegetable oil. These artificial fats oxidize immediately upon exposure to air, the moment you unseal the can or bottle, and they continue to oxidize inside your system, setting up a chain reaction of molecular mayhem that destroys cells and disrupts vital functions much faster than your body's natural capacity to defend itself from such damage.

All hydrogenated vegetable oils are free-radical bombs which explode the moment you ingest them. That includes margarine, bottled salad dressings, commercial cooking oils, shortening, and non-dairy creamers. Since high heat causes oils to oxidize even faster, all deep-fried foods are loaded with free radicals. According to Dr Harman and other scientists, oxidation of unsaturated fats in the human system is the primary cause of the cellular pathology associated with aging.

Of all the tissues in the human body, the brain contains the highest percentage of unsaturated fats, and therefore brain cells are the most vulnerable of all to free-radical damage caused by lipid peroxidation. Modern diets, especially in the Western world, have replaced most natural fats with artificial unsaturated fats made with hydrogenated vegetable oils that have been chemically altered and stripped of all nutrients. The body, which cannot function without fat molecules, gets fooled into accepting hydrogenated fat molecules as substitutes for the natural fatty acids it requires, and these artificial fat molecules thus become incorporated into the structural matrix of cells, particularly brain cells and white blood cells, which have the greatest need for fat molecules. Once they are built into the cell's structure, these denatured fat molecules oxidize and unleash wave upon wave of corrosive free radicals that attack cells and eventually cause genetic damage, either killing the cell or subverting it into aberrant behaviour. Many medical scientists now believe that this is one of the primary mechanisms that cause cancer. Dr Ross Pelton, a leading researcher in the prevention of brain aging, states: 'The process of partially hydrogenating fats and oils is so dangerous and harmful to health that no compromise can be made. Partially hydrogenated fats should not be added to any food used by humans or animals!'

Toxic metals such as aluminium and cadmium are also major sources of free-radical damage in modern environments. Aluminium is commonly added to food preservatives, antacid tablets, public drinking water, antiperspirants, and cosmetics. Aluminium cookware is another common source of aluminium poisoning. Autopsies performed on victims of Altzheimer's disease reveal abnormally high levels of aluminium in their brain tissues. In a region of England where the incidence of Altzheimer's disease was unusually high, it was discovered that public drinking water there was being treated with unusually high levels of aluminium salts, supposedly to 'purify' it for human consumption. When fluoride is added to water in which aluminium salts are present, the assimilation of aluminium from the water increases manifold. The chlorine added to drinking water is also a poison which produces free radicals. Public drinking water has thus become a primary source of free radicals throughout the world.

Other common sources include the hydrocarbons in smog, industrial pollutants, cigarette smoke, the toxic acetaldehydes produced in the liver from the breakdown of alcohol, and exposure to medical X-rays and microwave radiation.

What can we do to defend ourselves from this onslaught? The first step is to eliminate all unnecessary sources of free radicals, such as hydrogenated fats, tap water, microwave devices, and cigarettes. The second step is to fortify our bodies' own natural defences with the weapons forged for this purpose by latter-day alchemists, who have discovered that various nutrients, natural herbs, and a new family of pharmaceuticals, when taken in sufficient doses and correct combinations, arrest and disarm free radicals before they do serious damage.

Antioxidants to the rescue

Nature's defence against the biological warfare waged on us by free radicals is provided by an army of biochemical commandos called antioxidants, or 'free-radical scavengers', chief among which are the powerful antioxidant enzymes glutathione peroxidase and superoxide dismutase (SOD). At the annual meeting of the American Association for the Advancement of Science in 1992, the biologist Michael Ross of the University of California reported the discovery of what he calls the 'anti-aging gene'. This gene is responsible for regulating production of SOD.

Without SOD and other antioxidant enzymes, our tissues would quickly burn up in the biochemical brush fires constantly ignited throughout the body by free radicals. Many scientists believe that the aging process is simply a side effect of declining production of SOD and other antioxidant enzymes. Nature deliberately suppresses the genes responsible for producing antioxidant enzymes in those individuals whose health and vitality have declined to the point that they are no longer viable candidates for reproduction of the species. This is an evolutionary device designed to ensure that only the fittest specimens reproduce. Michael Ross states: 'Evolution doesn't care how long you live; it only cares about your fitness, which really means your reproductive fitness.' In other words, when you are no longer fit to produce healthy offspring, nature turns off your 'anti-aging genes'. This idea agrees with the traditional Taoist view that sexual vitality is a prime sign of flourishing health and a firm foundation for longevity, whereas sexual debility is the first forerunner of terminal decline.

Glutathione peroxidase and superoxide dismutase are the body's primary free-radical scavengers, and in order to produce them the body requires abundant supplies of the minerals selenium and zinc. Without sufficient selenium and zinc, it is impossible to synthesize these two vital antioxidant enzymes. As soon as a molecule of SOD mops up a free radical, it goes out of commission and must be replaced. Selenium has become virtually extinct in the human food chain due to modern farming and food-processing methods, and most of the world's population is also chronically deficient in zinc. Daily supplements of selenium and zinc are thus essential for ensuring adequate supplies of SOD and other antioxidant enzymes.

In addition to the body's internally produced antioxidants, there are also external agents which manifest potent antioxidant activity when ingested into the human system. Foremost among these external sources of antioxidants are various nutrients, especially vitamins A, C, E, B_1, B_5, B_6, and betacarotene (the precursor to vitamin A), and the amino acids taurine, cysteine, methionine, and glutathione. In the 'Health/Science' column of the 12 March 1992 issue of the *International Herald Tribune*, the protective antioxidant powers of these vitamins are described as follows:

> These enigmatic chemicals may help forestall or even reverse many diseases of aging, including cancer, heart disease, osteoporosis, a flagging immune system, neurodegeneration and other chronic disorders . . . Certain vitamins, particularly vitamins E, C and beta-carotene, may help prevent cancer by scavenging free radical molecules that might harm the cell's fragile genetic material . . . Antioxidant compounds may also battle cardiovascular disease . . . [and] prevent the body from turning otherwise innocuous cholesterol into a sticky and reactive form that can clog the arteries and set the stage for heart attacks . . . By disarming free radicals, vitamins seem to guard against cellular and genetic mayhem.

Antioxidant nutrients

Vitamin C
Humans are among only a handful of species on the planet who cannot manufacture there own supplies of vitamin C from glucose and must therefore replenish their supplies daily from dietary sources. Why daily? Because vitamin C is a water-soluble vitamin, which means that whatever supplies are not immediately used are quickly excreted in the urine. In fact, the biochemical activity of vitamin C lasts only six hours in the human system, regardless of whether it's ingested in food or as pills, so it's best to replenish your supplies three times per day.

The brain and central nervous system have such enormous needs for vitamin C that they actually operate 'vitamin-C pumps' to extract it from the circulating blood and concentrate it in the cerebrospinal fluid, where its level is ten times greater than in the blood. From the cerebrospinal fluid, another pump transfers vitamin C directly into the sheaths enveloping brain and nerve cells, concentrating it by another factor of ten, which means that the cells of the brain and central nervous system are bathed in a solution of vitamin C that is 100 times more concentrated than in blood plasma and other bodily fluids. Vitamin C is obviously very important to the health of brain and nerve cells.

The body concentrates vitamin C around brain and nerve cells specifically to protect them from oxidation and free-radical damage, because vitamin C is one of nature's most powerful antioxidants. The recommended daily amount (RDA) of 60 mg of vitamin C set by the US Food and Drug Administration is not even enough for normal nutritional needs, much less for viable protection from free-radical damage in the brain and spinal cord. Here again we see a link to the tenets of traditional Chinese medicine, which cites the spinal cord as a central pillar of the human immune system. Without sufficient supplies of vitamin C, the spinal cord deteriorates from chronic free-radical damage caused by lipid peroxidation, and the entire body then becomes vulnerable to disease and degeneration because of faulty communication between brain and body and impairment of biofeedback between the nervous and immune systems.

Vitamin C also protects other tissues from free-radical damage. Whenever it encounters a free radical, it sacrifices one of its own electrons in order to 'pacify' and neutralize the intruder, destroying itself in the process. This running battle between vitamin C and free radicals occurs hundreds of thousands of times per second, and if you fail to supply your body with adequate quantities of this friendly free-radical scavenger, the enemy will eventually erode your body by attrition.

Vitamin C may be taken in remarkably high doses without toxic side effects. You'd have to take about three pounds in one day to reach a lethal dose. Reports that large doses of vitamin C can cause kidney stones have been found to be without scientific basis. The easiest way to find your own individual limit for this vitamin is to take increasingly larger doses until you start to experience diarrhoea. This is known as the 'bowel tolerance' level and indicates that your tissues are saturated with vitamin C. By slightly reducing your dosage from bowel-tolerance level you will arrive at your own maximum therapeutic dosage. For most people, bowel tolerance is well over 20 grams per day, although in times of disease or distress, your body's capacity to assimilate and utilize vitamin C rises dramatically. Dr William Cathcart III of Nevada has successfully used megadoses of vitamin C up to 100 grams per day to treat AIDS, cancer, pneumonia, hepatitis, and other diseases regarded as 'incurable' by the medical establishment. For healthy adults, anywhere from 2 to 6 grams per day is a good maintenance dose, and this may be doubled during periods of extreme stress or disease.

Vitamin E

Vitamin E is a fat-soluble vitamin, which means that it operates primarily in fatty solutions, such as the cerebrospinal fluid. Scientific evidence suggests that vitamin E, unlike most other vitamins, does not function in any way as a nutritional building block. Instead, its sole role seems to be antioxidant defence against free-radical damage. It has also been shown that vitamin E works best in combination with selenium, and that the antioxidant protection provided by this synergistic team exceeds the sum of the two alone.

Since vitamin E is fat-soluble, it plays a primary role in protecting delicate brain and nerve cells from free-radical damage, and here it works synergistically not only with selenium, but also with vitamin C. The combination of vitamins E and C with the mineral selenium thus form a very powerful combination of free-radical scavengers, particularly in the brain and nervous system. The RDA of 15 IU (international units) of vitamin E set by the US FDA is regarded as absurdly low by most experienced nutritional scientists, who recommend instead a daily dosage range of 400–800 IU under normal conditions, and 1,200 IU under conditions of disease or distress.

Betacarotene/vitamin A

Vitamin A is a fat-soluble nutrient found only in foods from animal sources, whereas betacarotene ('provitamin A') is a plant-source nutrient from which the body produces its own vitamin A. Since vitamin A can be toxic at high dosages, it's best to take this nutrient in the form of betacarotene, which the body converts into vitamin A exactly according to requirements.

In addition to its role as a precursor of vitamin A, betacarotene itself has potent antioxidant properties and neutralizes two of the most dangerous types of free radicals: polyunsaturated-fat radicals and singlet-oxygen radicals. The latter variety of free radical, which is produced as a natural by-product of metabolism as well as by exposure to ultraviolet rays, is particularly reactive and highly destructive to cells, and betacarotene is the only known defence against singlet-oxygen radicals. Betacarotene is one of the prime defenders of the body's mucous membranes, especially in the lungs and gastrointestinal tract, which makes it an excellent preventive against lung and intestinal cancers.

The best dietary sources of betacarotene are the red pigment vegetables, such as carrots, papayas, pumpkins, and squashes, and the cruciferous family of vegetables, including cauliflower, broccoli, Brussels sprouts, and cabbage. Other potent dietary sources of betacarotene include chlorella, spirulina, wheat grass juice, and green barley-grass extract. Few people, however, consume sufficient quantities of these vegetables to provide adequate antioxidant protection, so it's a good idea to take daily supplements as well.

Nutritional scientists recommend that adults take a daily supplement of 20,000–50,000 IU of betacarotene, depending upon health conditions. For children, dosages are substantially lower and may be taken in the form of one or two teaspoons of cod-liver oil, which is a good source of prefabricated vitamin A. Adults using betacarotene should also take daily supplements of zinc, because the vitamin A produced by the body from betacarotene is stored in the liver, which requires zinc to mobilize it to other parts of the body. About 25 mg of zinc per day suffices for this purpose, but since zinc is also required for the synthesis of the antioxidant enzyme SOD, it's best to take about 50 mg per day.

Vitamin B complex
Certain of the B vitamins provide potent antioxidant protection, particularly to cells of the brain and central nervous system, but since they are part of a synergistic family that works best as a team, they should all be taken together.

Vitamin B_1 (thiamine) protects nerve cells and their connective fibres from free radicals produced by peroxidation of lipids as well as by alcohol abuse. B_5 (pantothenic acid) is a potent antioxidant as well as a highly effective enhancer of mental and physical stamina. B_6 (pyridoxine) functions as a radical scavenger and is also an important cofactor in the synthesis of vital neurochemicals from amino acids. The other major B vitamins are B_3 (niacin), which enhances cerebral functions and in high doses also lowers blood cholesterol, and B_{12}, which also improves cerebral functions and protects nerve cells from free-radical damage.

Adults should take 50–100 mg per day of each of the B vitamins, except for B_{12}, which should not exceed 1 mg (1,000 mcg) per day. Additional doses of specific B vitamins may be taken for specific purposes, such as 2–3 grams of niacin per day to lower serum cholesterol or treat schizophrenia, or 500 mg of B_5 to increase mental and physical stamina.

Amino acids

Amino acids are the building blocks with which the body synthesizes the various complex proteins it requires, including all neurochemicals. Some amino acids also function as potent antioxidants, particularly cysteine, taurine, glutamate, and methionine. A supplemental dose of one gram per day of these amino acids will significantly enhance your overall antioxidant defence system, especially if taken in conjunction with vitamins B_5 and B_6, which work as synergistic cofactors with most amino acids. As the precursors to neurochemicals, other amino acids such as choline, arginine, and phenylalanine, when taken in conjunction with synergistic vitamin cofactors, help sustain optimum cerebral functions by insuring adequate supplies of vital neurochemicals.

Antioxidant herbs

Besides vitamins, minerals, and amino acids, a variety of medicinal herbs also provide potent antioxidant protection to various tissues of the body. A few of these are briefly discussed below.

Ginseng

Known in Chinese medicine as the 'King of the Myriad Medicines', ginseng has been used in China since the dawn of history as a health and longevity supplement. Ginseng regulates heartbeat and blood pressure, controls blood sugar, stimulates memory, learning, and other cerebral functions, enhances digestion and assimilation of nutrients, increases resistance to stress, eliminates fatigue, and otherwise normalizes vital functions. It is also an effective free-radical scavenger throughout the system.

There are many different types of ginseng on the market, with varying degrees of potency and purity. People with high blood pressure should avoid using high dosages until their blood pressure has returned to normal. Generally speaking, the red variety is more potent and aggressive and is most appropriate for use in winter, while the white variety is milder and more suitable for use in summer or in hot tropical climates. Doses of 500–3,000 mg per day are recommended for therapeutic purposes.

Milk thistle

Silymarin, the active ingredient in a herb called milk thistle (*Silybum marianum*), is a remarkably potent antioxidant which specifically protects the liver from free-radical damage caused by liver toxins, including alcohol and drugs. It prevents the depletion of the antioxidant enzyme glutathione peroxidase, which is rapidly destroyed by alcohol, and stimulates the synthesis of the proteins the liver requires to mend itself.

Ginkgo

Ginkgo biloba, which at 300 million years old is the most ancient species of tree on the planet, has been used for thousands of years as a cerebral and cardiovascular tonic in Chinese medicine. It is extensively used in Europe, where physicians write over one million prescriptions per month for it. It is a potent antioxidant which specifically protects the brain and the liver. It also improves cerebral circulation, enhances brain metabolism, prevents hardening of the arteries, and increases the production of the universal energy molecule adenosine triphosphate (ATP). Some physicians have reported success in treating Parkinson's as well as Alzheimer's disease with ginkgo extracts.

Ginkgo is nontoxic even at very high doses and is inexpensive and readily available in healthfood shops. Extracts that contain a 24 per cent concentration of the active ingredient should be taken in doses of about 150 mg per day; lower-potency products require doses of up to 1 gram per day.

There are probably many other herbs in the Chinese pharmacopoeia with potent antioxidant properties, but so far not enough research has been conducted on this aspect of Chinese herbs to draw any firm conclusions. Many of the Chinese tonic herbs, which are used to enhance sexual potency, boost immunity, and improve cerebral functions, probably have potent antioxidant properties. Since tonic herbs are known to promote longevity, it stands to reason that they protect the body against its primary aging agents, free radicals. Antioxidant herbs work best in conjunction with synergistic antioxidant nutrients, such as vitamins A, C, and E, the minerals zinc and selenium, and various amino acids. The author's own herbal-nutrient antioxidant formula is available under the Vital Herb label.

Nootropics: Better living through neurochemistry

Like longevity, intelligence is not predetermined at birth, but can be enhanced by the judicious use of nutrients, antioxidants, and a new class of synthetic drugs called 'nootropics', which specifically stimulate and improve the functions of the brain. Derived from a

Greek root which means 'to influence the mind', the word 'noo-tropic' refers to a class of cerebroactive compounds, or 'smart drugs', which have been conclusively proven to improve memory and learning, enhance alertness and cerebral energy, stimulate cerebral circulation and metabolism, protect brain cells from free-radical damage, and increase the synthesis and activity of neurotransmitters, through which brain cells communicate with each other. Some amino acids and herbs also have nootropic properties. Nootropics are without question one of the most exciting discoveries of the New Alchemy.

Nootropics function in three ways:

● They stimulate the production, secretion, and activity of vital neurotransmitters, such as acetylcholine, noradrenaline, and dopamine.
● They enhance cerebral circulation of nutrients and oxygen by increasing the flow of blood to the brain.
● They stimulate the synthesis of the various complex proteins which the brain requires to repair dendrites, the long spindly fibres through which neurotransmitters carry messages between brain cells. Brain cells are irreplaceable once they die, but most cerebral impairments are caused by damage to dendrites, which can be repaired and regrown with proper nutrition and cerebral supplements.

All the body's biological clocks, which determine the rate at which the body ages and dies, are located in the brain, including the all-important pineal and pituitary glands. Nootropics can actually 'rewind' these clocks to set back the aging process and give you a new lease on life. The fact is that the body is only as healthy as the brain which commands it, and most degenerative conditions are either caused by cerebral malfunctions or else cause cerebral deficiencies which then further accelerate the degenerative conditions. Nootropic drugs can be important weapons in the battle against premature degeneration, senility, and death.

Below we'll take a brief look at five of the most promising new nootropic drugs developed by the Western pharmaceutical industry in Europe; then we'll discuss some of the most effective nootropic nutrients, or 'brain foods', as well as a few common Chinese herbs that have nootropic properties.

Nootropic drugs

Piracetum

Developed in Belgium and marketed under the label Nootropil, piracetum is the drug whose invention gave birth to the new category of cerebroactive pharmaceuticals known as nootropics. Virtually nontoxic (vitamin C is more toxic in megadoses than piracetum) and completely nonaddictive, piracetum may be taken in large doses over prolonged periods of time with no adverse side effects. It has been shown to improve memory, enhance learning capacity, and prevent senility. One of its most intriguing effects is to increase neural communication between the right and left hemispheres of the brain, thereby combining rational and intuitive cognition and stimulating creativity.

Piracetum is highly synergistic with the nootropic drug hydergine (see below) and the amino acid choline, which is the nutrient precursor of the neurotransmitter acetylcholine. Taken together, these three nootropics provide a potent boost to cerebral functions. Most people start out with a megadose of 3–4 grams for the first two days, then reduce the dosage to 1,600–2,400 mg per day, in three separate doses. When piracetum is taken in combination with hydergine and choline, the dosage may be further reduced to 800–1,600 mg per day.

Hydergine

Hydergine is the brainchild of Dr Albert Hofmann of Switzerland, one of the world's most gifted alchemists. It is refined from an extract of a rye mould called ergot, from which the same alchemist accidentally discovered the psychedelic drug LSD, which he calls his 'problem child'. Hydergine, however, has no psychedelic properties whatsoever. Instead, it has become the world's most widely used nootropic compound.

One of the most frequently tested pharmaceuticals, hydergine has been repeatedly proven to be nontoxic and safe for human use over long periods of time. Its proven effects include the following:

- Increases the supply of blood and oxygen to the brain.
- Stimulates cerebral metabolism.
- Inhibits the activity of free radicals in the brain.
- Protects the brain from damage during periods of oxygen deprivation.
- Removes deposits of lipofuscin ('age spots') from brain cells.
- Enhances memory, learning, and intelligence.
- Eliminates fatigue.

In France, hospital emergency rooms immediately administer an intravenous injection of hydergine to all patients who arrive in shock, coma, or other conditions which deprive the brain of oxygen. This increases the time physicians have to treat the patient before permanent brain damage occurs from about five minutes to forty-five minutes. When administered early enough, hydergine has been shown to alleviate the symptoms of Altzheimer's disease and other forms of senile dementia.

Hydergine seems to mimic the activity of a neurochemical called 'nerve growth factor', which stimulates synthesis of the cerebral proteins the brain needs to repair and regrow dendrites. When taken orally, about half the dosage ends up in the liver, where the drug's potent antioxidant properties help prevent free-radical damage. This makes hydergine an excellent supplement for recovering alcoholics and drug addicts.

Hydergine is available only by prescription in the USA, but it is sold over the counter almost everywhere else in the world. The standard US dosage of 3 mg per day is regarded as ineffective by physicians in Europe, where the standard dosage is 9 mg per day. It comes in oral and sublingual tablets, the latter delivering a higher concentration of hydergine to the brain. It is synergistic with piracetum, choline, and centrophenoxine.

Centrophenoxine

Marketed under the Lucidril label, centrophenoxine boosts intelligence, improves memory, removes lipofuscin deposits from brain cells, repairs synapses between nerve cells, and functions as a potent free-radical scavenger in the brain. Like hydergine, it also protects the brain from damage during periods of oxygen deprivation. It is nontoxic and easily tolerated, except by individuals with chronic hypertension or involuntary muscular convulsions. Centrophenoxine is usually administered in dosages of 1–2 grams per day, in two or three separate doses.

GH-3, KH-3

Originally developed as an anti-aging drug by Dr Ana Aslan in Romania, GH-3 (Gerovital) is composed of procaine hydrochloride, vitamin B_6, mesoinositol, and the neuroactive amino acid glutamic acid. It is also produced in Germany under the KH-3 label.

One of the most popular anti-aging compounds in the world, GH-3 has been shown to increase oxygen supplies to the brain, relieve chronic depression, enhance cerebral energy, and inhibit an enzyme called monoamine oxidase, which breaks down vital neurotransmitters such as dopamine, serotonin, and nora-drenaline.

The normal dosage schedule for GH-3 is to take one capsule in the morning every day for one month, then stop for a month or two, and resume again for another month, and so on.

Vasopressin

Vasopressin is a stimulating brain hormone secreted by the posterior lobe of the pituitary gland. A synthetic analogue of vasopressin is marketed in the form of a nasal spray under the Diapid label. Stimulant drugs such as cocaine and amphetamines produce their characteristic high by causing the pituitary rapidly to secrete its supplies of vasopressin, resulting in a brief rush of exhilaration followed by the familiar burnout syndrome. Conversely, marijuana, opium, and alcohol suppress vasopressin secretion in the pituitary, thereby causing the dopy feeling associated with excess use of these drugs. A few whiffs of Diapid usually suffice to eliminate either one of these side effects of recreational drug use.

Vasopressin is a cognitive enhancer which significantly increases the brain's capacity to assimilate and process new information. As such, it is a highly effective learning aid. It improves both long-term and short-term memory, increases attention span and concentration, and facilitates the imprinting of newly learned information. As a nasal spray, it is immediately absorbed by the mucous membranes in the sinuses and usually takes effect in about ten seconds. Three sprays in each nostril once or twice a day is an appropriate dosage level, but it's best not to use it on a daily basis, in order to avoid building up a tolerance to its effects. Use it whenever you need a quick mental lift, such as before an important meeting or exam, or whenever an extra cerebral boost is needed for prolonged periods of concentration, such as writing or memorizing new information.

Nootropic nutrients

Popularly known as 'brain food', nootropic nutrients are natural nutritional elements which enhance memory, cognition, and other cerebral functions. The key nutrients for this purpose are various amino acids – particularly arginine, choline, and phenylalanine – which are the building blocks the brain requires to synthesize neurotransmitters. However, in order for these amino acids to be converted into neurotransmitters, they must be taken together with the synergistic vitamin and mineral cofactors required to synthesize them.

In recent years, the American research scientists Durk Pearson and Sandy Shaw have decoded many of the nutritional formulas the brain uses to synthesize neurotransmitters. Based on their own extensive research and experimentation, they have formulated a series of cerebroactive nutrient drink powders with pronounced nootropic effects. These cerebral supplements are highly recommended by the author and may be ordered from the supplier listed in the Appendix.

Among the most effective nootropic nutrients are the following:

Arginine

In the 5 July 1990 issue of the *New York Times*, a front-page banner headline announced: 'Human Growth Hormone Reverses the Effects of Aging.' The article proceeded to describe how a synthetic form of growth hormone had dramatically reversed the symptoms of aging in an extensive scientific study. Unfortunately, the price tag for this therapy is $20,000–30,000 per year.

Pearson and Shaw, however, found an equally effective but far less expensive way to increase growth-hormone levels in the brain. By combining 6 grams of arginine with 600 mg of choline, 500 mg of vitamin B_5, and other nutrient cofactors, they created a formula that causes the pituitary to increase its secretions of growth hormone, thereby boosting immunity, increasing energy, and enhancing cerebral as well as sexual functions. This formula is particularly beneficial to body builders, professional athletes, and those who engage in hard labour. It is also strengthens the immune system and promotes rapid healing in cases of severe wounds such as broken bones, lacerations, and internal injuries.

Choline

Choline is the amino acid required by the brain to synthesize the neurotransmitter acetylcholine, which is the key neurochemical involved in memory and learning. Combined with the cofactors vitamin B_6, B_{12}, C, and others, choline increases the brain's supply of acetylcholine and thereby enhances cognition. It has also been shown to prevent rash emotional outbursts and improve sexual functions. Choline and its requisite cofactors are highly synergistic with all nootropic drugs, causing a manifold enhancement in their therapeutic benefits. You need to take about one gram of choline per dose, in combination with cofactors, to get the desired effects. A synergistically balanced choline drink formula is available from the supplier listed in the Appendix. The most common dietary source of choline is fish, which is why seafood is popularly known as 'brain food'.

Phenylalanine

Do you feel sluggish, fatigued, and foggy upon arising in the morning? If so, it may be due to a critical deficiency of the neuro-transmitter noradrenaline, which your brain produces from pheny-lalanine. Stumble into the kitchen and stir up a heaping tablespoon of Pearson and Shaw's phenylalanine nutrient powder in a glass of water, chug it down, and feel the cerebral power surge up from your stomach into your brain. The author likes to boost this formula with two teaspoons of bee pollen, two tablespoons of honey, a dropperful of DMAE (see below), and 25 drops each of liquid ginseng and *Ginkgo biloba* extract, all stirred together in warm (but not hot) water and taken first thing in the morning on an empty stomach, just before *chee-gung* practice.

Noradrenaline is the adrenaline of the brain, a stimulating neu-rotransmitter which greatly enhances cerebral energy and quickens cerebral response. This is another one of the neurochemicals released in the brain under the influence of caffeine, cocaine, amphetamines, and other stimulants, which rapidly use up the brain's supply of noradrenaline, leaving the user feeling wiped out. L-phenylalanine, plus its cofactors (chiefly vitamin B_6, also B_{12} and C), provides the raw materials required to synthesize and release fresh supplies of noradrenaline, without depleting the brain's own natural supply. Besides increasing cerebral energy, noradrenaline enhances memory and learning, heightens sensory perception, facilitates concentration, and has been shown to be a highly effec-tive remedy for chronic depression.

DMAE

Dimethylaminoethanol is a nutrient normally present in the brain. It occurs naturally in seafood, especially sardines and anchovies, and is known to be one of the most potent of all brain foods. It improves memory and learning, heightens intelligence, elevates mood, and increases both mental and physical energy. It accelerates the brain's synthesis of acetylcholine, which makes it a good syner-gist for choline supplements. It comes in powder, capsule, or liquid form and may taken in doses of 250–1,000 mg per day, preferably in the morning. An analogue of the DMAE compound is marketed as a nootropic drug under the Deaner label.

Niacin

Also called vitamin B_3, niacin increases circulation of blood to the brain and has been shown to enhance memory, learning, and other cerebral functions. It often causes a flushing sensation, causing the skin to itch and turn red, but this is a harmless side effect of its vasodilating properties. With prolonged use, this effect tends to diminish. A large dose of niacin is one of the most rapid and reliable ways to pull a person out of a bad trip on psychedelic drugs. A synthetic form of niacin called xanthinol nicotinate has been shown in several studies to be even more effective than ordinary niacin. It's best to start out on low doses of niacin for the first week or two, such as 50–100 mg per day, then gradually increase the dosage up to 250–500 mg per day. Daily amounts of 2–3 grams, taken in three separate doses with meals, are required for schizophrenia, chronic violence, and adverse drug reactions. These doses have also proven highly effective in lowering blood cholesterol. Xanithol nicotinate may be taken in daily amounts of 900–1,800 mg, divided into three separate doses with meals.

Nootropic herbs

Ginseng and *Ginkgo biloba* have already been mentioned as herbal antioxidants. Owing to the significant enhancement of cerebral circulation which they effect, they also have potent nootropic properties, for which they have been used for thousands of years in the Far East.

Another herb with strong nootropic properties is the Chinese tonic herb *Epimedium sagittatum*, commonly known as 'horny goat weed' because of its aphrodisiac effects. Epimedium dramatically increases blood circulation in minute capillaries, such as in the brain and genital organs. Besides sexual debility, Chinese physicians prescribe it as a remedy for absent-mindedness and poor memory. According to the *chee-gung* teacher Luo Teh-hsiou of Taiwan, one of this herb's primary benefits is direct stimulation of pituitary-gland secretions, including growth hormone, which regulates immune as well as sexual functions. Here we find another example of the ancient Chinese premise that immunity, sexual vitality, and cerebral functions are intimately related and mutually dependent.

The bronchial dilating herb ephedra, one of the oldest herbs in the Chinese pharmacopoeia, also has nootropic benefits. It is the model from which the Western pharmaceutical industry developed the synthetic analogue ephedrine, which is the base of many amphetamine compounds and should not be used owing to its deleterious side effects. However, natural ephedra may be safely used. In addition to its bronchial dilating and nootropic properties, ephedra has been shown to stimulate the body to burn off excess fat, which makes it a good remedy for obesity. If you're overweight, have respiratory problems, and need a cerebral lift, ephedra is the herb for you. Pearson and Shaw have developed a nutrient drink formula based on ephedra, available through the supplier listed in the Appendix. It's best not to use it after sunset, unless you wish to stay up till the crack of dawn.

Balancing cerebral energy

Our brains consist of about one billion neurons, all packed into the compact cranial case we carry around on our shoulders. These neurons communicate constantly with one another via electrochemical signals transmitted across their synapses by neurotransmitters. Like a computer that is never switched off, the brain continuously processes incoming data, monitors the body's vital functions, and orchestrates a multitude of biochemical activities every moment. All this cerebral activity requires a steady input of cerebral energy, just as a computer must remain plugged into a live electrical source in order to continue executing its programs.

As noted earlier, the brain's circuitry generates a constant flow of direct electrical currents, which is turn produce the 'halo' of an electromagnetic field around the head. As forms of pure energy, the electric currents and magnetic fields of the brain are influenced by and interact with any other energy fields which penetrate or overlap them by proximity. Just as a computer can go haywire when exposed to abnormal electric currents, magnetic fields, or microwave radiation, so the human brain can get short-circuited or overloaded by abnormal energy input. Whenever that happens, cerebral energy loses its natural balance and the brain malfunctions, invariably causing problems down the line of the central nervous system, such as loss of immunity, sexual debility, lack of energy, physical degeneration, mental confusion, aberrant behaviour, and so forth. One of the primary purposes of Taoist internal alchemy is to restore and maintain the natural balance of cerebral energy which the brain requires to function and fulfil the myriad tasks of regulating the body and protecting it against disease and degeneration. Nutrition, nootropics, and antioxidants all help maintain cerebral balance on the fundamental level of essence, while *chee-gung* and meditation work directly with energy to restore cerebral equilibrium.

According to Taoist alchemy, we have seen that emotions constitute a form of aberrant energy which severely disrupts the balance of the human energy system, particularly in the brain. Let's take a look at this traditional Eastern view from the angle of modern Western science. Western medical science has identified a family of neurochemicals called 'endorphins' and 'enkephalins', which in molecular structure and biochemical function are very similar to opiates. One type recently identified at Stanford University is 200 times more potent than morphine. These neurochemicals provide us with feelings of wellbeing, pleasure, comfort, and calm, and in times of traumatic injury they insulate us from pain. Whenever deficiencies in our supplies of these opiates of the brain occur, we suffer from anxiety, hypertension, malaise, depression, migraine headaches, pain, and other unpleasant symptoms.

It is a scientifically established fact that emotions directly influence the secretion of endorphins and enkephalins in the brain. Emotional agitation has been shown to inhibit these secretions, and if emotional imbalance is permitted to continue for days and weeks on end, as is so common in modern industrial societies, the somatic consequences can become quite severe. By contrast, emotional tranquillity and mental calm stimulate abundant secretions of these natural cerebral opiates, which may well account for the intense bliss that many meditators report whenever they manage to enter and sustain states of deep tranquillity. Many of the therapeutic benefits of meditation are achieved by enhancing the biochemical activity of cerebral essence and energy.

Chee-gung, meditation, and other traditional techniques for rebalancing cerebral energy are highly effective methods for counteracting and remedying the disruptive influence of electromagnetic pollution. The same modern technology that created these hazards has also given birth to high-tech devices for fighting fire with fire, and latterday Taoists would be well advised to include some of these tools in their practice.

Cranial electro-stimulation (CES) is one such method. CES works directly with the brain's own electromsgnetic energy to restore cerebral energy balance and counteract the effects of electropollution. Working through the same bioenergy systems used in *chee-gung* and meditation, CES stimulates the synthesis and secretion of the full spectrum of vital neurochemicals, including hormones, neurotransmitters, and endorphins. Among the problems which CES effectively corrects are emotional instability, poor memory, impaired learning, drug addiction, aberrant behaviour, fatigue, chronic depression, immune deficiency, and sexual dysfunction.

Another device which helps maintain optimum cerebral balance amid the aberrant electromagnetic fields of contemporary environments is the pulsed scalar field generator, a small battery-operated apparatus worn on the body or carried in a pocket to ward off abnormal electromagnetic fields and microwave radiation. Tuned to the earth's normal pulse of 7.83 cycles per second, these electromagnetic harmonizers create a shell of normal energy pulsations around you, protecting body and brain from the aberrant influence of electromagnetic pollution.

There are many other devices which work along similar lines, including copper and silk biocircuits, negative-ion generators, harmonically pulsed light and sound machines, flotation tanks, magnetic plates and patches, and so forth. These tools are worth exploring for their energy-balancing, cerebral-enhancing, and health-promoting benefits, for they represent the latest discoveries in the ongoing Taoist tradition of harnessing science to serve rather than enslave humanity.

Grafting Eastern and Western alchemy

Traditional Taoist alchemy cites food, water, and air as the sources of the postnatal Fire energy that causes human degeneration. Could this be the same agent of human aging that modern medical scientists identify as 'free radicals'? And is it not possible that the rejuvenating Water energy obtained from the 'original essence' of hormones and enzymes function similarly to what modern science refers to as 'antioxidants'? Free radicals are generated internally by the 'fire' of postnatal metabolism and are assimilated externally from polluted food, water, and air. Like a fire out of control, they 'burn up' human tissues, and the only thing that keeps them from totally incinerating our bodies is the cooling antioxidant activity of 'original essence' such as superoxide dismutase, glutathione peroxidase, and other enzymes, as well as various essential nutrients, which work like 'water' to quench free radicals and extinguish the biochemical brush fires they ignite in our tissues.

Whether you take ginseng or vitamin C, practise *chee-gung* or wear a pulsed scalar field device, meditate in the lotus position or lie in the stillness and silence of a flotation tank, it's all part of the Taoist alchemy of harmonizing the Three Treasures of essence, energy, and spirit to promote health, prolong life, and cultivate spiritual awareness. Latterday Taoists who insist on utilizing only 'traditional' methods are as prejudiced against progress and as blind to new ideas as conventional practitioners of modern science who sneer at ancient traditions simply because they do not conform to their own preconceived notions of 'science'. Far more research needs to be conducted in order to reveal the common denominators linking traditional Taoist and modern Western sciences, whose apparent contradictions may be more a matter of terminology than substance. In the meantime, Eastern and Western Taoists already share sufficient common ground to graft the various branches of their respective theories and practices and develop a hybrid tree of health, longevity, and spiritual development that produces far sweeter fruits than either one could possibly yield alone.

PART V

Precious Prescriptions:
Harvesting the Tree of Health

CHAPTER 24

Tonic Herbs and Formulas

With the aid of external tonics, we are better able to cultivate the internal elixir within.

Master Hui Ssu (sixth century AD)

The category of herbs known as 'tonic medicine' (*bu yao*) are called
'Superior Herbs' and are the most highly prized plants in the entire
Chinese pharmacopoeia. They also constitute the most important
type of supplement in traditional Taoist training programmes.

Western allopathic medicine doesn't even recognize tonics as a
legitimate class of medication, because allopathic medicine is
geared entirely towards using drugs to treat diseases that have
already developed, rather than preventing disease with tonic
supplements. If everyone learned the secrets of keeping their own
bodies healthy, allopathic doctors would go out of business.

The most important point to understand about tonic herbs is that
they are meant to be used exclusively by healthy people to maintain health and prevent disease, boost vitality and prolong life. In
China, Taoist adepts used to apply the extra essence and energy
derived from tonics to accelerate their progress in practice, while
wealthy gentlemen utilized them as sexual tonics to boost their
capacity to satisfy the many wives and concubines they kept in
their households. Because of the close connections between sexual
and neurological secretions, tonics may also be used to improve
memory, learning, concentration, mental stamina, and other
cerebral functions, and to enhance creativity. By nourishing essence
and stimulating its transformation into energy, tonic supplements
provide a potent and reliable source of vitality that may be applied
to whatever activities you choose.

If you fall ill, even if it's only a common cold, you should
immediately cease using tonics and resort instead to curative
remedies and nutritional supplements to correct your condition

and restore your health before resuming use of tonics. Tonic herbs are potent medicines that can be utilized only by strong, flourishing energy systems. If you're weak or ill when you take them, they'll overheat your system and compound your problems.

Tonic herbs and formulas have a wide range of beneficial effects in the human system. They stimulate production of hormone essence, enhance overall energy, increase surface resistance, improve internal immunity, boost cerebral functions, tonify tissues, strengthen sexual vitality, and prolong life. They stimulate, balance, and harmonize the major functional energy systems in the body: they balance yin and yang; harmonize the Five Elemental Energies of the organs; strengthen the Four Foundations of health (blood, energy, nourishment, resistance); and facilitate the internal alchemy of the Three Treasures. They are used with equal efficacy in the martial, meditational, and medical arts and are regarded as our greatest natural allies in the quest for health and longevity.

Owing to their stimulatory affinity for vital glands and organs, tonics simultaneously enhance the three basic energy systems that rely most on secretions of vital essence: immunity, sexual potency, and cerebral function. As we have seen, these three systems are closely related and mutually dependent. Strong sexual potency is associated with high immunity and mental clarity, while low immunity is almost always accompanied by sexual debility and poor cerebral function. This is due to biofeedback between the hormones of the endocrine system and the neurotransmitters of the nervous system. Tonics are a great way to maintain high levels of hormone secretions, which in turn have a positive influence on neurochemicals through biofeedback.

Another benefit of tonic supplements is that they enhance the body's ability to adapt swiftly to climatic and environmental changes and help human energies harmonize with the cyclic changes of nature. Through their associations with the Five Elemental Energies and their corresponding affinities to various internal organ-energy systems, tonic herbs amplify human energies with the basic forces of nature and harmonize the human system with the environment.

Types of tonic

There are four major categories of tonic herbs and formulas, each associated with a basic human system of essence and energy. Depending on your condition and requirements, you may select individual herbs or compound formulas which specifically boost one or two of these systems, or you may use formulas which tonify and balance all four systems. The four major types of tonic supplement are briefly described below.

Energy tonics

Energy tonics are used to increase the body's available supply of vital energy. They act primarily upon the lung and spleen organ-energy systems: the lungs extract energy from air, and the spleen extracts energy from food. By tonifying these organs, energy tonics enhance the body's production of energy from food and air.

Yang tonics

Yang tonics boost the body's supply of primal energy by stimulating and 'warming' the kidney organ-energy system. Yang deficiency is usually associated with impaired kidney function and includes such symptoms as cold hands and feet, impotence, premature ejaculation, urinary incontinence, poor memory, and low immunity.With their potent benefits for sexual vitality, yang tonics are renowned as highly effective aphrodisiacs. They also improve cerebral functions and enhance immunity. However, they should be used only by people with either yang deficiency or balanced yin/yang levels. If taken by people with yang excess and/or yin deficiency, they will overheat the system and cause energy imbalance. Owing to their heating properties, yang tonics are excellent winter supplements but should be used sparingly in hot weather.

Blood tonics

Blood tonics are used to nourish the blood in cases of weak blood (anaemia), insufficient circulation, and other blood deficiencies. They are of particular benefit to the female reproductive system, including fertility, sexual response, menstrual regularity, and related functions. They appear in almost all compound tonic formulas in order to insure optimum circulation of the other ingredients.

Yin tonics

Yin tonics nourish the yin energy of the kidneys, lungs, stomach, and liver and enhance the body's secretions of vital fluids. They supply the fluids required for production of blood plasma, semen, spinal fluids, lymph, and mucus. They are applied primarily in cases of excess heat and dryness, as well as for yin deficiency and/or yang excess.

Generally speaking, energy and yang tonics fall into the same basic category and primarily benefit men, while blood and yin tonics are related and are of most benefit to women. However, there are also women who require external supplements of yang and men who need to take yin supplements to maintain internal energy balance. It all depends on your individual condition, your external environment, and your practical requirements. A sexually active adept might wish to take daily doses of yang tonics, while an adept who is concentrating on solitary meditation practice would benefit more from soothing yin tonics. The best way to determine your personal preferences in tonics is to experiment with individual herbs as well as compound formulas under different conditions, until you discover the items and combinations that suit you best.

Methods of preparation

As noted earlier, traditional Chinese herbal formulas are blended according to the principle of synergy among the primary and secondary herbs used. The 'imperial' herb is the chief active ingredient, the 'ministerial' herb enhances the effects of the main ingredients and promotes circulation of the entire formula, the 'assistant' herb counteracts undesirable side effects, and the 'servant' herb synergizes and balances the various energies within the formula.

Chinese herbal formulas may be prepared either at home or at the pharmacy, and some may be purchased as ready-to-take patent medicines, usually in the form of tablets or liquid extracts. The latter are introduced in Chapter 26. There are four primary methods of preparing herbal formulas for ingestion.

Decoction

Empty a packet of blended raw bulk herbs into a glass or ceramic cooking vessel (do not use metal) and add three cups of water. Bring to boil, cover, lower heat, and simmer slowly until the liquid is reduced to about one cup. Strain fluid into a cup, then add two more cups of water to the herbs, bring to boil, and simmer again until reduced to about one cup. Total yield is two cups. Drink one cup in the morning and one in the afternoon or evening, on an empty stomach. Continue for up to thirty days.

Powder

Most herbal pharmacies will grind bulk herbs into a fine powder for you. The powder may be stirred into a cup of hot water and drunk as a tea, or put into large (00-size) gelatin capsules for convenient storage and ingestion. Each capsule holds about 1 gram of powder. Typical dosages for powders in 1-gram capsules are two caps two or three times daily, taken with a cup of warm water, preferably on an empty stomach. Loose powder should be stirred into a cup of hot water in 2-gram doses and taken twice a day. Powder is the most convenient form of herbal supplement for travelling.

Paste and pills

To make paste, the bulk herbs are finely powdered and placed in a glass or ceramic bowl. Honey is then added to the powder and stirred in until a thick paste is formed, similar in consistency to bread dough. The paste is stored in a glass jar in the refrigerator and taken as needed. Average dosage for herbal paste is one tea-spoon twice a day, taken with a cup of warm water.

To make pills, use the thumb and index finger to pinch a small quantity of paste and roll it into a little round pellet, about the size of a pea. Lay the pills on a baking sheet and place in the oven under very low heat, or set out in the sun, until they are dry. Store in air-tight containers away from heat and light; refrigeration is not necessary. Take 3–6 pills three or four times per day, with warm water.

Spirits

This is probably the best way of all to take herbal tonics on a long-term basis. The alcohol extracts and preserves the most potent elements from the herbs and facilitates their rapid absorption into the bloodstream. Herbal spirits may be stored indefinitely without losing potency and are very convenient to take.

Place the roughly chopped bulk herbs in a glass or ceramic vessel and pour your choice of spirits over them. Best choices in liquor are vodka, rum, or brandy. Use 30–60 grams (1–2 ounces) of bulk herbs per litre of spirits. For convenience, it's best to steep herbal spirits in large quantities, such as 6–8 litres. The longer you let them steep, the more potent they become (up to one year), and the better the flavours blend and mellow. The authors method is to steep about 300 grams (10 ounces) of herbs in 6 litres of spirits for four or five months, then decant half the brew through a cloth filter into clean bottles and pour another 3 litres of fresh spirits into the remaining mixture and let it steep for another six months, for a total yield of 9 litres per batch. You may add a little honey or raw sugar to each bottle of decanted herbal spirits to enhance flavour and provide another metabolic catalyst.

A standard dose is one fluid ounce, taken on an empty stomach. In hot weather, do not take more than one ounce per day; if it is cold outside, you may take 2–3 ounces per day. Taken before meals, herbal spirits strongly stimulate the appetite. It's a good idea to keep two or three different batches brewing both for variety and to ensure a steady supply.

Tonic herbs and formulas

Briefly described below are some of the main tonic herbs and formulas used in Taoist training as well as general health and longevity programmes. These herbs may be taken individually, in combination with one or two other tonic herbs, or as compound herbal formulas. Readers are advised to experiment first with individual herbs in order to determine which ones provide you with the most noticeable benefits, then move on to simple combinations and complex formulas. Alternatively, you could visit an experienced Chinese physician for a general diagnosis of your condition and a specific analysis of your individual energy requirements, and ask him to recommend appropriate herbs and formulas for long-term use as tonic supplements.

The herbs and formulas introduced below should suffice to get you started on a regular programme of tonic herbal supplements. For best results, you should first detoxify your body with an internal cleansing routine, then commence herbal tonification in conjunction with proper diet and nutrition, *chee-gung*, sexual discipline, and other Taoist health regimens. Readers who wish to delve more deeply into the theory and practice of herbal medicine may refer to the author's book *Chinese Herbal Medicine*, and to other books on the subject listed under 'Recommended Reading'. For additional tonic herbal formulas, see *Shaolin and Taoist Herbal Training Formulas* by James Ramholz and *Chinese Tonic Herbs* by Ron Teeguarden.

Single herbs

Western name: Panax ginseng (ginseng)
Chinese name: ren-shen
Energy: warm
Flavour: sweet, slightly bitter
Organ-energy affinity: spleen, lungs

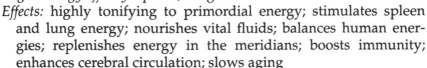

Effects: highly tonifying to primordial energy; stimulates spleen and lung energy; nourishes vital fluids; balances human energies; replenishes energy in the meridians; boosts immunity; enhances cerebral circulation; slows aging

Remarks: Known as 'King of the Myriad Herbs', ginseng is universally regarded as the best overall tonic for the human system. Generally, price reflects quality and potency in ginseng, although for long-term use as a tonic, ordinary grades suffice. The key to ginseng use is to take a small amount daily for prolonged periods of time; megadoses taken sporadically are of little benefit. You should avoid taking coffee, tea, soya beans, or turnips for at least two or three hours after using ginseng, because these items counteract its effects.

Western name: Astragalus membraneceus
Chinese name: huang-chi
Energy: slightly warm
Flavour: sweet
Organ-energy affinity: spleen, lungs, kidney

Effects: energy tonic; enhances protective *wei-chee* around the body; improves circulation in flesh and skin; regulates blood pressure and blood sugar; boosts immunity; promotes healing of wounds; increases kidney organ energy

Remarks: This herb is also a cardiotonic, which makes it a good choice for people with heart problems. Research has shown *Astragalus* to be a potent immune-system booster, especially in cancer patients undergoing radiation or chemotherapy. It also inhibits excess sweating and is an excellent supplement for controlling mild forms of diabetes.

Western name: Polygonum multiflorum (Chinese cornbind)
Chinese name: ho-shou-wu
Energy: slightly warm
Flavour: bitter, sour
Organ-energy affinity: liver, kidneys, heart

Effects: blood tonic; nourishes blood and semen; tonifies liver and kidneys; strengthens sinew, cartilage, and bone; mildly laxative; regulates blood pressure; prevents hardening of arteries

Remarks: This is a traditional Chinese anti-aging tonic found in many longevity formulas. It restores prematurely grey hair to its original colour and strengthens kidneys and entire lumbar region.

Western name: Cervus nippon (deer horn)
Chinese name: lu rung
Energy: warm
Flavour: sweet, salty

Organ-energy affinity: liver, kidneys

Effects: potent yang tonic; tonifies kidney yang; stimulates Fire energy; warms the Lower Elixir Field below the navel and the Gate of Life between the kidneys; nourishes semen, marrow, sinew, and cartilage; aphrodisiac; supports hormone production

Remarks: Deer horn is one of the most ancient and highly prized yang tonics in the entire Chinese pharmacopoeia. For full potency, the horn must be cut while it is still young and covered in velvet, when it is filled with blood and hormones. Mature, hard horn contains only about 10 per cent of the active essence found in soft young horn. The spotted sika deer native to northern China and Manchuria provides the best product, although other varieties are also used. In combination with ginseng, deer horn becomes an even stronger yang tonic and potent sexual elixir. High-grade deer horn is quite expensive and is therefore most economical when used as an ingredient in herbal spirits.

Western name: Epimedium sagittatum (horny goat weed)
Chinese name: yin-yang-huo (ARTWORK)
Energy: warm
Flavour: pungent

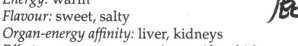

Organ-energy affinity: liver, kidneys

Effects: yang tonic; stimulates kidney-yang energy; dilates capillaries; enhances cerebral circulation; stimulates pituitary gland; aphrodisiac

Remarks: By dilating capillaries, this herb also lowers blood pressure. It simultaneously tonifies sexual, cerebral, and immune functions, both by enhancing circulation and by stimulating pituitary secretions. When included in formulas for tonic herbal spirits, it facilitates the circulation of other ingredients and amplifies their effects.

Western name: Schizandrae chinensis
Chinese name: wu-wei-dzu
Energy: warm

五 味 子

Flavour: sour, sweet, slightly salty, pungent, and bitter
Organ-energy affinity: kidneys, lungs
Effects: yin and yang tonic; astringent; tonic to kidney-yin energy; nourishes sexual fluids; boosts sexual stamina; stimulates hormone production; balances internal energies
Remarks: The name of this herb translates literally as 'five-flavour seeds'. Though primarily sour, it has traces of all Five Elemental Energies, which makes it an excellent general health tonic for men and women. A traditional method of using this herb is to take about 10 grams daily, either as decoction or powder, for 100 consecutive days, which is said to purify the blood, restore kidney energy, rejuvenate sexual vitality, clarify the mind and brighten the complexion.

Western name: Lycium chinensis (Chinese wolfberry)
Chinese name: gou-ji-dzu
Energy: neutral
Flavour: sweet

枸 杞 子

Organ-energy affinity: liver, kidneys
Effects: yin tonic; nourishes blood and semen, tonifies liver-yin and kidney-yin; improves vision, especially night vision; longevity tonic; builds strength in legs; calms heart and nervous system
Remarks: Decocted together with either ginseng or Rehmannia, this herb makes an effective sexual tonic. Included in most formulas for tonic herbal spirits for its synergy with other tonic herbs. Effective remedy in mild forms of diabetes. May be used as a tonic herb in cooking, especially in soups and stews.

Western name: Angelica sinensis (angelica)
Chinese name: dang-gui
Energy: warm
Flavour: sweet, pungent

當 歸

Organ-energy affinity: liver, spleen
Effects: blood tonic; tonifies spleen and liver; promotes circulation; sedative for nervous tension; controls internal and external bleeding; corrects menstrual disorders; promotes muscular endurance
Remarks: This is the most important blood tonic in Chinese herbal medicine, especially for women. Generally added to tonic herbal formulas to promote circulation and assimilation of other

ingredients. Combined with ginseng, it makes a well-balanced yin/yang, blood and energy tonic.

Western name: Eucommia ulmoides
Chinese name: du-jung
Energy: warm
Flavour: sweet

杜　　仲

Organ-energy affinity: liver, kidneys
Effects: yang tonic; tonifies liver-yang and kidney-yang; nourishes bones, sinew, and cartilage; corrects lumbago due to kidney deficiency; sedative to restless foetus; lowers blood pressure
Remarks: Women prone to miscarriage may use this herb as a preventive during pregnancy. For men, this herb is used mainly as a sexual tonic. It is one of the most effective natural remedies for high blood pressure and hypertension.

Western name: Rehmannia glutinosa
Chinese name: shou-di-huang
Energy: cold (raw); warm (steamed)
Flavour: sweet

熟　地　黄

Organ-energy affinity: heart, liver, kidneys
Effects: yin tonic (raw); blood tonic (steamed); purifies and nourishes blood; stimulates endocrine secretions; tonifies kidney-yin; the steamed herb is primarily used to nourish blood and marrow; the raw herb is used to cool the blood and to promote kidney functions; also tonifies small and large intestines and stimulates metabolism
Remarks: The raw herb helps restore kidney-yin and kidney fluids when kidneys become deficient through excess ejaculation in males. The steamed herb is a popular restorative tonic for women after childbirth. Popular anti-aging supplement among elderly Chinese. The raw herb also helps reduce fevers and inflammations.

Western name: Cnidium monnieri
Chinese name: she-chuang-dzu
Energy: warm
Flavour: pungent, bitter

蛇　床　子

Organ-energy affinity: kidneys
Effects: yang tonic; stimulates kidney-yang energy; aphrodisiac; astringent; stimulant; antiseptic
Remarks: This is a potent tonic for sexual insufficiency in both males and females and a major ingredient in many formulas for tonic

herbal spirits. A decoction of this herb makes a highly effective antiseptic wash for yeast infections, parasites, rashes and vaginal itching in women.

Compound formulas

The formulas given below are all classical combinations from the Chinese pharmacopoeia that have been used for thousands of years by Taoist adepts, martial artists, and ordinary people to guard the Three Treasures of life and cultivate optimum vitality. Ingredients are readily available at traditional Chinese pharmacies in Chinatowns through the world, or by mail order from the suppliers listed in the Appendix. All formulas can be easily prepared at home. If you prefer ready-made patent tonics, you'll find some excellent varieties listed in Chapter 26.

The quantities listed for the herbs in each formula are sufficient to prepare a one-day dosage by decoction (three cups reduced to one cup in first boiling; two cups reduced to one cup in second boiling), or to prepare one litre of herbal spirits. If you plan to take a particular formula by decoction for ten days, you should order ten packets of the formula in the proportions given below. To make six litres of herbal spirits in one batch, simply use six times the quantities specified. For powders and pills, the quantities given are sufficient for three to five days' dosage, so it's best to order bigger batches for long-term use. The quantities listed for each herb may also be used as general proportions when ordering larger batches of a formula.

Ten Complete Great Tonic

This is one of the oldest tonic formulas in Chinese medicine. It is regarded as one of the best overall health and longevity tonics for long-term use. Ingredients and proportions are perfectly balanced to make this formula an energy, blood, yang, and yin tonic all in one recipe. It promotes physical endurance, nourishes blood, boosts vital energies, and prolongs life.

Ingredients:

Panax ginseng	8 grams
Atractylodes macrocephala	8 grams
Poria cocos	8 grams
Glycyrrhiza uralensis or *G. glabra*	8 grams
Rehmannia glutinosa	8 grams
Ligusticum chuangxiong	8 grams
Angelica sinensis	8 grams

Paeonia lactiflora	8 grams
Cinnamomum cassia	4 grams
Astragalus membraneceus	4 grams

Preparation and dosage: Decoction, powder, pills, or spirits. Take two or three doses daily for two to three months.

Contraindications: Common cold, fever, respiratory ailments.

Longevity Tonic

This is a classical Taoist longevity tonic used by martial artists as well as meditators. It promotes internal alchemy among the Three Treasures, boosts vital energy, and tonifies the liver and kidneys. It is appropriate for long-term use by adepts as well as other men and women, young and old.

Ingredients:

Panax ginseng	8 grams
Polygonum multiflorum	8 grams
Lycium chinensis	8 grams
Schizandrae chinensis	8 grams
Asparagus lucidus	8 grams

Preparation and dosage: Decoction, powder, pills, or spirits. For spirits, use six times the quantities given above and steep in 6 litres of spirits. Two doses daily, morning and evening, for three to six months.

Contraindications: Cold, fever, respiratory ailments.

Deer-horn and Silkworm Tonic

This is a strong male sexual tonic, suitable for short-term use in cases of impotence in young and middle-aged men, or for long-term use by elderly males. Avoid coffee and tea within three hours of taking a dose of this tonic. Young deer horn is saturated with male hormones, which stimulate sexual glands and functions in those who take it.

Ingredients:

Cervus nippon (deer horn)	15 grams
Bombyx mori (silkworm)	15 grams

Preparation and dosage: Have your herbalist grind the ingredients to a fine powder and put it in size 00 gelatin capsules, or make honey pills. Take 3–5 grams of pills or capsules twice daily, on an empty stomach, preferably with some wine or liquor (no ice). Use for one month.

Primordial Energy Elixir

This is a very old formula designed to tonify primordial energy, enhance immunity and prolong life. It is balanced to build blood as well as energy and boost yin as well as yang. It harmonizes Fire and Water energies and infuses the lower abdomen with extra primordial energy, thereby improving sexual functions and strengthening the knees and lower back.

Ingredients:

Rehmannia glutinosa	24 grams
Panax ginseng	16 grams
Dioscorea japonica	8 grams
Cornus officinalis	8 grams
Angelica sinensis	8 grams
Lycium chinensis	8 grams
Zizyphus spinosa	8 grams
Eucommia ulmoides	8 grams
Glycyrrhiza uralensis	4 grams

Preparation and dosage: Powder, pills, decoction, or spirits. Twice daily on an empty stomach. Suitable for long-term use by men and women.

Contraindications: Respiratory ailments, fever. Avoid coffee, tea, soya beans, turnips, and shellfish.

Angelica Elixir

This is a renowned female tonic formula used for thousands of years in the wealthy households of ancient China. It purifies, balances, and tonifies blood and regulates menstrual functions. In cases of premenstrual syndrome, it should be taken for about one week prior to the onset of menstruation. As a general blood tonic, it may be taken in courses of two to three months.

Ingredients:

Angelica sinensis	8 grams
Rehmannia glutinosa	8 grams
Paeonia lactiflora	8 grams
Astragalus membraneceus	8 grams
Poria cocos	8 grams
Glycyrrhiza uralensis	8 grams
Codonopsis tangshen	8 grams
Ligusticum wallichii	8 grams

Preparation and dosage: Powder, pills, decoction, or spirits. This tonic is most commonly prepared in the form of herbal spirits. Twice daily, morning and night, on an empty stomach. Also suitable for use by men in cases of anaemia or other blood deficiencies.

Spring Wine
This is the author's own version of an old formula for health and longevity used by General Yang Sen in Taiwan. General Yang was a student of Lee Ching-yuen, the herbalist who lived for over 250 years. This is primarily a male formula and sexual tonic, but it may also be used by women who are deficient of yang energy. Yang-deficient women often have trouble reaching orgasm. This formula facilitates female orgasm by warming the sexual organs and enhancing blood circulation to the genitals. The formula is balanced to tonify energy, blood, yin, and yang, with an extra boost for kidney-yang. It is a very effective blood and body warmer during cold winter weather. Taken half an hour before dinner, it strongly stimulates the appetite.

Ingredients:

Cervus nippon (horn shavings)	60 grams
Cervus nippon (resin)	60 grams
Equus asinus chinensis (resin)	60 grams
Clemmys chinensis (resin)	60 grams
Epimedium sagittatum	60 grams
Rehmannia glutinosa	60 grams
Astragalus membraneceus	30 grams
Angelica sinensis	30 grams
Eucommia ulmoides	30 grams
Lycium chinensis	30 grams
Ligustrum wallichii	30 grams
Cynomorium coccineum	30 grams
dried human placenta	30 grams
Panax ginseng (red)	20 grams
Rubus coreanus	15 grams
Hippocampus coronatus (seahorse)	2 each
Phrynosoma cornuta (spotted lizard) (one male, one female)	2 each

Preparation and dosage: Place all ingredients in a large glass or ceramic vessel and pour 6 litres of vodka, rum, or brandy over it. Steep four months, strain off half the brew for use, then add another 3 litres of spirits and let steep for another six months. Keep vessel sealed air-tight while steeping. Add a little honey or sugar to each decanted bottle of tonic. In cold weather, take two 1-ounce doses daily, on an empty stomach. When it is warm, take only one. May be used long-term by men, especially after age forty. Women should use this tonic only as required: for example, to warm the body in very cold weather, for a boost of extra energy when needed, or to facilitate orgasm.

Contraindications: Fever, colds, flu, etc.; liver inflammation; extremely hot weather.

Wolfberry Wine

This is a simple but effective health tonic, especially for building blood and improving sexual functions. It nourishes vital fluids, boosts kidney-yin, and prevents premature aging. It may be used by both men and women and is suitable for long-term therapy.

Ingredients:

Lycium chinensis	10 grams
Rehmannia glutinosa	10 grams
Polygonum multiflorum	10 grams

Preparation and dosage: Steep the herbs in one litre of spirits for two months. Take 1 fluid ounce twice daily, on an empty stomach. For long-term use, increase the quantities to 60 grams each and use 6 litres of spirits.

Six-flavour Rehmannia Tonic

This ancient formula is one of the most famous yin tonifiers in the Chinese pharmacopoeia. It tonifies yin energy, builds strong blood, stimulates secretions of vital hormones, and promotes production of kidney fluids, including secretions of the adrenal glands. It cools the system and supplements the basic vital essences from which the body derives energy by internal alchemy. It is particularly effective in restoring and maintaining kidney-yin energy in males who deplete their kidney essence through excessive ejaculation. By building the Water energy of the kidneys, this tonic also helps calm and cool the excess Fire energy of overactive hearts (high blood pressure, palpitations, angina, etc.).

Ingredients:

Rehmannia glutinosa	12 grams
Cornus officinalis	7 grams
Dioscorea japonica	7 grams
Lycium chinensis	7 grams
Paeonia suffruticosa	4 grams
Poria cocos	4 grams
Alisma orientalis	4 grams

Preparation and dosage: Powder, pills, or decoction. Two or three doses daily for one to two months at a time. This formula is also available as pills in ready-made patent form.

CHAPTER 25

Therapeutic Food Recipes

> A truly good physician first finds out the cause of the ill-
> ness, and, having found that, he first tries to cure it by
> food. Only when food fails does he prescribe medication.
>
> Sun Ssu-mo (seventh century AD)

In Chinese medical tradition, diet and nutrition have always
formed the first line of defence against disease, and food has
always been regarded as a form of medicine. In fact, in the wealthy
households and imperial palaces of ancient China, herbal physicians rather than cooks formulated the recipes used to prepare the
daily fare, employing precisely the same principles of balance and
harmony used in blending herbal prescriptions. The great gourmet
recipes of classical Chinese cuisine are therefore potent prescriptions for health and longevity as well as culinary works of art. In
Chinese households, the kitchen is also the family clinic.

Perhaps the greatest defect of modern Western medicine is its
failure to recognize the vital role nutrition plays in human health.
American medical schools do not provide physicians with even
the most basic education in nutritional science. Yet the six leading
causes of death in the USA today have all been directly linked to
dietary factors: heart disease, cancer, stroke, diabetes, arteriosclerosis, and cirrhosis of the liver.

This has not always been the case. Before the triumph of allo-
pathy and the demise of preventative health care in Western
medicine during the early decades of the twentieth century,
Western physicians were well aware of the vital importance of diet
and nutrition in human health. Dr Charles Mayo, one of early
twentieth-century America's most renowned physicians, stated:
'Adequate food is the cradle of normal resistance, the playground
of normal immunity, the workshop of good health, and the laboratory of long life.'

The materials and methods used in preparing traditional Chinese cuisine lend themselves perfectly to transforming an ordinary kitchen into a health clinic and creating therapeutically beneficial dishes from ordinary ingredients. The keys to Chinese cooking are the same basic principles of balance and harmony, yin and yang, Five Elemental Energies, and other universal laws of nature which run throughout all the Taoist arts and sciences. By learning the culinary aspects of those basic principles and familiarizing yourself with the fundamental techniques of Chinese cooking, you may improvise and apply these methods to whatever materials happen to be available in your local markets.

A complete course in Chinese cookery is beyond the scope of this book. Instead, this chapter simply provides a small selection of recipes for foods and beverages that meet the two basic criteria of classical Chinese cuisine as well as traditional Taoist diet: therapeutic potency for human health and gourmet satisfaction for human pleasure. Some of the recipes given below are not even Chinese in origin, but they all conform to the same basic Taoist principles of balance and harmony and are therefore included here to illustrate how Taoist methods may be applied to any materials. Readers who wish to learn more about classical Chinese cuisine and how to prepare it at home may refer to the author's *Complete Chinese Cookbook*, which includes chapters on Chinese food history, traditional condiments and seasonings, cooking methods, kitchen utensils, and over 500 home-tested recipes from China.

Any kitchen may be converted into a Chinese kitchen and any food may be transformed into Chinese food with just a few fundamental utensils, condiments, and seasonings.

Utensils: round-bottomed Chinese cooking pan, or wok (black iron is best, stainless steel second best; avoid aluminium and Teflon), with cover; long handled spatula for stir-frying; stove with at least one intense high-heat burner, preferably gas.
Condiments: soya sauce; Chinese sesame oil; cooking wine
Seasonings: garlic; ginger; scallion (spring onion); chilli.

With these few basic, inexpensive, and readily available items at hand in your own kitchen, you can easily prepare any of the following recipes, as well as most other Chinese dishes, at home. Bear in mind that the essential spirit of Chinese cooking is spontaneous creativity and personal improvisation, not rigid adherence to recipes, so feel free to substitute ingredients, adjust proportions, and experiment creatively with the materials and methods introduced below, which are meant more to inspire you than to instruct you. All the recipes serve four or five persons. Some of these recipes show you how to compose culinary prescriptions for health from ordinary kitchen ingredients, while others illustrate how to use tonic herbal medicines from the Chinese pharmacopoeia to create delicious, nutritious, and therapeutically potent dishes and drinks. When composing entire meals with these and other recipes, be sure to follow the laws of trophology (food combining) in order to ensure smooth digestion of food, facilitate assimilation of nutrients, and establish pharmacodynamic synergy among the various foods on the table and in your stomach.

Food
Hunan fish (or chicken)

This is a classical Chinese recipe from Hunan province, which favours spicy cuisine. It's an excellent way to take your daily dose of garlic, ginger, scallions (spring onions), and chilli. Garlic boosts immunity and vitality and provides potent antibiotic and antiviral protection. Ginger warms the stomach, aids digestion, and facilitates assimilation. Scallions are cleansing, digestive, and benefit the respiratory system. Chillis stimulate metabolism, promote circulation, drive out internal heat and dampness, enhance energy, and kill intestinal parasites. The recipe may be applied to beef and lamb as well as fish and chicken, and vegetarians may prepare it with tofu.
Material:
● About 2lb of fresh deep-water fish such as tuna, *mahi-mahi*, or shark; or boneless chicken breast; or tenderloin of beef or lamb. You may also use scallops, prawns, or lobster.
● Soy sauce; white wine, rice wine, or sherry; sugar
● ½ cup each of finely minced fresh garlic, ginger root, and scallions, and ¼ cup of minced red chillis (fresh or dried)
Method:
● Cut the fish or meat into chunks about 1 inch wide and ½ inch thick.
● In a large bowl, stir together ⅓ cup soya sauce, ½ cup cooking wine, and 3 tbsp sugar and mix well. Add the cut fish and mix with sauce. Let marinate 15 minutes for fish, 30 minutes for chicken and meat.
● Divide the minced garlic, ginger, scallions, and chillis into two equal portions. Drain fish or meat and reserve marinade.
● Heat 3–4 tbsp cooking oil in a wok (or iron skillet) over medium heat. Add half the minced seasonings and stir quickly with spatula. Raise heat to high and add drained fish or meat to wok and stir-fry

till about half done (2–3 minutes). Add remaining half of minced seasonings and stir-fry. Then add half of the marinade sauce, plus 1 tbsp more soya sauce and 2 tbsp more wine, to the fish in the wok, stir together, then lower heat to medium and let simmer till done (about 4–5 minutes for fish, 6–9 minutes for chicken and meat).

Ginseng chicken

Ginseng and chicken form a classic combination in Chinese cuisine as well as medicine. This tonic food is frequently prescribed for women recovering from childbirth, patients recovering from prolonged illness, and to ward off the ravages of aging in the elderly. It is also a good general health tonic which stimulates energy, promotes hormone production, and boosts immunity. By the addition of 10–15 grams of sliced *Panax notoginseng* (*san-chee*) along with the regular ginseng, this dish also becomes a cardio-tonic, enhances blood circulation, and promotes rapid healing of wounds.

Material:
- 5–6 chicken legs, preferably organically raised
- 1 cup rice wine or dry sherry
- 3 scallions (spring onions), finely minced
- 6 thin slices of peeled ginger root
- 15 grams *Panax ginseng* root, any variety, thinly sliced
- 10–15 grams *Panax notoginseng*, thinly sliced (optional)

Method:
- Cut chicken legs at joint into thigh and drumstick, then use heavy cleaver to chop each piece in half through the bone. Place chopped chicken in Pyrex glass or heatproof ceramic bowl together with wine, ginger, and ginseng.
- Set bowl in a steamer basket or steamer-wok, cover steamer tightly, and steam over high heat for one hour.
- Sprinkle a bit of fresh ground pepper, sea salt, minced scallion, and a few drops of Chinese sesame oil into individual soup bowls, then ladle chicken, ginseng pulp, and broth into each bowl, stir, and serve.

Poissons crux

This is a traditional Tahitian way of preparing fresh raw fish for the dining table. For people who find Japanese *sashimi* a bit too 'fishy' for their taste, this is a great way to eat raw fish. Fresh raw deep-water fish is one of the richest sources of essential fatty acids, particularly the omega-3 fatty fish oils which so effectively prevent arteriosclerosis and heart disease. It is also an excellent source of essential amino acids, minerals, and trace elements.

Material:

● 2lb very fresh fillet of tuna, *mahi-mahi,* salmon, or other edible raw deep-water ocean fish, skinned and boned

● juice of 4–5 lemons or limes; 1 tsp sea salt

● ¾ cup coconut cream (the white liquid extract of coconut meat, available canned in the Oriental section of grocery shops)

● 1–2 white onions, carrots, and green bell pepper, finely sliced

Method:

● Cut fish into bite-size chunks, about 1 inch by ½ inch, and place in glass or ceramic bowl with lime juice and salt. Mix together well and let marinate 15 minutes for 'rare', 20 minutes for 'medium', or 25 minutes for 'well done', then drain off excess marinade and discard.

● Add sliced onion, carrot, and bell pepper to fish, pour on the coconut cream, mix together well, and serve.

Pearl barley and brown rice porridge

This is a traditional Chinese tonic breakfast food and a great dietary way to start the day. Easy to prepare, inexpensive, and packed with nutritional and tonic benefits, it makes a good staple breakfast for the entire family. Pearl barley is 17 per cent protein, tonifies yang energy, decongests the lungs, improves digestive functions, and is mildly diuretic. Brown rice provides a rich source of B vitamins, dietary fibre, and other nutrients and is regarded as the most perfectly balanced food in terms of the Five Elemental Energies. Optional extras are jujubes (Chinese dates), which are energy and nerve tonics, raw egg yolks for lecithin and amino acids, sliced bananas for potassium, and whatever else your imagination cooks up. If you prefer it sweet rather than salty, you may add some honey, barley malt, or maple syrup.

Material:

• 1 cup brown rice

• ½ cup pearl barley

• 6–8 dried jujubes (*Ziziphus jujuba*), squeezed with pliers until the kernel inside cracks (optional)

• 2 raw egg yolks (optional)

• Chinese sesame oil, sea salt

Method:

• Soak brown rice and barley in pure water for about 1 hour, then drain off the water.

● Put in pot, add 6–7 cups pure water, bring to boil, lower heat, cover but leave small opening for steam to escape, and simmer slowly for about 1 ½ hours, stirring occasionally. If it gets too thick, add a bit more water. If using jujubes, add them along with the rice and barley.

● Sprinkle a bit of sea salt and a few drops of Chinese sesame oil into individual soup bowls; if using egg yolks, whisk the yolks together with salt and sesame oil in each bowl; ladle porridge into each bowl, stir to mix, and serve. If you prefer sweet flavours, omit salt and sesame oil and use your choice of sweetners, dried fruit, bananas, etc.

Chinese wolfberry stew

Chinese wolfberries are one of the most popular longevity tonics in China. The 250-year-old Lee Ching-yuen consumed them daily for most of his life in the form of a tasty soup. Wolfberries are tonic to the kidneys and liver, nourish blood and semen, improve vision, promote hormone production, enhance sexual stamina and increase physical endurance. They also help remedy mild forms of diabetes. Lamb is the richest dietary source of carnitine, the amino acid which delivers fat molecules into cells for conversion into energy, and *shiitake* mushrooms are an ancient Oriental longevity tonic that have been shown by recent studies to enhance immune functions and inhibit growth of cancerous cells.

Material:
● 2lb fresh beef or lamb, tender
● 15–20 dried *shiitake* mushrooms
● 1 cup rice wine or dry sherry
● 1 ounce Chinese wolfberry (*Lycium chinensis*)
● Sea salt, pepper, sesame oil

Method:
● Cut the beef into 1-inch chunks and brown quickly by stir-frying in a few tbsp oil in wok for 1 minute, then remove; if using lamb, blanch briefly by dropping into rapidly boiling water for 1 minute, then drain.

● Pour 2 cups boiling water over dried mushrooms in a bowl and soak for 20 minutes, then drain, reserving water.

● Put meat, mushrooms, and wolfberries into pot, add wine, half of the water from the soaked mushrooms, plus 2½ cups pure water and bring to boil. Lower heat, cover pot, and simmer 2 hours.

● Sprinkle some sea salt, pepper, and a few drops sesame oil into individual bowls, ladle stew on top, stir, and serve. Eat the wolfberries along with the soup.

Steamed fish

For nutrition, steaming is by far the best way to prepare fish, short of eating it raw. Steaming retains moisture, which in turn protects nutrients from damage by excess heat and dryness. Steaming requires no extra fat or oil for cooking and permits creative improvisations, such as adding various different sauces to the steamed fish. You may apply this method to whole fish, fish steaks and fillets, shrimp, and shellfish.

Material:
● Fresh fish, prawns, or other seafood
● Garlic, ginger, scallions (spring onions), chillis
● Soya sauce; white wine or sherry
● Other sauces and seasonings, as desired

Method:
● For whole fish, scale and gut the fish and score each side three times with a sharp knife. For steaks, cut them thick. Shellfish may be steamed in or out of the shell. Before cooking, place fish on a platter, sprinkle both sides well with wine, and let sit for 30 minutes, then drain off the wine.
● Place fish on a heatproof plate and sprinkle with some fresh wine. Finely chop some ginger root and sprinkle over fish. Bring steamer to boil and set the fish inside, covering tightly. For whole fish, steam 7–8 minutes for a small one, 10–12 minutes for medium size. For steaks and fillets, 7–9 minutes. Prawns and shellfish, 6–7 minutes. Steam on high heat. When done, remove from steamer and drain off excess fluids from the plate.
● Prepare a sauce separately and either dribble it over the fish before serving, or set it on table in a bowl so that each person can use it as desired. You can also prepare a selection of two or three different sauces. Here are some suggestions:

Garlic chilli sauce Finely mince ⅓ cup garlic, ⅓ cup ginger, ⅓ cup scallion, ¼ cup chillis; heat 2 tbsp cooking oil and 1 tbsp sesame oil in wok on medium (not high) heat, add minced seasonings, and stir-fry quickly. Add salt, wine, dash soya sauce, dash sugar, stir and simmer 1 minute, then remove from heat. Pour it over the fish, or serve separately.

Sweet soya sauce Heat 2 tbsp sesame oil in wok on medium heat, add 3 tbsp wine, 2 tbsp soya sauce, 1 tbsp sugar, 1 tsp vinegar. Blend well, then pour it over the fish or serve separately.

Ginger and vinegar Finely shred 8–10 thin slices ginger root and put in a bowl with 1 tsp sugar and ⅓ cup vinegar (rice vinegar or apple-cider vinegar is best); stir well and let sit about an hour prior to cooking the fish. This should be served separately in the bowl, not poured over the fish.

Beverages

Beverages are a quick and convenient way to get your daily nutrition from foods and herbs without going to the trouble of cooking a whole meal. They are readily digested and their nutrients easily absorbed. However, it's best not to mix these beverages with solid food, to avoid indigestion and also to insure maximum assimilation of their nutrients. The drinks introduced below should serve as guidelines to inspire you to create other beverages with your own favourite ingredients.

Almond milk

The Chinese have recognized the nutritional value of almonds for thousands of years. Almonds are a rich source of essential fatty acids and amino acids and therefore an excellent substitute for meat and other animal products for vegetarians, but they must be eaten raw for nutritional benefits. They are the only nut that provide the complete range of required protein elements. However, they are difficult to digest and should therefore be soaked in water overnight. Eat them whole after soaking, or make delicious almond milk.
Material:
• 1 cup raw almonds
• 1 tbsp vanilla extract
• 2 tbsp honey
• pure water and ice cubes
Method:
• Soak almonds overnight in refrigerator in pure water.
• Drain off water, place almonds in a blender, add vanilla, honey, 4–5 cracked ice cubes, and 1½ cups water, and blend at high speed for 2–3 minutes.
• Pour into glasses, let dregs settle to bottom, and drink. For a smooth, dreg-free texture, you may run the almond milk through a sieve or strainer. However, it is better to drink it with the dregs, which are a good source of dietary fibre.

Banana fig shake

This is an excellent energy and nutrition beverage. Bananas are a rich source of potassium, which balances the excess sodium most of us ingest, and figs are not only highly nutritious, they are also very beneficial to lower bowel functions. Molasses is the best source of organic iron, which builds haemoglobin in blood plasma and is also a mild laxative. This is a good, quick, liquid breakfast for those in a hurry in the morning, as well as an effective energizer in the afternoon.

Material:
• 1 large or 2 small bananas, 2–3 figs (fresh or sun-dried), 1 tbsp molasses
• 3–4 ice cubes, pure water

Method:
• Put bananas in blender; dice the figs and add to bananas; add molasses, cracked ice cubes, and water.
• Blend at high speed until smooth.

Ginger and scallion-root tea

This hot beverage is a traditional Chinese remedy for colds, flu, and other bronchial ailments, as well as for indigestion and winter chills. It is effective only against colds accompanied by chills, not fevers, because its effect is warming. Ginger is tonic to the stomach, spleen, and lungs. It dissolves phlegm, aids digestion, relieves nausea (including seasickness), and is an antidote in seafood poisoning. Scallions are warming, digestive, antiseptic, and diaphoretic (induce sweating).

Material:
• 5–6 thin slices ginger root
• white rootlets of 5–6 fresh scallions (spring onions; buy only scallions that still have the roots attached)
• Raw sugar or honey to taste

Method:
• Put ginger, rootlets, and sugar in a pot with 1 ½ cups water, bring to boil, and simmer for 6–7 minutes. Strain into cup.

Hot hibiscus toddy

This is a hot drink that is cooling to the body and makes a good summer cooler. Its action is astringent, and it has natural affinity for the sexual organs. For men, it helps retain semen during intercourse and also relieves discomfort in the urinary tract. For women, it helps relieve premenstrual syndrome and other menstrual disorders. Its astringent properties also help control diarrhoea.

Material:
• 10–12 buds of dried hibiscus flower
• Raw sugar or honey to taste
Method:
• Preheat a large mug or glass with hot water, then put the hibiscus buds and sugar or honey into the mug. Pour boiling water over it, cover, and let steep for about 10 minutes.

Pollen and honey

Bee pollen is a potent source of essential fatty acids, amino acids, zinc, and trace elements. It is one of the best natural remedies for prostate problems, skin disorders, and allergies. Honey acts synergistically with pollen, lubricates the digestive tract, benefits skin, and provides quick energy. You may use this blend as a base for other ingredients, such as ginseng extract, ginkgo extract, phenylalanine powder, and other 'eye-openers' for an effective early-morning boost.
Material:
• 2 tsp bee pollen
• 2 tbsp honey
Method:
• Put pollen and honey into a large mug, add whatever other ingredients you wish to use, then fill mug with medium-hot (but not boiling) water. Stir well.

Barley water

Barley is highly nutritious, aids digestion, decongests the lungs, and cools the system. It is also diuretic and benefits the eyes. It relieves ailments associated with excess dampness, such as rheumatism. Barley water is a popular traditional beverage in Korea, Japan, and other northern Asian regions, and is a very good dietary supplement for bottle-fed infants. It may be drunk as a refreshment throughout the day, either hot or cold, and sweetened to taste with a bit of honey, though most people drink it plain.
Material:
• 2–3 tbsp barley
• 2 cups pure water
Method:
• Put barley and water in a pot, bring to boil, and simmer for about one hour. Strain into cup and serve hot, or else let it cool first.

Lotus root cooler

This drink makes a great summer cooler, hot or cold. It expels excess Fire from the system, cools the blood, and pacifies 'rebellious ascending energy' from overworked livers. It helps detoxify the liver and relieves the itching of summer heat rashes. For quick relief of heat rashes, mash the fresh root to a pulp and apply it externally.
Material:
• 1 large fresh lotus root (available at Oriental groceries), cut into sections at the joints
• Raw sugar or barley malt (not honey, which counteracts the effects of the root)
• Pure water
Method:
• Put the sections into a pot and add 2 litres water; bring to boil and boil briskly over medium-high heat for 45 minutes.
• Remove roots, add sugar and stir. Serve hot or cold. Large batches may be kept in refrigerator for several days.

Ginseng liquorice tea

A traditional tonic tea that is usually prepared in the morning and kept hot all day by adding more boiling water to the herbs as the brew is consumed, this herbal elixir may be used on a daily basis by the whole family. Unlike most ginseng formulas, it uses the least expensive form of ginseng. The brew tonifies energy, detoxifies the organs, balances internal energies, is soothing to the lungs, and improves digestive functions. Liquorice is the most widely used herb in Chinese medicine, appearing in almost all prescriptions. It enters all twelve meridians and organs, and prolongs the effects of other herbs. Its flavour improves the taste of all prescriptions, and in this recipe its natural sweetness eliminates the need for sugar or honey.
Material:
• One handful of small tendril rootlets of white ginseng roots (*Panax ginseng*). These are sold separately from the roots and are not expensive.
• 10 long thin slices of liquorice root (*Glycyrrhiza uralensis* or *glebra*)
Method:
• In an ordinary ceramic teapot of 1 litre capacity, or a thermos, put the ginseng tendrils and liquorice root. Add boiling water, cover, and steep for 15–20 minutes. If brew is not drunk within half an hour, pour it off into a separate pot or thermos, then add more boiling water to herbs and steep again, as needed. Pot may be refilled up to six times throughout the day.

CHAPTER 26

Remarkable Remedies

> Chinese herbal patent formulas . . . are of significant
> benefit in a variety of health complaints, without side
> effect, and relatively inexpensive . . . Often, patents are
> used alone in acute problems at recommended package
> doses with remarkable effect . . . In chronic problems
> of deficiency (*chee*, blood, yin, yang), they are often the
> therapy of choice.
>
> Jake Fratkin, doctor of Oriental medicine (1986)

Traditionally Chinese herbal remedies were prepared at home by
the decoction method, or at the pharmacy in the form of honey pills
or powders. In recent years, however, pharmaceutical technology
has permitted large-scale production of concentrated, highly
refined extracts of medicinal herbs, blended precisely according to
the tried-and-true classical formulas used for thousands of years in
China. Produced and packaged in the form of pills or liquid
extracts, these patent herbal formulas are far more convenient to
take than traditional prescriptions made from bulk herbs, and
thanks to mass production they are relatively inexpensive.

People in the Western world spend billions of dollars every year
buying synthetic over-the-counter remedies for common ailments
and chronic deficiencies. These drugs are made with chemicals
rather than herbs, conflict rather than cooperate with natural
human energies, are of dubious efficacy, often lead to drug dependency, and have undesirable side effects. For a lot less money, far
greater therapeutic efficacy, and no dangerous side effects,
Westerners could purchase the remarkable herbal remedies currently being produced in China, Hong Kong, and Singapore and
distributed worldwide through health shops, herbal pharmacies,
and mail-order suppliers. In addition, many classical Chinese
formulas are now being manufactured by herbal suppliers in the

USA, and the quality of these Western-made Chinese formulas is consistently reliable. Chinese patent herbal remedies work very well when properly applied to the indicated conditions, and the only reason they are not more widely used in the West is that very few people know about them. Allopathic doctors are certainly not going to tell you, so it's up to you to obtain these products yourself and try them on your own conditions. Once you do, you'll never go back to the nasty Western chemical nostrums.

This chapter introduces a selection of various patent herbal remedies for a wide range of ailments. All of them are classical Chinese formulas that have evolved over many centuries based on practical clinical experience and empirical observation. The great advantage of using classical Chinese combinations is that these formulas have been continuously refined and adjusted over many centuries of practice in order to obtain maximum therapeutic results with minimum risk of unwanted side effects. Unlike modern pharmaceuticals, whose long-term side effects are still unknown and which often cause more problems than they cure, traditional Chinese herbal formulas are virtually fail-safe owing to thousands of years of practical application in millions of patients.

The first section of this chapter introduces Chinese patent formulas manufactured in China, Hong Kong, and Singapore and widely distributed in the Western world. They are generally available in herbal pharmacies and Oriental grocery shops in the Chinatowns of major Western cities such as Los Angeles, San Francisco, New York, Chicago, London, and Paris, as well as many smaller towns with Chinese communities. They are also sold in health shops throughout the USA and Europe, or may by ordered by mail from the suppliers listed in the Appendix.

The second section introduces a variety of Chinese patent formulas produced by herbal suppliers in the USA. Formulated according to the orthodox Taoist principles which govern Chinese herbal medicine, these American-made Chinese remedies generally use only the highest-grade herbs and therefore are sometimes more expensive than similar products imported from China. Many of them come in the form of highly refined liquid concentrates which, despite their higher cost, are ultimately very cost-effective because of their purity and potency.

There are well over 300 different Chinese patent herbal remedies on the market today, but only a few dozen of the most renowned formulas are introduced below. These should suffice to deal effectively with most of your common ailments and chronic deficiencies, while also providing you with a sufficient range of choices for personal experimentation and familiarization. For a more complete guide to the field of Chinese patent remedies, readers may refer to Jake Fratkin's *Chinese Herbal Patent Formulas* and *Chinese Classics*.

Made in China

The following patent formulas are listed according to the type of ailments and deficiencies they remedy. Both the English and the Chinese names are given (the name printed in capital letters is the one which appears on the label), as well as a brief description of each formula's particular properties and applications. They should be used according to the instructions on the label.

Colds, flu and fever due to 'external wind' invasion

GAN MAO LING
('Common Cold Tablet')   感 冒 灵
Main ingredients: ilex root   Vitex fruit
                        Evodia fruit   Lonicera flower
                        Isatis root   menthol
                        chrysanthemum

Actions: An excellent remedy for common cold and flu, including chills, fever, swollen lymph glands, sore throat, stiff neck and shoulders. Sedates excess heat and dispels external-wind invasions, both hot and cold. May be used in higher doses to cure colds, low doses to prevent colds.

BI YAN PIAN
('Nose Inflammation Pills')   鼻 炎 片
Main ingredients: magnolia   forsythia
                        Xanthium   angelica
                        Phellodendron   Anemarrhena
                        liquorice   chrysanthemum
                        Platycodon   Siler root
                        Schizandrae   Schizonepeta

Actions: Effective against head colds caused by wind-heat or wind-cold invasion, including sneezing, watery eyes, sinus congestion, and related headache. Also good for chronic rhinitis, sinusitis, hay fever, and general mucus congestion in the face. Should be taken immediately upon contracting a cold.

YIN CHIAO TABLETS
('Honeysuckle and Forsythia Tablets')   銀 翹 片

Main ingredients: *Lonicera*   *Soja* seed
                         forsythia   liquorice
                         Arctium   *Lophatherum*
                         Platycodon   *Schizonepeta*
                         mint

Actions: Highly effective remedy for colds with toxic heat symptoms, such as flu, sore throat, swollen lymph nodes, fever, headache, stiff neck and shoulders. Expels toxins by inducing sweating. To be effective, it must be taken on the first day that symptoms appear, for two or three days.

Coughs, phlegm and respiratory congestion

CHUAN KE LING
('Asthma and Cough Remedy')   喘 咳 靈

Main ingredients: *Platycodon*   *Armeniaca*
                         liquorice   pig bile

Actions: Stops coughing, dissolves phlegm, and tonifies lung energy. Facilitates breathing. Effective remedy for chronic asthma, bronchitis, and emphysema.

CLEAN AIR TEA   清氣化痰丸
(*Ching Chee Hua Tan Wan*)

Main ingredients: *Pinellia*   *citrus ganpi*
                         Arisaema   *citrus xiangyuan*
                         Trichosanthes   *Armeniaca*
                         Scutellaria   *Poria* fungus

Actions: This is a classical prescription for clearing phlegm and heat from the lungs, throat, and sinuses. Remedies congestion and excess phlegm in the bronchial passages and sinuses and provides relief for chronic asthma and emphysema. This formula is most effective for chronic conditions and the later stages of serious colds that have become entrenched in the respiratory system, not for the early stages of external wind invasion.

TUNG HSUAN LI FEI PIEN
('Decongest and Regulate Lungs Tablets')

通宣理肺片

Main ingredients: liquorice   *Tussilago*
                        Perilla   citrus peel
                        Peucedanum root   *Pueraria* root
                        Aurantium   lily bulb
                        Platycodon root

Actions: Decongests lungs by dissolving phlegm, relieving heat, and dispelling wind. Relieves coughing due to wind invasion and asthma. Effective against both thick and watery nasal discharge. Also relieves headache, fever and chills, sneezing, and body aches caused by wind invasion.

NATURAL HERB LOQUAT FLAVOURED SYRUP
('Honey Refined *Fritillaria* and
Eriobotrya Syrup')

蜜煉川貝枇杷膏

Main ingredients: *Fritillaria* bulb   *Platycodon* root
                        Eriobotrya leaf   *Pinellia*
                        citrus peel   *Armeniaca*
                        mint   ginger
                        Trichosanthes   honey
                        liquorice   sugar

Actions: This is a herbal syrup for relieving acute coughs, sticky phlegm, and excess lung heat due to external wind invasion. It tonifies lung energy, dissolves phlegm, and relieves sinus congestion. Useful for acute coughing due to emphysema and bronchitis.

Internal toxicity and excess heat in organs

HERBAL TORTOISE JELLY
('Tortoise and Smilax Syrup')

藥制龜苓膏

Main ingredients: golden coin tortoise   *Lonicera*
                        smilax   *Desmodium*
                        Rehmannia   *Tribulus*
                        liquorice

Actions: A honey-based herbal syrup for internal use in cases of inflamed or infected skin lesions, such as abscesses and carbuncles, or chronic skin inflammations. Also relieves painful lesions in urinary and gastrointestinal tracts. Dispels internal toxic heat, nourishes blood and yin, and promotes tissue regeneration.

LUNG TAN XIE GAN PILL
('Gentian Liver Purging Pills')

龍胆泻肝丸

Main ingredients:

Gentiana root	angelica
Bupleurum root	*Scutellaria* root
gardenia	clematis root
Plantago seed	*Rehmannia*
Alisma	liquorice

Actions: This is a classical formula used to purge excess heat from liver and gall bladder, as well as damp heat from the Triple Burners. Relieves symptoms caused by rising liver Fire, such as headache, bloodshot eyes, ringing in ears, sore throat, fever blisters on mouth. Also good for damp heat in liver and gall bladder, with symptoms of leukcorrhea, urinary-tract infections, and rashes in groin. Provides relief in oral and genital herpes. Cools the liver and stimulates liver energy.

BEZOAR ANTIPYRETIC PILLS
(*Niu Huang Jie Du Pian*)

牛黄解毒片

Main ingredients:

rhubarb	liquorice
gypsum	borneol crystal
Scutellaria root	ox gallstone
Platycodon root	

Actions: This is one of the many patent remedies for internal toxic heat in the liver and gall bladder based on ox gallstone. This formula relieves symptoms of congestion and toxic heat in liver, heart, and stomach, including fever, sore throat, inflamed gums, bloodshot eyes, earache, swollen glands, headache, and oral ulcers. May be safely used for fevers in children. This formula should be used only for toxic-heat syndromes caused by excess Fire in the organs, not by deficiencies.

Stagnant blood, internal bleeding

FARGELIN FOR PILES
('Potent Haemorrhoid Dissolving Remedy')

强力化痔靈

Main ingredients:

pseudoginseng root	*Callicarpa* root
Succinum resin	*Sanguisorba* root
Sophora	*Corydalis*
Scutellaria	bear gallbladder

Actions: Provides rapid relief of swelling in cases of acute and chronic haemorrhoids due to blood stagnation and heat. Stimulates blood circulation, breaks up blood stagnation, dispels heat congestion, and relieves pain.

HSIUNG TAN TIEH TAH WAN
('Bear-Gall Sport Injury Pill')

熊胆跌打丸

Main ingredients:

angelica	*Amomum* fruit
rhubarb	*Carthamus*
Inula root	pseudoginseng root
Curcuma root	bear gall

Actions: Stimulates blood circulation, breaks up blood stagnation, reduces swelling, dispels heat, and promotes rapid healing of injured blood vessels. Particularly effective for severe bruises, sprains, swelling, and inflammation due to traumatic injuries. This is a popular remedy in China for injuries sustained in sports and martial-arts training.

YUNNAN PAIYAO
('Yunnan White Medicine')

雲南白藥

Main ingredient: pseudoginseng root
(other ingredients are secret)

Actions: This is one of the most highly prized medicines among China's martial artists and military forces. A powder that may be used internally or externally, it swiftly stops bleeding, disperses stagnant blood, relieves pain, and promotes rapid healing of wounds. May be applied directly to external wounds. Also effective against bleeding ulcers, excessive menstrual bleeding, menstrual cramps, and festering skin infections The small red pill in each bottle is meant to be taken internally with a little wine in cases of severe bleeding, such as gunshot wounds. This powder was standard issue in the field kits of the North Vietnamese army during the Vietnam War.

Heart disease

DAN SHEN TABLETS
('Salvia Root Tablet')

複方丹參片

Main ingredients: *Salvia* root
borneol crystal

Actions: This formula relieves pain in the heart due to blood stagnation and stimulates circulation in the coronary blood vessels. Effective remedy for angina pectoris, heart palpitations, pain running down left arm, and chest pains. Also reduces blood cholesterol and lipids.

REN SHEN ZAI ZAO WAN
('Ginseng Restorative Pills') 人 參 再 丸

Main ingredients:

ginseng root	*Coptis*
cinnamon bark	mantis egg case
angelica	tortoise plastron
Ligusticum	myrrh resin
Rehmannia	frankincense resin
Gastrodia	dragon's-blood resin
Agkistrodon pit viper	*Carthamus* flower
Succinum resin	

Actions: Tonifies blood, yin, and energy, stimulates blood circulation, and dispels stagnation. This formula is used primarily for symptoms related to stroke, including speech impediments, contractive or flaccid muscle tone in extremities, numbness and tingling in limbs, and facial paralysis. Should be administered immediately after stroke occurs.

Indigestion and intestinal congestion

PO CHAI PILLS
('Protect and Benefit Pill') 保 劑 丸

Main ingredients:

Gastrodia elata	*Saussurea* root
Poria cocos	chrysanthemum
mint	angelica
tangerine peel	*Lophanthus rugosus*
Halloysite	*Atractylodes*
Pueraria lobata	*Oryza* malt
Trichosanthes root	magnolia
Coix seed	

Actions: Regulates spleen and stomach functions, facilitates digestion, dispels wind and damp from stomach. Effective for a wide range of digestive problems, including nausea, vomiting, cramps, abdominal distension, gas, food stagnation, and indigestion associated with travelling. Safe for children. This highly effective digestive remedy is made in Hong Kong, but a similar product is also made in mainland China under the name China Po Chi Pills.

APLOTAXIS CARMINATIVE PILLS
('*Saussurea* Harmonize Energy Pills')　木香順氣丸

Main ingredients:	angelica	*Poria cocos*
	magnolia	*Pinellia*
	Alpinia	*Alisma*
	Saussurea	ginger
	Amomum	citrus peel
	Atracylodes	*Cimicifuga*
	Aurantium	*Bupleurum*
	Evodia	

Actions: This formula remedies indigestion and food stagnation in stomach due to congestion and energy stagnation in the liver, including such symptoms as abdominal distension, poor digestion, belching, constipation, and accumulation of phlegm and dampness in the stomach. Disperses stagnant liver energy, cools over-heated gall bladders, nourishes liver blood, and tonifies the spleen. Effective remedy for food stagnation caused by excess consumption of ice-cold food and drink, overeating, and eating immediately prior to sleep.

SIX GENTLEMEN TEA PILL
('*Shiang Sha Liu Jun Wan*')　香沙六君子丸

Main ingredients:	*Codonopsis*	citrus peel
	Pinellia	liquorice
	Atractylodes	*Amomum*
	Poria cocos	*Saussurea*

Actions: This is a classical formula for correcting indigestion due to deficient spleen energy, stagnation of stomach energy, and excess cold in the Middle Burner. Improves poor appetite due to insufficient digestive energy, relieves nausea, stops diarrhoea, and may also be used for morning sickness by pregnant women. This formula was also traditionally used to enhance physical stamina in children.

Tonics

Blood tonics

EIGHT TREASURE TEA
('Women's Eight Treasure Pill')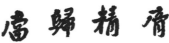

Main ingredients:

Paeonia root	*Rehmannia*
angelica	*Atractylodes*
Poria cocos	*Codonopsis*
Ligusticum	liquorice

Actions: A classical combination that nourishes blood and tonifies energy. Excellent general health tonic for women. Regulates menstruation, relieves fatigue, dizziness, and heart palpitations, improves appetite, and restores health and vitality after childbirth or illness.

REHMANNIA GLUTINOSA COMPOUND PILLS 婦科種子丸
('Women's Seed Pill')

Main ingredients:

Rehmannia	*Dispsacus* root
Eucommia bark	*Artemisia*
Cyperus	donkey-skin glue
Ligusticum	*Scutellaria*
angelica	*Paeonia* root

Actions: Nourishes blood and stimulates circulation, warms the uterus and cools the liver. Used in cases of female blood deficiency, including symptoms of cold uterus, infertility, amenorrhaea, miscarriage, menstrual cramps, cold hands and feet.

TANG KWE GIN 當婦精膚
('Angelica Syrup')

Main ingredients:

angelica	*Poria cocos*
donkey-skin glue	*Paeonia* root
Codonopsis	*Ligusticum*
Astragalus	liquorice
Rehmannia	sugar

Actions: This formula contains 70 per cent angelica, which is the best blood tonic in the Chinese pharmocopoeia. Nourishes blood, improves circulation, and tonifies the spleen. Good general tonic for women, but may also be used by men in cases of blood deficiency due to illness, surgery, trauma, or fatigue.

Yin tonics

DA BU YIN WAN
('Great Yin Tonic Pill') 大 補 陰 丸

Main ingredients: Rehmannia Anemarrhena
tortoise plastron Phellodendron

Actions: A traditional formula to correct severe deficiency of kidney yin, accompanied by such Fire symptoms as night sweats, insomnia, hot palms and soles, hot flushes, and burning sensation over the kidneys. Effective for acute hot flushes due to menopause. May also be used by men with deficient kidney yin.

LIU WEI DI HUANG WAN
('Six-Flavour *Rehmannia* Pills') 六 味 地 黄 丸

Main ingredients: Rehmannia Paeonia
Cornus fruit Poria cocos
Dioscoria root Alisma

Actions: A popular classical formula for tonifying kidney, liver, and spleen yin; also boosts kidney and spleen energy. Effective for such yin-deficiency symptoms as insomnia, lower-back pain, chronic fatigue, night sweats, dizziness, ringing ears, impotence, and high blood pressure. In men, high blood pressure can easily be caused by excess ejaculation, which depletes kidney yin. When kidney yin is weak, Water energy of kidney loses its control over Fire energy of heart, which flares up and causes high blood pressure. This formula is also helpful in mild forms of diabetes and may be taken for prolonged periods of time.

Energy tonics

PANAX GINSENG EXTRACTUM 吉 林 人 參 精
('*Ren Shen Jing*')

Main ingredient: ginseng root

Actions: A highly concentrated, pure liquid extract of Kirin ginseng from northern China, this product is a good bargain. Kirin ginseng is relatively inexpensive and mild, but taken regularly over a period of time, it is a very effective energy tonic. Builds energy, boosts immunity, stimulates the endocrine system, regulates blood pressure and blood sugar.

GINSENG ROYAL JELLY VIALS
('*Ren Sheng Feng Wang Jiang*')

Main ingredients:	royal jelly	honey
	ginseng	

Actions: A nutrional tonic that enhances spleen and lung energy and improves assimilation of nutrients. Stimulates appetite and facilitates digestion. Particularly beneficial for the elderly, and for those recovering from illness or childbirth. This pleasant-tasting liquid comes in convenient single-dose vials.

JEN SHEN LU JUNG WAN
('Ginseng and Deer-Horn Pills')

Main ingredients:	longan fruit	*Morinda* root
	angelica	ginseng
	Astragalus	deer horn
	Eucommia	honey
	Achyranthes	

Actions: Tonifies kidney and spleen energy, as well as kidney yin and yang. Effective restorative tonic after prolonged illness, surgery, or childbirth, including symptoms of anaemia, poor appetite, fatigue, insomnia, sciatica, lumbago, and poor memory. Improves sexual, cerebral, and immune functions.

Yang tonics

GOLDEN LOCK TEA
('*Jin Suo Gu Jing Wan*')

Main ingredients:	lotus seed	lotus stamen
	Astragalus seed	'dragon tooth'
	Euryale seed	oyster shell

Actions: Potent classical prescription for tonifying kidney yang energy. Astringent properties help restrain male emission of semen during intercourse as well as sleep, and may be used to control vaginal discharge in women. Useful male supplement for cultivating ejaculation control.

GEJIE BU SHEN WAN
('Gecko Kidney Tonic Pills')

Main ingredients:	gecko lizard	*Eucommia*
	Poria cocos	deer horn
	Atractylodes	ginseng
	Lycium	dog penis and testes
	Astragalus	*Coridceps fungus*

Actions: Excellent general tonic for boosting kidney yang and kidney energy, especially in males. Effective remedy for such symptoms of kidney deficiency as chronic fatigue, physical weakness, cold hands and feet, excessive urination, poor circulation, and poor memory. Useful tonic for male impotence and for restoring vitality after a period of excessive ejaculation.

NAN BAO CAPSULES
('Male Treasure')

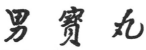

Main ingredients:

donkey kidney	sea horse
dog kidney	donkey-skin glue
ginseng	*Astragalus*
angelica	*Rehmannia*
Eucommia	*Poria cocos*
cinnamon	*Atractylodes*
deer horn	*Paeonia* root
Cornus fruit	*Epimedium*
Cuscuta	Aconite
Psorelea	*Lycium*
Cistanche	*Morinda* root
Rubus	*Ophiopogon* root
Trigonella	*Cynomorium*
Dipsacus	*Curculigo*
Achyranthes	*Scrophularia*
liquorice	

Actions: This is a potent male tonic for deficiency of kidney yang, kidney energy, spleen energy, and blood. Popular tonic remedy for impotence, premature ejaculation, insufficient erection, loss of sexual drive. Also a good geriatric tonic for men, providing relief from chronic fatigue, lower-back pain, poor memory, indigestion, and other symptoms of kidney yang deficiency due to age. The high ratio of animal parts in this formula gives a strong boost to the male endocrine system.

General tonics

TIN HEE PILLS
('Celestial Happiness Pills')

Main ingredients:

ginseng	deer horn
angelica	ginger
Amomum	cinnamon
liquorice	nutmeg

Actions: A very effective general tonic for women, with specific benefits for menstrual disorders and postnatal problems. Dissolves and eliminates clotted blood from uterus after childbirth or abortion. Relieves discomfort of menopause. Improves circulation and appetite, relieves insomnia and irritability due to insufficient circulation, and balances blood. A good travel tonic for women on the move; helps body adapt to changing conditions. This patent is made in Hong Kong, based on a famous formula popular among the women of wealthy households during the Ching dynasty.

GEJIE TA BU WAN 蛤 蚧 大 補 丸
('Great Gecko Tonic Pill')

Main ingredients:

gecko lizard	*Morinda* root
Rehmannia	*Atractylodes*
Polygonum	*Codonopsis*
Dioscorea root	*Eucommia*
Ligustrum	*Astragalus*
Poria cocos	*Lycium*
Dipsacus	*Drynaria*
Cibotium	angelica
Chaenomeles fruit	liquorice

Actions: This formula tonifies blood, energy, and yang and strengthens the kidneys, lung, spleen, and heart. It may be used as a long-term general tonic by men or women, or as a restorative remedy after surgery, prolonged illness, or childbirth. Particularly useful in building kidney energy.

GINSENG TONIC CAPSULES 人 參 補 丸
('*Ren Shen Bu Wan*')

Main ingredients:

ginseng	*Achyranthes*
Cistanche	*Poria cocos*
Adenophora root	sea horse
Cornus fruit	

Actions: Tonifies energy, strengthens internal organs, and benefits kidney yin as well as yang. May be used as a general long-term tonic, or as a restorative after illness, surgery, and childbirth. Particularly beneficial as a geriatric tonic.

TEN FLAVOUR TEA
('*Shih Chuan Da Bu Wan*') 十 全 大 補 丸

Main ingredients:

angelica	*Paeonia* root
Rehmannia	*Poria cocos*
Codonopsis	liquorice
Astragalus	cinnamon
Atractylodes	*Ligusticum*

Actions: This is a patent version of the classical formula introduced in Chapter 24. It has a wide range of tonic benefits, including spleen and heart energy, kidney and spleen yang, and blood. It promotes circulation, improves appetite and digestion, warms the kidneys, boosts protective *wei-chee* energy, strengthens the legs, and eliminates fatigue. May be used as a long-term general tonic by men and women, or as a restorative after illness, surgery, and childbirth.

TZEPAO SANPIEN JING
('Precious Three-Whip Essence') 至 寶 三 鞭 精

Main ingredients:

dog penis	gecko lizard
deer penis	deer horn
seal penis	sea horse

plus other tonic herbs, minerals, and animal parts, for a total of 42 ingredients

Actions: 'Whip' is a Chinese euphemism for penis, which is a potent male sex and vitality tonic. This broad-spectrum formula tonifies energy as well as blood, strengthens kidney, spleen, and lung energy, and tonifies protective *wei-chee* as well as nourishing *ying-chee*. Primarily a male potency tonic, it may be used in the long term to enhance mental and physical functions, strengthen legs and lower back, boost sexual potency, counteract chronic fatigue, and remedy insomnia, asthma, profuse spontaneous sweating, and poor memory. Packaged in vials as a liquid extract. Avoid cold food and cut down on raw food when taking this tonic.

Insomnia and restlessness

AN MIEN PIEN
('Peaceful Sleep Pills') 安 眠 片

Main ingredients:

Zizyphus seed	*Poria cocos*
Polygala root	liquorice
gardenia fruit	

Actions: Remedy for insomnia due to excess heat or congestion in the liver, resulting in 'rebellious ascending energy' that agitates the heart and disturbs the mind, including symptoms of anxiety, nightmares, poor memory, dizziness, bloodshot eyes, and mental exhaustion.

AN SHEN PU SHIN WAN
('Pacify Spirit and Tonify Heart Pills') 安神補心丸

Main ingredients: mother-of-pearl   *Albizia* bark
                         Polygonum   *Cuscuta*
                         Ligustrum   *Schizandrae*
                         Eclipta leaf   *Acorus*
                         salvia root

Actions: This popular formula calms the spirit, tonifies the heart, clears obstructions from blood vessels, and harmonizes energy connection between heart Fire and kidney Water. Remedy for insomnia caused by deficient kidney and/or heart energy, as well as related symptoms of dizziness, restlessness, excessive dreaming, and heart palpitations. Also helps remove plaque deposits from arteries, thus preventing their hardening. This formula is known for its soothing, tranquillizing effects.

Made in USA

A wide range of classical Chinese herbal formulas are now manufactured and distributed as patent remedies in the USA. Established and operated by American entrepreneurs who are trained in traditional Chinese herbal medicine, these companies utilize the latest pharmaceutical technology and the highest-quality medicinal herbs to produce classical Chinese formulas that are at least as pure and potent as the patents currently coming out of China. These patent formulas are available in many health shops throughout North America and in some parts of Europe, and may also be ordered by mail. A list of suppliers and their addresses is provided in the Appendix.

Some of the better American manufacturers of traditional Chinese herbal formulas, as well as a few of their most outstanding remedies, are briefly introduced below. Readers may write to these companies, or to suppliers of their products, for complete catalogues of the full range of herbs and formulas they produce.

East Earth Herb Company

Based in Oregon, East Earth produces herbal products made from imported Chinese herbs. Their line of labels include Turtle

Mountain, Dragon Eggs, Jade Pharmacy, and Jade Medicine. Their products are distributed by Health Concerns, listed in the Appendix, and carried by some health shops.

DETOX: This formula helps purge the system of accumulated toxins and thereby relieves such toxic symptoms as tissue inflammation, allergic reactions, boils and carbuncles, constipation, hepatitis, bloodshot eyes, and sore throat. It acts primarily on the liver, sedating excess Fire, reducing inflammation, and dispelling wind, and secondarily on the lungs and stomach. Should not be used for more than one week at a time.

EXPRESS: Stimulates circulation of blood and energy, nourishes yin and blood, and clarifies the mind. Boosts cerebral functions and eliminates fatigue. Good substitute for coffee and tea as a morning eye-opener. Contains the stimulant herb *Ephedra*, as well as ginseng, jujube, bee pollen, and other tonics. Should not be used by people with weak hearts.

DRAGON'S BREW: An excellent general tonic for blood and energy, yin and yang, based on a classical formula. Tonifies the energy of lungs, kidneys, spleen, and liver, promotes circulation of blood and energy, assists digestion, and harmonizes the functions of the Middle Burner. May be used daily on long-term basis. Contains a live enzyme ferment which facilitates absorption and metabolism of the thirty-six herbal components in the formula.

Health Concerns

Located in California, Health Concerns has recently launched a new line of patent remedies called Chinese Traditional Formulas, selected and designed by Dr Subhuti Dharmananda. They are made from powdered herbs pressed into tablets.

ASTRA-GARLIC: An excellent blood cleanser and purifier, this formula detoxifies the bloodstream, promotes circulation, stimulates blood production, and clears up blood stagnation. It also helps eliminate bacterial, fungal, and amoebic infections. Contains garlic, *Astragalus*, angelica, and other blood tonics.

STOMACH TABS: A digestive aid that disperses stagnant energy in the Middle Burner, clears food stagnation in the stomach, and relieves abdominal bloating, gastritis, flatulence, headache, and other symptoms caused by overeating and improper food combinations. Also helpful in obesity and stomach ulcers.

ASTRAL DIET TEA: This formula suppresses appetite, regulates stomach and spleen functions, and clears stomach phlegm. May be used in weight-reduction programmes, both to curb appetite and to provide extra energy while dieting. Take thirty minutes before meals.

Dragon River

Dragon River, located in New Mexico, produces a wide range of individual herbs as well as compound formulas from cultivated, wild, and imported herbs. Their products come in the form of tincture extracts with high purity and potency. For those who like to blend their own formulas, the individual herbs produced by Dragon River are very convenient to use, and dosages may be precisely measured and blended by the drop. This company will also custom-blend any formula you send them.

MIND AND BODY ENERGIZER: A formula that promotes mental clarity and physical stamina. Increases overall energy and endurance. A good morning eye-opener. Contains ginseng, ginkgo, *gotu kola*, bee pollen, and other energizing herbs.

LIGHTS OUT: A remedy for insomnia, this formula calms overactive nerves, relieves stress, and quiets the brain. Also good for muscular spasms and cramps due to physical strain, nervous tension or menstrual disorders.

GINSENG COMPOUND: A blend of four varieties of ginseng that boosts peak physical and mental energy for intense short-term performance. Good for sports competitions, exams, and other endeavours that require high energy levels and intense concentration.

LIVER TONE: This formula stimulates the liver to flush out accumulated wastes and toxins. Relieves liver congestion and related symptoms, such as constipation, poor fat metabolism, insufficient bile production, bloodshot eyes.

McZand

Located in California, McZand Herbal produces a line of traditional Chinese formulas called Zand Chinese Classics in liquid-extract form. Pure, potent, and convenient to carry and use, these extracts are highly suitable for the fast pace of modern life. McZand produces a wide variety of classical Chinese formulas, and their quality is consistently high.

MINOR BUPLEURUM FORMULA: This formula corrects chronic disorders due to liver stagnation and/or toxicity, including hepatitis, hyoglycaemia, insomnia, poor appetite, and anxiety. It is also useful for relieving the discomfort and accelerating the rate of withdrawal from smoking and drugs.

GINSENG NUTRITIVE FORMULA: A general health tonic, especially for the elderly, this formula tonifies deficiencies of blood and energy in the internal organs, relieving such common symptoms as fatigue, insomnia, anxiety, heart palpitations, and loss of appetite.

CURING FORMULA: A classical combination of herbs to remedy a wide range of digestive complaints, including gastritis, abdominal distension, flatulence, irregular bowels, food poisoning, hangovers, morning sickness, nausea, and motion sickness.

K'an Herb Company

K'an Herb offers a wide range of herbal products and related services to health professionals, including two lines of formulas: K'an Herbals and Chinese Modular Solutions. K'an also distributes products made by Health Concerns, Phytotherapy, and MycoHerb, and supplies various other individual herbs and patent formulas. They will also arrange special educational seminars on various aspects of Chinese herbal medicine anywhere in the USA on request.

COMFORT SHEN: A quick and effective remedy for extreme nervous tension due to acute or chronic stress. Sedates excess liver yang and overactive heart spirit, restores equilibrium, promotes restful sleep.

CONSOLIDATE BLOOD: A classical Chinese formula to regulate, nourish, and circulate blood. Effective remedy for excessive uterine bleeding during menopause, bleeding haemorrhoids, heavy bleeding after childbirth or surgery, and other blood disorders.

ESSENCE CHAMBER: A special formula for preventing and curing prostate disorders in men. Disperses the excess dampness, yin, and stagnant energy which often accumulate in the prostate, causing swelling, infections, and other disorders.

HARMONIZE KIDNEY AND HEART: Many mental and emotional disorders, including chronic depression, are caused by disharmony between heart Fire and kidney Water. This formula harmonizes heart and kidney energies, thereby establishing basic systemic balance in the body as well as the mind.

APPENDICES

Tao Centres, Teachers and Schools of Traditional Medicine

Readers who wish to delve more deeply into the Tao and cleave more closely to the Taoist way of life should seek centres, teachers, and schools for direct transmissions of the Taoist teachings which appeal to you most. Reading is a good way to get acquainted with the Tao, but personal transmission from teacher to student and master to disciple provides the vital spiritual spark which illuminates the teachings in the student's mind and inspires you to follow the well-trod path of the ancient sages in your own daily life. For those who wish to earn a living practising a 'Taoist profession', traditional Chinese medicine is the most logical choice, especially in the light of its growing popularity as an alternative therapy.

Personal transmission can take many forms, and masters come in many guises. Without uttering a word, a traditional healer might impress you so deeply with his art as well as his attitude that his example inspires you to take up traditional medicine as a vocation. In that case, he's your master, your guru, the one who propelled you onto the path, and those from whom you subsequently learn the technical skills of the trade are your subsidiary teachers. A chance encounter with a professor, a writer, a herbalist, or anyone else who practises the Tao may provide a few gems of personally transmitted insight that shed light on your most deeply rooted concerns and change your life for ever. You may spend years searching in vain for the master you've always dreamed about, complete with long white beard and Chinese robes, only to discover later that your own wife or husband can teach you everything you need to know about cultivating the Tao. Some of the best teachers of all are children, but few adults are willing to learn from them. The Way can be found anywhere, but it's not always easy to recognize it.

In Taoist tradition, one of the primary conditions for cultivating the Way is the company of like-minded friends and fellow travellers on the path. Camaraderie among adepts of all schools of

Taoism is a grand old tradition that provides encouragement, support, and reliable companionship to those on the Great Highway of Tao, regardless of their vehicle and pace of progress. By hanging around Tao centres, Chinese temples, public parks (especially at dawn), herb shops, and other places where Taoists tend to congregate for practice as well as for leisure, you'll cultivate contacts that pave the way to whichever Taoist arts and sciences you wish to explore.

The centres, teachers, and schools listed below are drawn from the author's own circle and represent only a small selection of the available sources. Taoists tend to change addresses frequently and without notice, so if you cannot get any information from one source, try another, and always ask for references to other centres, teachers, and schools.

Centres

Yang's Martial Arts Association (YMAA)
38 Hyde Park Avenue
Jamaica Plain, Massachusetts 02130
Fax 617/524–4184
Master: Dr Yang Jwing-ming
(martial arts, *chee-gung*, healing massage, books, equipment)

Sung-Yang Taoist Meditation Center
Taiwan: No. 33–8, Ta-Lin Village
Ping Ling, Taipei County
Taiwan
Tel 8862/2665–6995, 2665–6555
Canada: c/o Claude Gravel
7284 Cordner
Ville La Salle, Quebec
Canada, H8N 2WB
Fax 514/652–8449
Master: Han Yu-mo
(Taoist meditation, *feng shui*, Taoist astrology, spirit channelling, Taoist philosophy)

Living Tao Foundation
P.O. Box 846
Urbana, Illinois 61801
217/337–6113
Master: Chungliang Al Huang
(brush calligraphy, *I Ching* philosophy, East-West cultural synthesis)

Healing Tao Center
P.O. Box 1194
Huntington, NY 11743
Tel 516/367–2701
Master: Mantak Chia
(martial arts, *chee-gung*, healing massage, internal alchemy)

Teachers

Master Han Yu-mo (address above): One of Taiwan's most renowned geomancers and astrologers, Master Han also teaches Taoist meditation and related spiritual practices at his centre in Taiwan, and he plans to open centres in Canada, Europe, and the USA as well. He is also available for private consultations in geomancy and astrology, both to individuals and corporations.

Dr Yang Jwing-ming (address above): Master of *tai-chi*, *Shao-lin*, and other forms of Chinese martial arts, both internal and external, Dr Yang has established his own centre in Massachusetts, where he teaches martial arts, *chee-gung*, and other Taoist skills. He also has branches in Europe. He has written a dozen books on various forms of *chee-gung* and martial arts, available by mail order from YMAA.

Master Luo Teh-hsiou (136, Lung Men St, San Chung City, Taipei County, Taiwan): A highly advanced adept of internal martial arts and *chee-gung*, Master Luo conducts private classes in Taiwan for students who have already achieved basic proficiency. His speciality is a rare internal form called *Ba Gua* ('Eight Trigrams'). Master Luo and his senior students are available for private workshops overseas by arrangement on a case-by-case basis.

Chungliang Al Huang (address above): Trained in *tai-chee*, *chee-gung*, and other internal forms, Huang has been teaching Taoist health regimens and philosophy to American students for many years. Author of several books on the Tao, he has been instrumental in bringing Taoism to the Western world and also organizes annual retreats in China for his Western students.

Mantak Chia (address above): Mantak Chia and his wife Maneewan teach *chee-gung*, healing massage, internal alchemy, and other Taoist skills at their Healing Tao Center, which has many branches throughout the USA and Europe. He has written numerous books on various aspects of *chee-gung* and internal alchemy, available by mail order.

Schools of traditional medicine

Academy of Chinese Culture and Health Sciences
1601 Clay Street
Oakland, California 94612

American College of Traditional Chinese Medicine
455 Arkansas Street
San Francisco, California 94107

Oregon College of Oriental Medicine
10525 SE Cherry Blossom Drive
Portland, Oregon 97216

Oriental Medical Institute of Hawaii
181 S. Kukui St, Suite 206
Honolulu, Hawaii 96813

Pacific College of Oriental Medicine
702 W. Washington Street
San Diego, California 92103

Center for East-West Medicine
University of Hawaii at Manoa
Hawaii

China Medical College
Taichung, Taiwan

Chinese University
Hong Kong

Foundation of East-West Medicine
210 Hsin Yi Rd, Sec 4, 12th Floor
Taipei, Taiwan

(There are also numerous schools of traditional Oriental medicine
in China, Japan, and Korea, but you must be fluent in the spoken
and written languages of those countries in order to attend classes.
In Taiwan and Hong Kong it is possible, though difficult, to find
English-speaking teachers.)

Supplemental Supply Sources

Various products mentioned in this book may be ordered by mail from the suppliers listed below. The author recommends these suppliers for the consistently high quality of their products and the reliability of their services. The addresses given here are current as of January 1993, but are subject to change. Readers who order products from these suppliers should mention this book as their source of information.

Vitamins

Bio-San Laboratories
P.O. Box 325
Organic Park
Derry, NH 03038 USA
Fax 603/434–4736
(Bio-San produces three lines of vitamins and minerals, as well as digestive enzymes and other supplements: Mega-Food, Essential Organics, and Aller-Guard; top quality)

Neuroactive amino acid formulas

Life Services Supplements
3535 Highway 66
Neptune, NJ 07753 USA
Fax 908/922–5329
(Life Services produces the amino acid plus cofactor formulas designed by Pearson & Shaw: Memory Fuel, Fast Blast, and Power Maker; also vitamins and antioxidants)

Nootropics (smart drugs)

Inhome Health Services
Box 3112

CH-2800 Delemont
Switzerland

Interlab
BCM Box 5890
London WC1N 3XX
United Kingdom

(These companies supply a wide range of nootropic compounds not available in the USA and UK, or available only by prescription, particularly hydergine, piraceturn, vasopressin, KH-3, and centrophenoxine. Perversely, people in the UK must order from the address in Switzerland.)

Chinese herbs and formulas

McZand Herbal
P.O. Box 5312
Santa Monica, CA 90409 USA
Tel 800/800–0405
(Producers of the Zand Chinese Classics line of traditional formulas)

Health Concerns
2415 Mariner Sq. Drive #3
Alameda, CA 94501
Tel 800/233–9355
(Supplier of Zand Chinese Classics and several other lines of herbal supplements, including East Earth)

K'an Herb Company
2425 Porter Street
Soquel, CA 95073
Fax 408/479–9118
(K'an herbal products are sold only to professional health practitioners)

Mayway Trading Company
780 Broadway
San Francisco, CA 95073
Tel 415/788–3646
(Suppliers of Chinese patent herbal formulas from China, as well as single herbs)

Dragon River Herbal
P.O. Box 28
El Rito, NM 87530
Tel & Fax 505/581–4441
(Produce and supply their own line of single herbs and formulas, as fluid tincture extracts; pure and potent)

Kanpo Formulas
P.O. Box 60279
Sacramento, CA 95860
Tel 916/487-9044
(Herbs and formulas as concentrated granular extracts)

Fasting supplements

Arise & Shine
P.O. Box 901
Mt. Shasta, CA 96067
Tel 916/926-0891
Fax 916/926-8866
(Suppliers of a wide range of effective herbal supplements for fasting, detoxification, and intestinal restoration)

Colema Boards, Inc
P.O. Box 1879
Cottonwood, CA 96022
Tel 916/347-5868
Fax 916/347-5921
(Producers and suppliers of Colema Board colonic equipment, plus intestinal cleansers and other supplements for therapeutic fasting)

Electromagnetic and audiovisual 'brain machines'

Tools for Exploration
4460 Redwood Highway
Suite 2
San Rafael, CA 94903 USA
Tel 415/499–9050 or 800/456–9887
Fax 415/499–9047
(Suppliers of a wide range of New Age electronic brain enhancers, audiovisual machines, negative ion generators, full-spectrum lights, and other high-tech health tools, plus book)

Raw nuts, dried fruits, wild rice, etc.

Sunnyland Farms
Willson Road at Pecan City
P.O. Box 8200
Albany, GA 31706–8200
Tel 912/883–3085
Fax 912/432–1358
(Supplier of premium quality pecans, almonds, figs, dates, apricots, etc.; also wild rice, honey, maple syrup and other health foods; excellent mail-order service)

Celtic sea salt

Grain & Salt Society
14351 Wycliff Way
P.O. Drawer DD
Magalia, CA 95954
Tel 916/873–0294

(For information regarding benefits of Celtic sea salt and how to obtain it)

Recommended Reading

The books listed below are recommended for further background information on the topics covered in this book. In order to avoid repetition, the books listed here are different from those listed in *The Tao of HS&L*, to which readers may refer for additional recommended reading on these subjects.

Taoist philosophy

Cleary, Thomas, *Awakening to the Tao*, Shambhala, Boston, 1988.
Cleary, Thomas, *I Ching: The Book of Change*, Shambhala, Boston, 1992.
Cleary, Thomas, *The Inner Teachings of Taosim*, Shambhala, Boston, 1988.
Cleary, Thomas, *Vitality, Energy, Spirit*, Shambhala, Boston, 1992.
Porter, Bill (Red Pine), *Road to Heaven*, Mercury House, San Francisco, 1993.
Wong, Eva, *Cultivating Stillness*, Shambhala, Boston, 1992.

Chee-gung and internal alchemy

Chia, Mantak, *Chi Nei Tsang: Internal Organs Chi Massage*, Healing Tao Books, New York, 1990.
Yang, Jwing-ming, *The Eight Pieces of Brocade*, YMAA, Jamaica Plains, 1988.
Yang, Jwing-ming, *Muscle/Tendon Changing and Marrow/Brain Cleansing Chi Kung*, YMAA, Jamaica Plains, 1989.
Yang, Jwing-ming, *The Root of Chinese Chi Kung*, YMAA, Jamaica Plains, 1989.
Yang, Jwing-ming, *Chinese Qigong Massage*, YMAA, Jamaica Plains, 1992.

Chinese Herbal Medicine

Fratkin, Jake, *Chinese Herbal Patent Formulas*, Shya Publications, Boulder, 1986.
Fratkin, Jake, *Chinese Classics*, Shya Publications, Boulder, 1990.
Lee, William, *Herbal Love Potions*, Keats, New Canaan, 1991.
Mowrey, Daniel, *The Scientific Validation of Herbal Medicine*, Keats, New Canaan, 1986.

Mowrey, Daniel, *Next Generation Herbal Medicine*, Keats, New Canaan, 1991.
Ramholz, James, *Shaolin and Taoist Herbal Training Formulas*, Silk Road Books, Chicago, 1992.
Reid, Daniel, *Chinese Herbal Medicine*, Shambhala, Boston, 1987.
Teeguarden, Ron, *Chinese Tonic Herbs*, Japan Publications, Tokyo, 1984.

Diet and Nutrition

Balch, James and Phyllis, *Prescription for Nutritional Healing*, Avery, New York, 1990.
Colbin, Annemarie, *Food and Healing*, Ballantine, New York, 1986.
Deal, Grady, *Dr Deal's Delicious Detox Diet*, Wellness Lifestyle (P.O. Box 1147, Kapaa, Kauai, Hawaii 96746), 1991.
Garrison, Robert and Elizabeth Somer, *The Nutritional Desk Reference*, Keats, New Canaan, 1989.
Howell, Edward, *Food Enzymes for Health and Longevity*, Omangod Press, Woodstock Valley, 1980.
Igram, Cass, *Eat Right or Die Young*, Literary Visions, Cedar Rapids, 1989.
Reid, Daniel, *The Complete Chinese Cookbook*, Weldon Publishing, Willoughsby, 1990.
Shelton, Herbert, *Food Combining Made Easy*, Willow, San Antonio, 1982.
Shelton, Herbert, *The Science and Fine Art of Nutrition*, Natural Hygiene Press, Tampa, 1984.

Fasting and excretion

Anderson, Rich, *Cleanse and Purify Thyself*, Arise and Shine (3225 N. Los Altos Avenue, Tucson, Arizona 85718), 1988.
Gray, Robert, *The Colon Health Book*, Emerald Publishing (Box 11830, Reno, Nevada 89510), 1986.
Jensen, Bernard, *Tissue Cleansing through Bowel Management*, Jensen Enterprises, Escondido, 1981.

Sexual Yoga

Douglas, Nik and Penny Slinger, *Sexual Secrets*, Destiny Books, Rochester, 1989.
Reid, Daniel, *The Tao of Health, Sex, and Longevity*, Simon & Schuster, New York and London, 1989.

Electromagnetic and human energy systems

Becker, Robert & Gary Selden, *The Body Electric*, William Morrow, New York, 1985.

Becker, Robert, *Cross Currents*, Jeremy Tarcher, Los Angeles, 1990.
Schwarz, Jack, *Human Energy Systems*, E. P. Dutton, New York, 1980.

Nootropics and neuroscience

Dean, Ward and J. Morgenthaler, *Smart Drugs and Nutrients*, B&J Publications, Santa Cruz, 1990.
Hutchinson, Michael, *Megabrain*, Ballantine, New York, 1986.
Pearson, D. and S. Shaw, *Life Extension: A Practical Scientific Approach*, Warner Books, New York, 1982.
Pelton, Ross, *Mind Food and Smart Pills*, T&R, San Diego, 1986.

INDEX